American Academy of
Ambulatory Care Nursing

Real Nurses. Real Issues. Real Solutions.

Telehealth
Nursing Practice
Essentials

Maureen Espensen, MBA, BSN, RN
Editor

Copyright © 2009

Telehealth Nursing Practice Essentials

Editor
Maureen Espensen, MBA, BSN, RN

Contributors
Traci Haynes, MSN, BA, RN, CEN
Marlene Glasser, RN
Pam Lursen, RNC
Sherri Smith, MBA, MSN, RN
Lynn Smith-Cronin, BSN, RN
Gina Tabone, MSN, RNC
Eugene Young, MS, RNC
Carol Zeek, MBA, BSN, RNC
James "Jay" Cronin (graphic artist)

Managing Editor: Katie R. Brownlow
Director of Editorial Services: Carol M. Ford
Cover Design: Robert Taylor
Art Director: Jack M. Bryant

AAACN Board Liaison: Traci Haynes
AAACN Executive Director: Cynthia Nowicki Hnatiuk
AAACN Director of Association Services: Pat Reichart
AAACN Education Director: Sally S. Russell

Publication Management:
Anthony J. Jannetti, Inc.
East Holly Avenue/Box 56, Pitman, NJ 08071-0056

This publication is based on and includes information previously published by the American Academy of Ambulatory Care Nursing in the *Telehealth Nursing Practice Core Course Manual* (1st and 2nd editions), with contributions from:
Martha Barstow, MBA, RN; Betty Jo Dennis, BSN, RN; Darla Dernovsek, BS; Maureen Espensen, MBA, BSN, RN; Denine Gronseth, BSN, RN; Aurelia Marek, BSN, RN; Diane Maxwell, MSN, RN; Penny Meeker, MHA, BS, RN; Ruth Rea, PhD, RN; Lisa Schwarzentraub, BS, RN; Terri Spiegel, MS, RN

Copyright © 2009 American Academy of Ambulatory Care Nursing
ISBN 978-0-9819379-0-8

DISCLAIMER
The authors, contributors, editors, and publishers of this book have made serious efforts to ensure that treatments, practices, and procedures are accurate and conform to standards accepted at the time of publication. Due to constant changes in information resulting from continuing research and clinical experience, reasonable differences in opinions among authorities, unique aspects of individual clinical situations, and the possibility of human error in preparing such a publication, the reader should exercise individual judgment when making a clinical decision, and if necessary, consult and compare information from other authorities, professionals, or sources.

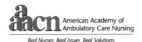

American Academy of Ambulatory Care Nursing
Real Nurses. Real Issues. Real Solutions.
East Holly Avenue/Box 56, Pitman, NJ 08071-0056
Phone: 800-262-AMBNURS (262-6877); Fax: 856-589-7463
Web site: www.aaacn.org; Email: aaacn@ajj.com

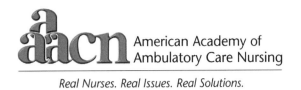

American Academy of
Ambulatory Care Nursing

Real Nurses. Real Issues. Real Solutions.

Introduction

Telehealth Nursing Practice Essentials provides information necessary for safe, competent practice of telehealth nursing. It includes a culmination of topics which are essential for nurses new to telehealth practice, experienced in telehealth, and for those interested in expanding their knowledge base. Key information is presented, including the nursing process, focus, roles, legal issues, communication, customer service, technology, clinical decision tools, documentation, and clinical information for the nurse to have an in-depth understanding of the telehealth nursing scope of practice.

The concept for this book was developed from the *Telehealth Nursing Practice Core Course (TNPCC) Manual* by the American Academy of Ambulatory Care Nursing (AAACN). When the *TNPCC Manual* was written in 2001, it was not known that it would have such sustainability over nearly a decade of telehealth nursing practice. Over the years, there have been considerable changes in telehealth practice. Roles have expanded and evolved from telephone triage. A myriad of telecommunication devices are now used for the encounter: the nurse-patient interaction. Roles include telehealth triage, consultation, follow-up, and monitoring. Although roles have evolved, the patient remains the center of focus. The patient expects the care, and the nurse is the provider of care.

No matter what the telehealth setting, nurses reading this book should be able to identify issues relative to their particular situation and apply the information in order to enhance practice. It is with this goal in mind, and on behalf of my AAACN telehealth nursing colleagues, that we present the first edition of *Telehealth Nursing Practice Essentials*, a valuable information source for telehealth nursing.

Maureen Espensen, MBA, BSN, RN
Editor

AAACN's Vision for Telehealth Nursing

Telehealth will be recognized as an integral part of ambulatory care and AAACN will be the industry leader for telehealth nursing practice.

AAACN strongly encourages all telehealth nurses to become certified in ambulatory care nursing. Because telehealth nurses provide nursing care to patients who are in an ambulatory setting, they must possess the knowledge and competencies to appropriately provide ambulatory care.

Ambulatory care nursing certification, especially with the enhanced telehealth component, is the career credential for all ambulatory care nurses. Ambulatory certification is and will continue to be the gold standard credential for any nursing position within ambulatory care.

Corporate Sponsorship

AAACN would like to thank LVM Systems, Inc. for their sponsorship of this book.

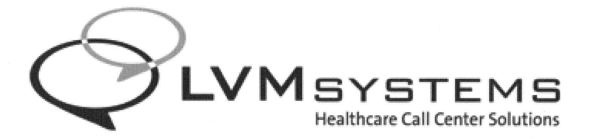

See page 288 for a complete profile of LVM Systems, Inc.

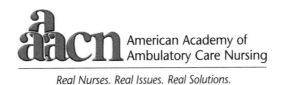

American Academy of
Ambulatory Care Nursing

Real Nurses. Real Issues. Real Solutions.

Telehealth Nursing Practice Essentials

TABLE OF CONTENTS

✆ *Earn 1.4 contact hours!*

✐ *Earn 1.3 contact hours!*

. ▪ . ▪ . ▪ . ▪ . ▪ . ▪ . ▪ . ▪ . ▪ . ▪ . ▪ . ▪ . ▪ . ▪ . ▪ .

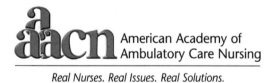

American Academy of
Ambulatory Care Nursing

Real Nurses. Real Issues. Real Solutions.

Section 1

Telehealth Nursing Systems and Professional Practice

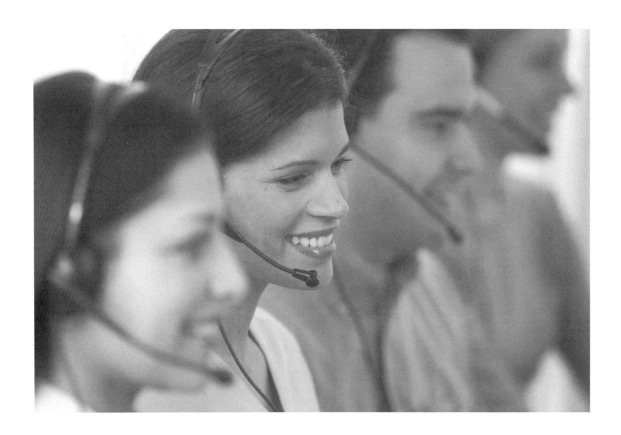

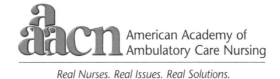

American Academy of
Ambulatory Care Nursing

Real Nurses. Real Issues. Real Solutions.

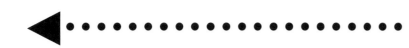

CHAPTER 1
Telehealth Nursing Practice: An Overview

In the ever-changing environment of health care, methods of delivering patient care and interacting with patients continue to evolve. One example is the increased use of telecommunications and its support of improved access, quality, and cost-efficiency of health care delivery in providing patient care (Becker & Haynes, 2006).

As early as the 1970s, nurses began to formally use the telephone to interact with patients. Telephone triage services were developed to help handle the symptom-based calls coming into emergency departments. Over time, services expanded to include physician referral services and "ask a nurse" type services for local communities. Pediatricians and family practice physicians were the first to discover the value of using nurses to answer their patient's off-hour telephone calls. These after hour calls helped decrease the work load of the on-call physicians while providing consistent responses to frequently asked questions.

Telephone triage services were developed to help handle the symptom-based calls coming from emergency departments.

TELEHEALTH PRACTICE

Telehealth nursing practice is recognized as a nursing subspecialty of ambulatory care nursing by the American Academy of Ambulatory Care Nursing (AAACN) and the American Nurses Association (ANA) (AAACN, 2005).

As the nurse's role in telehealth increased in breadth and scope, the need for practice standards emerged. When AAACN published its first set of *Telephone Nursing Practice Administration and Practice Standards* in 1997, the focus was on telephone nursing. These standards were the first of their kind published by a national nursing organization. In 2001, the second edition of the standards was written, and the term *telehealth* was used instead of *telephone*. The fourth edition, published in 2007, was titled *Telehealth Nursing Practice Administration and Practice Standards*. AAACN plans to support a biannual review to assure that the telehealth nursing practice standards continue to articulate expectations for nurses engaged in telehealth practice.

AAACN also recognized the void of formal education programs for the nurse involved in telehealth patient care. As a result, AAACN organized and financially supported a team of telehealth nurses to develop the *Telehealth Nursing Practice Core Course*. Additionally, an active AAACN special interest group exists to address professional issues and educational needs of nurses engaged in telehealth practice. In 1997, ANA sponsored the formation of the Nursing Organization Telehealth Committee, which serves as a forum

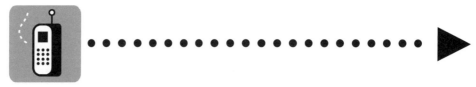

for groups involved in telehealth practice to address emerging issues from a multidisciplinary perspective.

Both AAACN and ANA recognize the professional registered nurse (RN) as the appropriate provider of telehealth nursing services. The application of the nursing process when providing patient care has always pointed to professional nursing practice. This chapter supports and maintains that the nursing process is clearly demonstrated by the RN providing telehealth patient care.

AAACN has developed a model that illustrates the interactive, circular relationship of the nursing process for telehealth nursing practice. The core reflects the interaction between the nurse and the patient/caregiver. The nurse prioritizes the urgency of the situation based on assessment data, utilizes decision support tools, and collaborates with other health care professionals and the patient/caregiver to develop a plan of care, implement appropriate interventions, and evaluate the outcome. The telehealth nursing practice model is described and shown in Chapter 2, "Focus and Roles."

> *The application of the nursing process when providing patient care has always pointed to professional nursing practice.*

TELEHEALTH NURSING SUPPORTS HEALTH CARE IMPROVEMENT

Telehealth nursing practice supports the achievement of the six specific Institute of Medicine (IOM) aims for health care quality improvement (safe, effective, patient-centered, timely, efficient, and equitable) (IOM, 2001). The aims state that health care must be safe ("first do no harm"), which when applied to telehealth nursing, means that the nurse will provide safe care. The second aim is that health care must be effective. For telehealth nursing, services must use the most appropriate and best available technologies, knowledge, and clinical information to effectively deliver the care. Third, the delivery of health care must be patient-centered. The application of this concept in telehealth means that the service will be convenient to the patient, easy to use, and focused on meeting the individual's culture, social, and specific needs. The fourth aim defined by the IOM is that care will be timely. For telehealth nursing, this means providing services to patients within appropriate timeframes and within hours convenient to the patient (and not just when convenient to the telehealth staff). The IOM expects that the health care system be efficient and seeks to reduce waste, supplies, equipment and time. With this in mind, the telehealth nursing service must always look for opportunities to improve the delivery of care. And last, the IOM expects that health care be equitable irregardless of race, ethnicity, income, or gender. The telehealth service and individual nurse shall provide care to all individuals without differentiation to their background or health care beliefs.

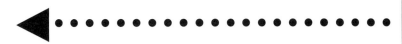

TELEHEALTH DEFINITIONS

The term *telehealth* will be used frequently in this chapter. The base, *tele,* is Latin and means "at a distance." Using the term *telehealth* encompasses all the current technology used by nurses and consumers. These include the telephone, email, Internet, facsimile, telephone devices for the hearing impaired (TTD/TTY), and any telecommunication equipment that will be developed in the future.

The AAACN Special Interest Group on Telehealth Nursing Practice has developed and approved the following definitions relative to telehealth nursing practice:

1. **Telehealth:** "The delivery, management, and coordination of health services that integrate electronic information and telecommunications technologies to increase access, improve outcomes, and contain or reduce costs of health care." *Telehealth* is used as an umbrella term to describe the wide range of services delivered across distances by all health-related disciplines.

2. **Telehealth nursing:** "The delivery, management, and coordination of care and services provided via telecommunications technology within the domain of nursing." Telehealth nursing is a subset of telehealth, encompassing all types of nursing care and services delivered across distances. *Telehealth nursing* is a broad term encompassing practices that incorporate a vast array of telecommunications technologies (for example, telephone, fax, email, Internet, video monitoring, and interactive video) to remove time and distance barriers for the delivery of nursing care.

3. **Telephone nursing:** "All care and services within the scope of nursing practice that are delivered over the telephone." A component of telehealth nursing practice restricted to the telephone.

4. **Telephone triage:** "An interactive process between nurse and client that occurs over the telephone and involves identifying the nature and urgency of client health care needs and determining the appropriate disposition." Telephone triage is a component of telephone nursing practice that focuses on assessment, prioritization, and referral to the appropriate level of care. Definitions were approved and adopted by the Telehealth Nursing Practice Special Interest Group (Greenberg, Espensen, Becker, & Cartwright, 2003).

Additional terminology will be defined throughout the remainder of this book.

Telehealth is the delivery, management, and coordination of health services that integrate electronic information and telecommunications technologies to increase access, improve outcomes, and contain or reduce costs of health care.

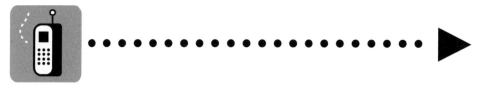

TNPE Setting and Scope

The *Telehealth Nursing Practice Essentials* addresses telehealth nursing practice across a broad range of settings, including physician offices, clinics, and contact centers. Recognizing that specific details of practice differ from a single-physician office to large contact centers, it addresses extensive issues related to this nursing activity. Nursing process, communication techniques, use of guidelines, documentation issues, and clinical knowledge are common across all practice settings. The course has been developed for nationwide distribution and provides general guidance related to various practice issues. Practice variations occur from state to state and within organizations. It is the professional nurse's responsibility to know the variations and how they impact nursing practice.

TNPE Language

Certain language has been adopted in the TNPE to keep the length of this book reasonable. These terms and their expanded definitions are as follows:

Patient	The person who is seeking health care or health information, whether for him/herself or on behalf of the patient (such as a family member, mother, father, guardian, or significant other).
Family	Identifies the multiple blends that are present in society, which include spouse, children, guardians, significant others, partners, etc.
Nurse	Refers specifically to the registered nurse performing telehealth nursing, regardless of the practice setting.
Contact Center	Refers to the particular place where a registered nurse practices telehealth nursing. A contact center may be a registered nurse providing telehealth services in a solo practice provider office or a setting that employs a large group of nurses. This manual is not geared toward one telehealth practice setting; however, the universal term *contact center* will be used to define the *space* where the nurse practices telehealth nursing.
Encounter	Interaction with the patient via any telecommunication device including, telephone, fax, email, Internet, video monitoring, and interactive video.

Nursing process, communication techniques, use of guidelines, documentation issues, and clinical knowledge are common across all practice settings.

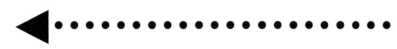

OVERVIEW OF THE
TELEHEALTH NURSING PRACTICE ESSENTIALS (TNPE)

The information provided in the *Telehealth Nursing Practice Essentials* (TNPE) is available as a live course (Telehealth Nursing Practice Core Course [TNPCC]), recorded course, or via this book to address the knowledge and key information for telehealth nursing practice. During the live course, information is presented during lecture and reinforced in interactive sessions. A Post Activity Learning Assessment is offered to measure acquisition of knowledge. Nurses may receive a different number of continuing nursing education hours for attending the live course, listening to the recorded course, and/or completing the book. Each methodology will offer a different learning experience to the participant.

Telehealth Nursing Practice Core Course (TNPCC) Participants

Congruent with AAACN's *Telehealth Nursing Practice Administration and Practice Standards*, attendees of the Telehealth Nursing Practice Core Course (TNPCC) must be registered nurses. The course is designed to provide core information in telehealth nursing. The course does not require the nurse to have prior experience in telehealth nursing; however, it is recommended to have exposure to telehealth nursing. The TNPCC is beneficial for those new to telehealth practice and those interested in adding to their knowledge, as well as a resource for those studying for the certification examination in ambulatory care nursing through the American Nurses Credentialing Center. Certification does not demonstrate competency in ambulatory care nursing. Actual competency demonstration is the responsibility of the individual and his/her employer.

Certification does not demonstrate competency in ambulatory care nursing. Actual competency demonstration is the responsibility of the individual and his/her employer.

SUMMARY

Telehealth nursing roles and opportunities will continue to increase during the 21st century. In the innovative spirit of Florence Nightingale, nurses will continue to influence the quality of care given within the telehealth environment.

References
American Academy of Ambulatory Care Nursing (AAACN). (1997). *Telephone nursing practice administration and practice standards*. Pitman, NJ: Author.
American Academy of Ambulatory Care Nursing (AAACN). (2001). *Telehealth nursing practice administration and practice standards* (2nd ed.). Pitman, NJ: Author.

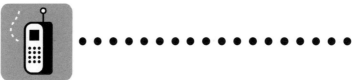

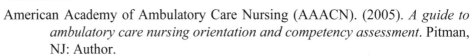

American Academy of Ambulatory Care Nursing (AAACN). (2005). *A guide to ambulatory care nursing orientation and competency assessment.* Pitman, NJ: Author.

American Academy of Ambulatory Care Nursing (AAACN). (2007). *Telehealth nursing practice administration and practice standards* (4th ed.). Pitman, NJ: Author.

American Nurses Association (ANA). (1997). Telehealth: A tool for nursing practice. *Nursing Trends Issues, 2,* 1-7.

Becker, C.A., & Haynes, T.S. (2006). Telehealth nursing practice. In C. Baker Laughlin (Ed.), *Core curriculum for ambulatory care nursing* (pp. 137-148). Pitman, NJ: American Academy of Ambulatory Care Nursing.

Greenberg, M., Espensen, M., Becker, C., & Cartwright, J. (2003). Telehealth nursing practice SIG adopts teleterms. *AAACN Viewpoint, 25*(1), 8-10.

Institute of Medicine (IOM). (2001). *Crossing the quality chasm: A new health system for the 21st century.* Washington, DC: National Academies Press.

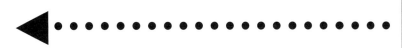

CHAPTER 2
Focus and Roles

Objectives

1. Describe the use of the nursing process as related to telehealth practice.
2. Explain how specific nursing foci are demonstrated in telehealth practice.
3. Summarize the four major roles of the nurse in telehealth practice.
4. Describe ways that life-long learning enhances telehealth nursing practice.

Whether providing care in a direct patient contact setting or remotely through telephone lines, the expectation of the nurse remains the same – to use the nursing process to determine the needs of the patient and to provide for the delivery of care. In addition to using the nursing process in a telehealth practice setting, the nursing skill set includes excellent communication skills, logical problem-solving skills, and critical thinking skills. Depending on the patient's presenting symptoms and/or needs, the use of each key component will vary as the nurse analyzes the situation. After interviewing the patient to assess the presenting symptoms and/or needs, the nurse should formulate a nursing plan of action and then use this analysis to determine the appropriate interventions using decision support tools, nursing expertise, and other resources as indicated.

Within most telehealth care settings (for example, a primary care office or a contact center), time with the patient is very limited compared to other health care settings (such as inpatient or rehabilitation facilities). The telehealth nurse is expected to establish an instant, trusting relationship with the patient using appropriate communication and interpersonal skills. This trusting relationship is essential to allow the nurse to ask the patient for graphically detailed explanations of body functions that they may never before have verbalized to anyone. Patients will provide response, with the expectation that the nurse will process the information and initiate a patient plan of care, all during a 5 to 10-minute telehealth encounter.

As telephones and computers continue to play a greater role in the delivery of patient care, it is essential that nursing education programs provide student nurses with baseline technical competencies. Nursing education programs are beginning to recognize the expanded role of the professional nurse due to the use of telecommunications and computer technology in the ambulatory care setting. Currently, the hiring

Within most telehealth care settings, time with the patient is very limited compared to other health care settings. The nurse is expected to establish an instant, trusting relationship with the patient using communication, charisma, and appropriate interpersonal skills.

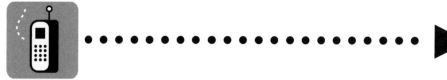

organizations are responsible for providing graduate nurses with opportunities to develop or expand the technical competencies necessary for the delivery of telehealth nursing practice. The nurse in any care delivery environment must exhibit core interpersonal and intellectual competencies as evidenced by critical thinking skills, effective verbal communication, a systematic approach in history-taking and assessment, and thorough documentation of the entire patient encounter. Despite the significant variability, both in the delivery of care and in the tools used in telehealth practice versus bedside practice, components of the nursing process remain the same.

NURSING PROCESS

Originally, telehealth nursing was offered only as a triage service to support patients needing assistance in matching their health needs to the resources available (telephone triage). With the acceptance and growth of the concept of a nurse providing care through telephone or other remote technology, the role of telehealth practice nursing has grown.

Originally, telehealth nursing was offered only as a triage service to support patients needing assistance in matching their health needs to the resources available (telephone triage). Limited nursing services were provided to the patient during a typically brief, single-contact event. With the acceptance and growth of the concept of a nurse providing care through telephone or other remote technology, the role of telehealth practice nursing has grown. Through telehealth practice, the nurse is providing care to patients during telehealth encounters in the same way that a hospital nurse might provide direct, hands-on care. The telehealth care plan is monitored for effectiveness, just as a hospital nurse checks on the patient to monitor for changes in health status. Therefore, a telehealth nurse may have several contacts with the same patient during a single working shift. The plan of care in either setting should be evaluated and modified based on the patient response to the intervention provided. The fine details of the nursing process will vary slightly depending on the practice setting, but the same general nursing process must be used by all nurses to maintain patient safety and to support nursing care delivery.

Telehealth nursing practice does not absolve the nurse of any traditional nursing responsibilities or accountabilities, but rather requires demonstrated use in a unique setting. The nursing process provides the blueprint for the consistent delivery of patient care in all settings. Typically, the nursing process is composed of the following elements: *Assessment, Analyze and Plan, Implementation,* and *Evaluation.* The nursing process is demonstrated in telehealth nursing as follows:

Assessment
Interview
Collect data
Assess
Prioritize

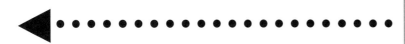

Analyze and Plan
Determine and use most appropriate decision support tool(s)
Reference other resources as appropriate
Collaborate

Implementation
Problem solve
Apply intervention and/or activate disposition
Educate the patient and/or family
Provide support
Coordinate resources
Facilitate appropriate follow-up care

Evaluation
Documentation
Communication
Follow-up
Analysis

The American Academy of Ambulatory Care Nursing (AAACN) has developed a model of telehealth nursing practice which reflects the ideal interactive, circular relationship of the nursing process within telehealth practice (see Figure 2-1). As demonstrated in this model, the core is the interaction of the nurse with the patient and/or family. With the help of this interaction, the nurse should be able to prioritize the urgency based on assessment data, utilize decision support tools and collaboration with other health care professionals to arrive at a plan of care, implement appropriate interventions, and evaluate the outcome. The activity is bound by the continuous flow of the nursing process – *Assess, Analyze, Plan, Implement,* and *Evaluate.* This is not a linear process, but is characterized by continuous movement and overlapping of components during the telehealth encounter.

The nurse should be able to prioritize the urgency based on assessment data, utilize decision support tools and collaboration with other health care professionals to arrive at a plan of care, implement appropriate interventions, and evaluate the outcome.

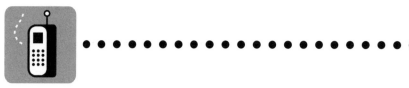

Figure 2-1.
Telehealth Nursing Practice

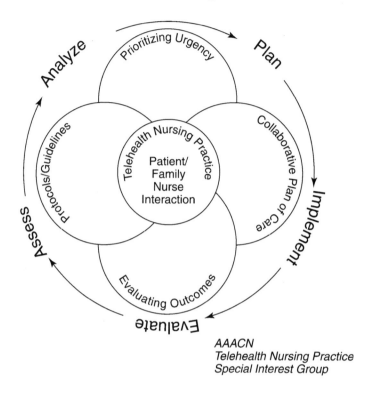

AAACN
Telehealth Nursing Practice
Special Interest Group

Assessment

Telehealth interactions that are symptom-based will incorporate all levels of the nursing process. With more advanced technology, the nurse's assessment may not be limited to verbal telephone communication. Patient information may also be transmitted to the nurse via telephone lines from remote monitoring devices located in places such as the patient's home. As previously outlined, the assessment step consists of the following components:

❖ **Interview**
❖ **Collect data**
❖ **Assess**
❖ **Prioritize**

Interview: Effectively interviewing the patient may be the most difficult component of telehealth nursing. To effectively communicate using only verbal processes demands a skill set that goes beyond what nursing education typically prepares nurses to do. Questions should be asked in a logical sequence sensitive to the acuity level of the presenting need, and in a matter that does not cause the patient to become defensive or evasive. During the initial interview process, the nurse must maintain

> *Telehealth interactions that are symptom-based will incorporate all levels of the nursing process. With more advanced technology, the nurse's assessment may not be limited to verbal telephone communication.*

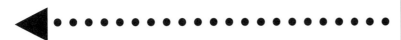

awareness of presenting symptoms that would indicate an emergency situation to avoid delays in activating emergency assistance, if required. The nurse must also review health history, chronic conditions, medications, and drug allergies with the patient. Effective communication techniques will be discussed in more detail in later chapters.

Collection of the data: Data collection to support the nursing process begins the moment the nurse asks: "Hello, how may I help you?" The nurse must be aware not only of the verbal response to that question, but of all the other indicators that can be heard over the telephone. For example, is the patient speaking in complete sentences? The nurse is required to analyze if the patient is hysterical or calm, coherent or confused (Briggs, 2007). The nurse should be alert for background noise(s) that would indicate other people are around. Is it a party or panic? Is there a child crying, another adult shouting, or outdoor noises? Is there too much static on the line for the nurse to clearly understand and be understood?

Any of these factors may alter how the nurse proceeds with interviewing the patient to collect additional information, assess the presenting symptoms and/or needs, and prioritize the acuity of the patient.

Assess: The key to proceeding with the interaction is the nurse's assessment of the patient's presenting symptoms and/or needs. Not only must the nurse consider the true acuity of the need presented, but he/she must also interpret the patient's perceived acuity of need. These two views may not agree. Patient anxiety may indicate a hidden agenda, or poor coping with the situation at hand. In addition, the nurse must be aware of stereotyping and prejudice as a potential risk to accurately assessing patients. The patient's tone of voice, perceived social-economic status, communication style, community location, gender, and/or ethnic traits can all be potential traps for the nurse, and can all trigger preconceptions of the significance of the patient's need.

With face-to-face assessment, the nurse is able to use all physical sensory input – auditory, visual, olfactory, and tactile – along with verbal and non-verbal communication to assess the patient's current state. The telehealth encounter restricts use of these senses. The nurse must be particularly sensitive to auditory, verbal, and emotional cues communicated through speech.

During telehealth assessment, the patient shares greater accountability in assisting the nurse with the assessment, intervention, and evaluation of outcome. The patient truly is partnered with the nurse in the nursing process. Patients may have confused or ambiguous expectations if they are not experienced in telehealth practice interactions. With this in mind, the nurse must stay sensitive to the patient's ability to communicate his/her current situation accurately. If the nurse is unable to fully assess the current situation from the information provided, it is the nurse's

During telehealth assessment, the patient shares greater accountability in assisting the nurse with the assessment, intervention, and evaluation of outcome. The patient truly is partnered with the nurse in the nursing process.

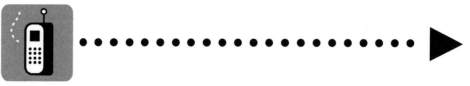

responsibility to continue asking open-ended questions or prompting the patient until all necessary assessment information has been gathered.

Prioritize: Prioritizing means that the nurse should immediately identify emergent situations and initiate the necessary interventions. The nurse's prioritization of the need for care is based on the patient's stated reason for the contact with the nurse, presenting symptoms and/or needs, and patient risk factors (including health history and potential outcomes). This process focuses on establishing the level of seriousness or urgency indicated by the presenting circumstances. At this stage, the nurse should attempt to resolve the patient's current situation instead of engaging in a lengthy discussion of behaviors that may have contributed to the current situation. After ruling out emergent calls, the nurse should use the assessment and planning components of the nursing process to determine the urgency of non-emergent presenting symptoms.

The prioritizing process in telehealth practice differs significantly from direct patient contact because of the complex interviewing skills necessary to complete a telehealth assessment. Triage decision support tools are highly useful to determine level of urgency, support nursing practice, and provide a framework that identifies essential interview information.

Analyze and Plan

During the course of patient assessment, the nurse should continuously analyze the information gathered to develop an effective plan of care. After a life-threatening emergency is ruled out, the plan of care is initiated with the following:

❖ Determine and use the most appropriate decision support tool(s)
❖ Reference other resources as appropriate
❖ Collaborate

Determining the most appropriate decision support tool(s) is based on the nurse's identification of the chief presenting symptom of the patient, using the interview and assessment process to support this decision. At this point, other important underlying symptoms may be uncovered that are determined to be of greater significance than those initially reported as the primary complaint by the patient. Decision support tool selection is not always direct, especially when the patient presents with a history of chronic disease or other risk factors. Considering all information gathered, the nurse should select the most appropriate decision support tool to direct the nursing care plan. Supported by the decision support tools, nurses can advise patients on options for intervention and/or referral.

The nurse may *reference other resources* if decision support tools are unavailable or the patient's presenting need is not fully addressed by the approved decision support tools. These situations might include patients seeking information regarding a particular medication, general medical

The nurse's prioritization of the need for care is based on the patient's stated reason for the contact with the nurse, presenting symptoms and/or needs, and patient risk factors (including health history and potential outcomes).

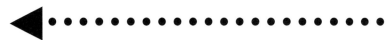

information, clarification of procedure preparation, and pre-arrival or post-discharge instructions. Other resources to consider are not limited to written materials, but should include consulting with other health care professionals when appropriate, such as physicians or pharmacists.

It may be necessary for the nurse to **collaborate** with other individuals in order to provide effective patient care. For example, the nurse is in a key position to access a collaborative continuity of care, particularly if working in the physician office setting. This collaboration effort may include the patient, family and/or care provider, physicians, and other health care or community service team members as needed. Group decision-making allows the presenting problem to be considered from multiple points of view, rather than solely from the viewpoint of a single nurse. Interdisciplinary collaboration may also be necessary with home health care or community service individuals, ensuring that the patient will have the support services necessary to maintain health care delivery in the home. A care conference involving any number of individuals from across the continuum of care, including telehealth nurses, may be required in the more complex patient care situations.

Telehealth nurses working in contact centers may also include other individuals in a collaborative effort to help patients understand and follow through with advised disposition and care. HIPPA laws require patients to give consent for other individuals to have access to their medical records (Protected Health Information – PHI). The telehealth nurse must always consider this when speaking with someone other than the patient.

An unexplained frequency of activity from a particular patient with a chronic disease process may indicate unmet patient needs. Following inpatient discharge, the telehealth nurse may be the first to recognize a need to investigate and evaluate appropriateness of the care plan. When these types of situations are identified (based on the patient's needs identified during a telehealth encounter), the telehealth nurse could serve as the initiator or coordinator of a care conference to implement and evaluate the comprehensive patient care plan. Therefore, the telehealth nurse is able to influence and enhance complete care across the continuum. Some institutions have technology that allows the telehealth nurse access to patient records in both the hospital and clinic settings. The electronic medical record provides immediate information and the nurse is able to reinforce physician directives. Involvement in the total patient care team provides the telehealth nurse with the opportunity to participate at a potentially higher level of the decision-making process.

During discharge planning, it is important to consider the role of the telehealth nurse. Depending on the facility and practice setting of the nurse, the telephone may be the identified support mechanism provided for the patient upon discharge from outpatient or inpatient services. If the nurse is the main support contact for the patient, he/she must be well

It may be necessary for the nurse to collaborate with other individuals in order to provide effective patient care.

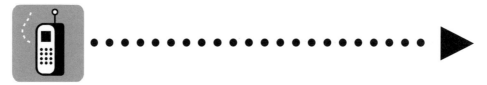

versed on the standards and directives provided to the patient for self-care following discharge.

Implementation

Implementation of the nursing plan involves the following components:

- ❖ Problem-solving
- ❖ Applying the intervention and/or activating the disposition
- ❖ Educating the patient and/or care provider
- ❖ Providing support
- ❖ Coordinating resources
- ❖ Facilitating follow-up care as indicated

This implementation process is seldom a linear progression. The nurse may need to modify the care plan often while working through the implementation phrase. Obstacles may present in each of the steps of implementation that will require the nurse to use problem-solving and critical-thinking skills to successfully conclude the encounter.

Problem-solving is a key component in the nurse's skill set and is used from the moment the telehealth encounter starts until its conclusion. Problems to be addressed can range from providing a quantitative measure for the patient to use when describing a presenting symptom to finding a drugstore open so that the patient can obtain needed home care supplies. For an indigent patient, the nurse may even have to facilitate transportation to a non-urgent care center or find financial resources to purchase necessary medication. The role of the nurse may at times appear to be more of a case manager or social services coordinator when no other support mechanism is available for the patient.

Problem-solving may also include sorting through the information provided by the patient to arrive at an accurate set of symptoms. The nurse should be sensitive to, but not led or influenced by, the patient's self-diagnosis. The patient may be influenced by what was wrong with a friend or relative last week, or what was reported on their local newscast (Briggs, 2007). In addition, the nurse should be cautious if the patient gives minimal details about symptoms, has difficulty in identifying the presenting symptoms and/or needs, or provides an inconsistent or cloudy history. The patient may be masking a more serious medical condition, sometimes due to fear of disease based on family history, or have a hidden agenda. The suppression of information may or may not be a deliberate, conscious act on the patient's part. Recall that a classic symptom of possible myocardial infarction is denial. It is the nurse's responsibility to verify and inquire further about the patient's presenting circumstances without offending the patient, to assure that the patient is not either

The patient may be masking a more serious medical condition, sometimes due to fear of disease based on family history, or have a hidden agenda. The suppression of information may or may not be a deliberate, conscious act on the patient's part.

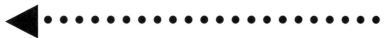

masking or enhancing his/her presenting symptoms in an attempt to influence the nurse's decision-making process toward a desired end.

Consider a patient who initially presents to the telehealth nurse with a set of symptoms that would warrant emergency room care. The patient strongly indicates that they do not want to go to the emergency room and would rather see their physician in the office. As the nurse interacts with the patient, the patient continually downgrades their presenting symptoms in an effort to persuade the nurse to agree to an office appointment. The nurse in this situation is challenged to ascertain accurate information and determine the appropriate disposition of the patient, not the patient's desired disposition.

Applying the intervention can include a composite of any of the following options necessary to support the appropriate disposition.

- ❖ Providing emergency directions or first aid instructions
- ❖ Teaching health principles to the patient
- ❖ Instructing on self care
- ❖ Scheduling appointment(s)
- ❖ Counseling
- ❖ Acting as a liaison in securing resources

These activities may include the patient, immediate caregivers, or family members as needed to ensure compliance with the disposition. All information provided for the patient should be in accord with organization-approved guidelines. The nurse must counsel the patient so he/she understands the need for timely intervention, the anticipated outcome, and the consequences of non-compliant activities. The nurse should provide complete information to the patient regarding when to contact the nurse again, specifying detailed instructions about symptom changes or new symptoms that may develop, and the urgency associated with those changes. For example, a small laceration typically heals very well with only home care interventions. However, the patient must be alert during the healing process. This includes not only how the normal healing process should progress, but also how changes would indicate a need for additional and timely interventions.

Patient education is dependent on the nurse's communication skills. It is essential for the patient to fully understand the directions provided for self-care during the telehealth encounter. In a clinical setting, the nurse has the opportunity to demonstrate self-care and have the patient return the demonstration until executed properly. A telehealth nurse must rely solely on his/her ability to verbally communicate the steps in self-care. In addition, the nurse must test the patient's understanding by having the patient repeat the instructions in his/her own words. This can be time-consuming, and the patient should take written notes for future reference. In some situations, it may also be necessary to instruct family members in

The nurse must counsel the patient so he/she understands the need for timely intervention, the anticipated outcome, and the consequences of non-compliant activities.

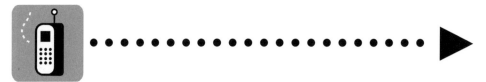

care delivery techniques so they may provide necessary support for the patient. It is easier to instruct a patient in a self-care skill by demonstration rather than by a step-by-step description. Additional variables that a nurse may encounter include the patient's high anxiety level, feeling ill, and/or being sleep deprived, as well as other factors, which make it difficult for the patient to understand the nurse's explanations. Therefore, patience is one of the most important attributes the nurse can exhibit in this type of encounter.

Providing accurate and complete information to the patient is essential. Hesitantly providing information or miscommunicating even a small element of information may undermine the patient's confidence in following the care plan implemented by the nurse. The nurse should not make assumptions about a patient's baseline knowledge, but should provide complete information in lay terms. The patient must fully understand all information provided to avoid either misapplication of instructions leading to potential negative outcomes or additional patient-initiated telehealth encounters merely to clarify information.

Providing support may be the most critical element of the nursing process if self-care has been determined to be the most effective plan for the patient. The support offered by the nurse may be primarily psychological in some cases, such as a parent with a new baby or an adult with a new chronic disease diagnosis attempting to cope with the changes in his/her daily living. The telehealth nurse can be instrumental in "making or breaking" the situation. A calm, empathetic listener that offers the reassurance needed by the patient may be decisive to the patient's ability to successfully manage a difficult situation. The nurse may provide the confidence that enables the patient to continue to do what is necessary. If the patient senses lack of concern by the nurse, the result may be frustration and a perceived sense of the nurse not caring.

When a chronic disease is newly diagnosed, the telehealth nurse can be a great value to the patient by lending support and reassurance, thereby resulting in greater compliance of disease management. An example could be a newly diagnosed insulin-dependent diabetic.

The nurse may provide patient support by **coordinating resources**. This may involve interactions with medical suppliers, home care services, and/or social agencies to determine what support is available to the patient as his/her needs are identified. Key questions for the nurse to consider are:

- ❖ What alternatives are available in the community?
- ❖ Are cash funds available to assist in the short-term with patient needs?

Depending on what support services are available, it may fall to the nurse to find answers to these questions and to see that the patient is connected to the appropriate resource.

Providing accurate and complete information to the patient is essential. Hesitantly providing information or miscommunicating even a small element of information may undermine the patient's confidence in following the care plan implemented by the nurse.

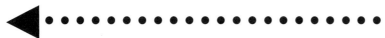

Facilitating appropriate follow-up care may involve scheduling follow-up office visits, scheduling nurse-initiated follow-up phone calls for progress reports, or making referrals to other agencies that can provide the appropriate support. This could also involve reinforcing to the patient why the follow-up care is indicated and enhance compliance.

Evaluation

Evaluation reviews the entire nursing process from assessment through implementation. This step consists of the following components:

❖ Documentation
❖ Communication
❖ Follow-up
❖ Analysis

Documentation of the nurse's assessment of the patient and the intervention is fundamental in maintaining the patient's written health records across the continuum. Documentation also facilitates evaluation of the nursing interaction for quality monitoring and may be reviewed if indicated by a legal inquiry. All written documentation must be complete, objective, accurate, timely, legible, and concise as defined by the organization's policy for nursing documentation and by state practice acts. The nurse should always be on the alert to recognize and avoid common documentation errors that have the potential for liability in the advent of a negative outcome. Good documentation is essential when historically reviewing information to determine quality of care and when looking for opportunities for improvement. If there are gaps in the documentation or the information is unclear, the documentation must be considered incomplete or inaccurate, thus posing potential legal risks to the nurse and the employer. Systematic evaluation will identify documentation patterns as well as suggest areas for quality improvement. Management review of nurses' documentation should occur at regular intervals. When the documentation is reviewed, all information that was shared between the nurse and patient must be noted and clear. Documentation will be covered more fully in later chapters.

Communication in telehealth nursing practice has two components, *verbal* and *written*. These communication skills are critical so that the nurse and the patient are able to effectively understand each other. Communication might also include collaboration with a physician regarding the presenting symptoms of a particular patient so as to determine the appropriate directive. The nurse will also need to be efficient and concise when communicating information to other members of the health care team, such as relaying pertinent patient information to an emergency department prior to the patient's arrival. Managers of institutions that have technology available to listen to nurses calls should

Documentation of the nurse's assessment of the patient and the intervention is fundamental in maintaining the patient's written health records across the continuum.

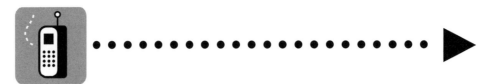

do so regularly. This is an effective way to evaluate the verbal communication component of telehealth nursing practice. Written and verbal communication will be covered in more detail in other chapters.

Follow-up can take on a variety of meanings, depending on the need that initiated the encounter and the action taken. For a directive to seek emergency care, follow-up could involve contacting the emergency room to determine if the patient arrived at the estimated time of arrival (ETA). If the patient has not arrived by the ETA, the nurse may attempt to contact the patient. This is especially important if the nurse has any reservations regarding patient compliance. A follow-up encounter may also be initiated if the nurse feels a lack of closure in a particular interaction, or if nursing judgment suggests that the patient's commitment to instructions may be weak. Despite the patient's agreement to follow a directive to go to an emergency room, there may be hesitancy, denial, or other factors (such as transportation problems) that the patient does not openly communicate with the nurse. During a follow-up, if the nurse finds that the patient did not take appropriate action, there is an opportunity to support the need for intervention and potentially avoid further delay of care. For non-emergent situations, a nurse can provide a follow-up 24 to 48 hours after the initial encounter to evaluate the effectiveness of the nursing process and to determine if there is further opportunity to improve the process.

Analysis of the encounter provides an opportunity for re-examination of each component of the nursing process as applied during the telehealth encounter. It is the nurse's responsibility (not the patient's) to ensure that telehealth practice effectively meets the patient's needs. For this reason, it is critical that the telehealth nurse continually evaluates the effectiveness of personal practice. Self-evaluation may occur concurrently during the encounter or retrospectively after the encounter is concluded. Questions to consider during this review include:

> *It is the nurse's responsibility (not the patient's) to ensure that telehealth practice effectively meets the patient's needs. For this reason, it is critical that the telehealth nurse continually evaluates the effectiveness of personal practice.*

- ❖ Did the assessment gather adequate information from the patient?
- ❖ Was the patient screened for all symptoms that would be considered emergent?
- ❖ Was the most appropriate decision support tool used to support the nursing process?
- ❖ Was the level of urgency or directive for care at the most appropriate level?
- ❖ Were all the appropriate and available resources considered in developing the plan?
- ❖ Did the implemented plan provide the desired result?
- ❖ Was documentation complete, concise, and accurate?
- ❖ Was communication made to other parties as appropriate to enhance quality of care?
- ❖ What could the nurse have done better?
- ❖ What was the patient's level of satisfaction with the care provided?

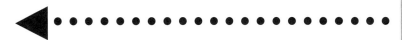

Evaluation of information gathered through follow-ups and other quality assurance initiatives may indicate the need to make changes in components of a guideline or a disposition if consistent weaknesses are identified. To consistently deliver quality care to the patient population, each nurse is responsible to continually monitor care outcomes, both in real time and in historical perspectives. Review of past telehealth encounters provides the individual nurse with opportunities for continuous improvement in delivery of patient care. Patient follow-ups, coordinating peer review with coworkers, and/or requesting physician feedback are a few examples of various methods to facilitate care review. Manager review of documentation and actual listening to calls are excellent ways to assess the quality of patient care provided by each nurse. These have been previously discussed in the communication section. Also the most recent release of the AAACN *Telehealth Nursing Practice Administration and Practice Standards* (2007) has further information regarding quality management in telehealth practice.

NURSING FOCI

While sharing many foci with the larger nursing profession, the nature of telehealth nursing practice modifies the manner in which the foci are operationalized. These foci are:

- ❖ Human response
- ❖ Patient support
- ❖ Patient respect
- ❖ Patient advocacy

Human Response Focus

In telehealth practice, patients frequently present with a cluster of symptoms, rarely reporting a medical diagnosis. Even when patients have a chronic disease, and they assume that the current problem is related to that disease, the nurse must elicit the current symptoms (or responses).

As the telehealth nursing practice role has expanded to include consultation and monitoring, increased emphasis is needed to support the patient who needs assistance in maintaining integration on the health care continuum. In addition to the initial disease/triage focus of the telehealth practice, an increased focus on behavior and psychological integration is occurring. The telehealth nurses may engage in teaching preventive self-care strategies as well as monitor cardiac status in support of home care services.

For example, a patient presents with a chief complaint of chest pain. Further interviewing reveals that it is associated with deep breathing and coughing. Using this information, the nurse develops a plan of action to address the patient's concerns. The depth of patient questioning is

As the telehealth nursing practice role has expanded to include consultation and monitoring, increased emphasis is needed to support the patient who needs assistance in maintaining integration on the health care continuum.

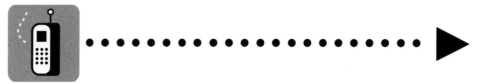

different if the patient has a chronic cardiac or respiratory disease, but the nurse still focuses on the patient's current symptoms or responses, not just on the medical diagnosis as reported by the patient.

Patient Support Focus

A patient may contact a telehealth nurse simply for reassurance that he/she is doing what is right for a home care situation. Supporting these patients is an important focus in telehealth practice. An experienced telehealth nurse may refer to some of these calls as "common sense" calls. When the traditional nuclear family was more common, a family member would have met the needs of these types of calls. These "common sense" calls may simply be the patient seeking a human response to a need when other, more traditional resources are no longer available to offer such reassurances.

Patient Respect Focus

The nurse needs to be aware of patient ethnicity factors. It is important for the nurse to know the cultural, ethnic, or spiritual groups within the specific community served by the telehealth practice.

The nurse needs to be aware of patient ethnicity factors. It is important for the nurse to know the cultural, ethnic, or spiritual groups within the specific community served by the telehealth practice. Certain ethnic groups dictate that the female members observe a subservient role; therefore, the male will provide all the information during a telehealth interaction regarding the health concerns of the female. This is in direct contradiction to good telehealth practice in that the nurse should always interact directly with the patient whenever possible. Knowledge of these groups and their cultural beliefs and values will assist the nurse in working with various populations without inadvertently offending the caller and while still being able to direct the encounter in a manner that enhances good patient outcomes.

Patient Advocacy Focus

As health care delivery becomes increasingly complex, nurses are more often involved in patient advocacy. Patients may present without any knowledge of how to proceed in obtaining the care and medical assistance they need, especially when new to a particular community or facility. As an advocate for the patient, the nurse must actively facilitate access to appropriate medical care and supplies. Within the telehealth practice environment, the nurse may also serve as the link between various health care professionals and health care delivery sites for patients.

ROLES

The nurse has an essential role in total patient care, and has become empowered to act with a greater level of autonomy in making decisions and in managing patient care within the nursing scope of practice. Telehealth nursing practice affords a nurse the opportunity for the same

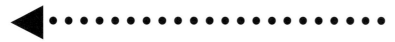

level of independence in practice as would be experienced in a nurse-run ambulatory clinic. The knowledge and skills needed for the successful telehealth practice nurse are no less than those needed for the ambulatory clinic nurse. In fact, the telehealth practice nurse and ambulatory clinic nurse may even be the same individual in varying circumstances. The distinction is in how the patient presents for care. The ambulatory clinic nurse traditionally has a patient physically present, with sight often being the primary sense used by the nurse for initial assessment. When delivering care via telehealth methods, either as a sub-role for the physician office nurse or as a primary role for a nurse in a contact center, active listening and communication skills become the primary tools that allow the nurse to create an image of a "virtual" patient.

The nurse draws upon various skill sets and knowledge bases to fully meet the patient's needs. If providing services as a component of an integrated delivery system, the nurse in a single telehealth encounter may draw upon multiple roles. Examples include providing triage, counseling, demand management, education, self-care support, insurance pre-certification, physician referral, and customer service. The patient may consider the nurse to be a general resource directory for any need that can be met by the health care system. This is more commonly known as the "when all else fails, ask the nurse" syndrome. The range of services can be narrowed down to a single focus if the organization's mission is to provide only a triage service that determines the patient's level of acuity and then directs them to the appropriate level of care. As true in any developing practice, the activity needs to be precisely defined so that the standards can be set, and so that the nurse knows and understands the expectations of professional practice. With standards in place, the consumer of the service also knows what to expect as an end result. AAACN (2007) has actively worked to this end by publishing *Telehealth Nursing Practice Administration and Practice Standards* and by sponsoring the development of this program. Consequently, additional efforts have been made to identify nursing roles or interventions within the realm of telehealth nursing practice. According to Haas and Androwich (1999), the four major telehealth nursing practice roles are telephone triage, telephone consultation, telephone follow-up, and telephone surveillance. During any given telehealth encounter, these roles may be used singularly or in combination to achieve the desired outcome.

Telephone Triage Role

Telephone triage is best defined as the matching of patient need to the most appropriate use of health care resources at the most important time. This should not be confused with triage as implemented in an emergency environment, where medical staff determines level of acuity to prioritize the order in which patients are treated. Typically, the patient initiates telephone triage by contacting a recognized medical unit (for example, the

Telehealth nursing practice affords a nurse the opportunity for the same level of independence in practice as would be experienced in a nurse-run ambulatory clinic. In fact, the telehealth practice nurse and ambulatory clinic nurse may even be the same individual in varying circumstances.

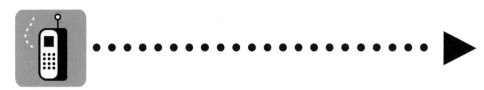

primary care provider or a nursing contact center). The nurse working in either of these settings responds by using the nursing process and interviewing skills to assess the patient's need, to apply organization-approved decision support tools to determine the urgency for intervention, and to consider other factors that would place the patient at risk. The nurse must separate chronic health concerns from acute needs. Through use of a strong knowledge base, critical-thinking skills, and utilization of formal nursing guidelines, the nurse is able to advise the patient of the appropriate plan of care, instruct the patient in self-care as appropriate, and offer other measures necessary to ensure the best outcome. At the conclusion of this interaction, depending on the disposition of care, the nurse may arrange a time and date for follow-up to monitor the patient's outcome.

Telephone triage can be very challenging and quite rewarding. Consider the amount of time involved to triage a patient who presents to the nurse in person for treatment of a rash. Consider the same patient presenting with the very same complaint to a telehealth nurse. The time to arrive at the same conclusion is significantly lengthened because many more questions must be asked to elicit the same information that the eye could register in seconds.

Telephone Consultation Role

The telephone consultation role focuses on providing health education and advice, and sharing information regarding health services. The patient or the nurse may initiate the contact. The primary role of the nurse in this encounter is educator or referral coordinator. The patient may not have an immediate health problem, but may recently have heard of a particular health issue through the media or an acquaintance, and calls the nurse as an easily accessible and reliable source of health information. In counseling the patient, effective education of health care principles can lead to greater maintenance of wellness. With the anonymity and confidentiality that a telehealth encounter can provide, the patient may have a sense of confidence and control of the interaction that would not be present if meeting with a physician or nurse face-to-face to discuss the same need for information. Difficult issues can be openly discussed without fear of recognition. The telehealth nurse can thus function as a health educator when the patient presents with a need for knowledge regarding health maintenance or disease avoidance. Some nurse contact centers are focused on this role primarily as a health education and service referral service, rather than as a triage service.

With this role, the nurse must give careful consideration to the information the patient is requesting and determine if there is a hidden agenda. These calls may start with simple opening statements such as, "What can you tell me about…" or "What are the symptoms of…" With further interviewing and by gaining the trust of the patient, the nurse may

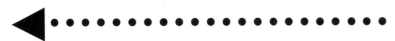

determine that the patient has an active medical concern that warrants further discussion or triage, or possibly need immediate care.

Telephone Follow-up Role

Telephone follow-up is typically a nurse-initiated contact with the patient. This scenario can be created by two different patient needs. The need for follow-up could be determined either at the conclusion of a prior telephone triage interaction or as a result of a consultation request. When completing a prior encounter, the nurse contracts with the patient for a time when the follow-up will occur. This is a controlled demand on the nurse as opposed to triage and consultation activities, which are patient-driven and consequently often unpredictable or variable demand.

Follow-up to a telephone triage encounter can be used as a tool to evaluate the effectiveness of the entire nursing process and to determine if further intervention is necessary. This is particularly useful for the nurse providing support to an individual who is hesitant or unsure of his/her ability to provide home care successfully, such as parents of young children. Acceptance and compliance with home care instructions are enhanced when the parent knows they are not isolated and that the nurse's involvement and support will continue. Ongoing telehealth contacts over the course of several hours may be needed to provide support for symptoms that meet home management criteria, such as fever or vomiting. Follow-up can also be used to gather patient satisfaction and quality indicators, with the follow-up occurring after the patient's initial request for assistance.

Follow-up to a telephone triage encounter can be used as a tool to evaluate the effectiveness of the entire nursing process and to determine if further intervention is necessary.

Follow-up to a consultation request may be used to determine patient follow-through with earlier information or to see if there are additional services that can be provided. Such an encounter could also occur if the nurse is unable to provide full information during the initial contact. Due to the complexity of the patient's request or the specificity of information needed, the nurse may need to do additional research and contact the patient at a later time to share what has been learned. This type of follow-up is more of a marketing initiative compared to a follow-up from triage, which evaluates quality of a previous encounter and brings closure to a symptom-based situation.

Telephone Surveillance (Monitoring) Role

Telephone surveillance or monitoring is perhaps the most recent development in telehealth nursing roles. With the continued sophistication of developing technology, the patient is now supported in their home environment with a variety of monitoring devices. The patient and his/her family or care provider are partnered with a nurse (or nurses) whose responsibility includes monitoring the patient and the equipment for any reportable change in the patient's health status.

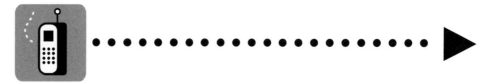

Available monitoring devices provide a variety of clinical information devices (for example, vital signs, EKGs, laboratory test results) along with video monitoring of the patient in their home environment. The depth of information reported will depend on the type of device installed in the patient setting. The telehealth connection, typically initiated by the nurse, is made at scheduled times to review the data received and to make general inquiries regarding the patient. However, unscheduled contacts may be needed to advise the patient that the devices indicate that a change in care management is required. The patient may also initiate the contact with concerns they have regarding the technology or his/her health status. Utilization of these monitoring devices typically allows the patient to remain in his/her home environment and promotes a more active role in self-care. In this type of situation, the patient should feel that he/she is less isolated and that support is provided as needed. For the provider, these devices permit more frequent monitoring and earlier intervention without putting the patient through the strain and risk of traveling from his/her home. With active monitoring, it is anticipated that there will be improved therapy compliance, better outcome tracking, and enhanced clinical decision-making. As this type of technology becomes more advanced, a need for centralized nurse monitoring centers will develop, analogous to work centers telemetry created in the hospital environment.

With active monitoring, it is anticipated that there will be improved therapy compliance, better outcome tracking, and enhanced clinical decision-making.

LIFE-LONG LEARNING

In general, nursing practice and telehealth practice are constantly evolving in response to technology and the ever-changing demand of the patient population that presents for care. Nursing is an applied profession and one in which knowledge is dynamically changing. Life-long learning is key to maintaining all competencies. Examples of clinical changes that demonstrate the need for life-long learning might include:

- ❖ *Female chest pain.* It is now documented that women do not follow the typical presentation pattern as evidenced in male patients. The telehealth nurse must know how the symptoms of the female patient presenting with chest pain vary from those experienced by the male patient population.
- ❖ *Outpatient or "short stay" surgical procedures.* Patients are often discharged to home following procedures that would have previously warranted at least overnight hospitalization, such as cholecystectomy. The telehealth nurse may be providing all post-procedure nursing support for self-care at home.
- ❖ *Postpartum care.* Providing mother and infant postpartum care instructions and support includes newborn care as well as breast-feeding guidance, because the mother's milk is not likely to be in before discharge to home.

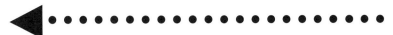

❖ *Newly released medications or treatment standards.* Patients may contact the telehealth nurse to obtain more detailed information about new medical practices they have heard about through the media or friends, or did not have fully explained while in the physician's office.

Several external mechanisms exist to ensure society of continued competency by nurses. After initial licensure requirement, several states require mandatory continuing nursing education hours for licensure renewal. Accreditation agencies place requirements on organizations to address the learning needs of employees. Finally, certifications address competency within a given specialty of nursing, and ambulatory nursing certification is available through the American Nurses Credentialing Center.

In addition to the external factors supporting life-long learning, individuals should be internally motivated to maintain the high standard of ongoing competency that warrants the trust of patients. Within the health care environment, nurses are increasingly valued as knowledgeable workers who manage change and provide innovative solutions. Critical-thinking skills are a necessary part of life-long learning. Employment of critical-thinking skills requires that nurses actively question and think about their nursing actions, and strategize ways to improve patient outcomes. Use of critical-thinking strategies empowers nurses to move beyond being merely competent to becoming nurse experts. The telehealth nurse might consider the following in the quest for nursing expertise.

Several external mechanisms exist to ensure society of continued competency by nurses. After initial licensure requirement, several states require mandatory continuing nursing education hours for licensure renewal.

❖ Describe personal ability to affect specific outcomes related to telehealth advice provided to patients.
❖ Determine that individual telehealth practice is based on evidence-based practices versus tradition.
❖ Analyze methods to improve personal telehealth practice.
❖ Describe ways that individual telehealth nursing actions make a positive difference to the patient.
❖ Outline actions to become an expert in telehealth practice.

SUMMARY

When all is considered, whether practicing in a telehealth environment or in a direct patient care setting, the nurse must bring to the role an appreciation for the patient and the opportunity to provide nursing care to each unique situation. There is never an occasion to lessen the nursing process in any practice setting. The competent nurse keeps the complete situation in mind from the moment patient contact is made and continually seeks to clarify the patient's need. During the interaction, the nurse implements interviewing and assessing skills to more sharply focus on the

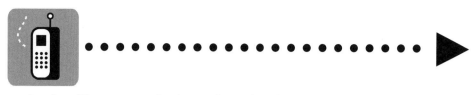

patient's dilemma and determine the intervention needed with the assistance of appropriate decision support tools. Telehealth practice places no greater or lesser strain on a nurse than any other nursing role. Every element of the nursing process is used as the nurse processes information received from the patient. All nursing environments demand competency, critical judgment, problem-solving, effective communication, and an ongoing desire to deliver to each patient the very best outcome possible.

Telehealth practice places no greater or lesser strain on a nurse than any other nursing role.

TIPS & PEARLS

☎ Demonstrate the nursing process with each encounter, along with responsibility and accountability for each encounter.

☎ Demonstrate competencies in communicating, logical problem-solving, critical thinking, professionalism, and accountability. In telehealth, these competencies are extremely important because the patient cannot see these skills – only hear them.

☎ Always ask the patient/caregiver to repeat back or summarize the care instructions to verify his/her understanding of the next steps.

☎ Reinforce to the patient why follow-up care is indicated. By educating the patient on why this care is important, there is a higher likelihood that the patient will comply with the instructions.

☎ It is your responsibility (not your employer's) to seek out new learning opportunities and commit to life-long learning.

☎ Challenge yourself to look for opportunities to demonstrate the four major roles of telehealth practice (triage, consultation, follow-up, and surveillance [monitoring]), and practice the necessary skill sets effectively.

References
American Academy of Ambulatory Care Nursing (AAACN). (2007). *Telehealth nursing practice administration and practice standards* (4th ed.). Pitman, NJ: Author.

Briggs, J.K. (2007). *Telephone triage protocols for nurses.* Philadelphia: Lippincott, Williams, & Wilkins.

Haas, S.A., & Androwich, I.A. (1999). Telephone consultation. In G.A. Bulechek & J.C. McCloskey (Eds.), *Nursing interventions effective nursing treatments* (pp. 670-684). Philadelphia: W.B. Saunders Company.

Answer/Evaluation Form
AMBP9c01
Continuing Nursing Education Activity
Telehealth Nursing Practice Essentials
Chapter 2: Focus and Roles

This activity provides 1.4 contact hours of continuing nursing education (CNE) credit in nursing.
(Contact hours calculated using a 60-minute contact hour.)

This test may be copied for use by others.

COMPLETE THE FOLLOWING:

Name: _____

Address: _____

City: _____ State: _____ Zip: _____

Telephone number: (Home)_____ (Work)_____

Email address:_____

AAACN Member Number and Expiration Date: _____

Processing fee: AAACN Member: $12.00
                 Nonmember: $20.00

Answer Form: (Please attach a separate sheet of paper if necessary.)
1. What did you value most about this activity?

_____
_____
_____
_____

2. If you could imagine that you have fully integrated your learning into practice, what would be different about your present practice?

_____
_____
_____
_____

Evaluation	Strongly disagree				Strongly agree
3. The offering met the stated objectives.					
a. Describe the use of the nursing process as related to telehealth practice.	1	2	3	4	5
b. Explain how specific nursing foci are demonstrated in telehealth practice.	1	2	3	4	5
c. Summarize the four major roles of the nurse in telehealth practice.	1	2	3	4	5
d. Describe ways that life-long learning enhances telehealth nursing practice.	1	2	3	4	5
4. The content was current and relevant.	1	2	3	4	5
5. The content was presented clearly.	1	2	3	4	5
6. The content was covered adequately.	1	2	3	4	5

7. How would you rate your ability to apply your learning to practice following this activity? (Check one)
   ☐ Diminished ability ☐ No change ☐ Enhanced ability

8. Time required to complete reading assignment and answer form: ___ minutes
Comments _____

I verify that I have completed this activity:

_____
Signature

Objectives
This educational activity is designed for nurses and other health care professionals who provide telehealth care for patients. This evaluation is designed to test your achievement of the following educational activities.
1. Describe the use of the nursing process as related to telehealth practice.
2. Explain how specific nursing foci are demonstrated in telehealth practice.
3. Summarize the four major roles of the nurse in telehealth practice.
4. Describe ways that life-long learning enhances telehealth nursing practice.

Evaluation Form Instructions
1. To receive continuing nursing education (CNE) credit for individual study after reading the indicated chapter(s), please complete the evaluation form (photocopies of the answer form are acceptable). Attach separate paper as necessary.
2. Detach (or photocopy) and send the answer form along with a check, money order, or credit card payable to *AAACN* East Holly Avenue/Box 56, Pitman, NJ 08071-0056. You may also send this form as an email attachment to ambp401@ajj.com.
3. Answer forms must be postmarked by December 31, 2011. Upon completion of the answer/evaluation form, a certificate for 1.4 contact hours will be awarded and sent to you.

Payment Options
☐ Check or money order enclosed (payable in U.S. funds to AAACN)

☐ MasterCard ☐ VISA ☐ American Express

Credit Card #:_____

Expiration Date: _____ Security Code:_____

Card Holder (Please print):

_____

Signature:

_____

This educational activity has been co-provided by the American Academy of Ambulatory Care Nursing (AAACN) and Anthony J. Jannetti, Inc. (AJJ).
AAACN is a provider approved by the California Board of Registered Nursing, Provider Number CEP 5336.
AJJ is accredited as a provider of continuing nursing education by the American Nurses Credentialing Center's Commission on Accreditation.
This book was reviewed and formatted for contact hour credit by Sally S. Russell, MN, CMSRN, AAACN Education Director, and Maureen Espensen, MBA, BSN, RN, Editor.

American Academy of Ambulatory Care Nursing
East Holly Avenue/Box 56, Pitman, NJ 08071-0056
Phone: 800-AMB-NURS; Fax: 856-589-7463
Web: www.aaacn.org; Email: aaacn@ajj.com

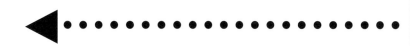

CHAPTER 3
Customer Service

Objectives

1. Describe the impact of customer service as it relates to health care.
2. Explain how the telehealth practice nurse provides high-quality customer service.
3. Offer key customer service interventions to quickly improve customer satisfaction.

Consumers seeking health care service have the:

- ❖ Expectation that quality service will be provided.
- ❖ Expectation that service will meet or exceed the perception.
- ❖ Expectation that if the service standard is not met, the situation will be remedied.
- ❖ Expectation that their symptoms and health concerns will be kept private and confidential.

Consumers are demanding high-quality service and attention to detail in every aspect of the service and production industries. The ability to compare prices, the desire for timely service, and the importance of name recognition are several of the driving forces behind consumer choices. Customers today have more options and less time than ever before. They are more technologically skilled than in the past and know that if their expectations are not met, they can walk down the street or surf the Internet and happily do business with a competitor within only hours or days (Zemke, 2003).

The primary consumer driving force is customer satisfaction and customers are satisfied when their expectations are met or exceeded. Because of the high importance of customer service, patients should be seen not only as patients, but also as customers.

While so much focus is given to providing good service to hospitalized patients, the same consideration must be given to internal and external telehealth customers. These customers include:

- ❖ The caller and patient.
- ❖ The patient's family, significant other(s), and/or friends.
- ❖ Members of the health care team, which may include providers, midlevel practitioners, co-workers, health plans, outpatient services, and case managers.

Consumers are demanding high-quality service and attention to detail in every aspect of the service and production industries. The ability to compare prices, the desire for timely service, and the importance of name recognition are several of the driving forces behind consumer choices.

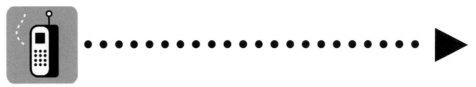

If a customer is unhappy with the service received, the customer will tell 9 or 10 people, and if satisfied, the customer will only tell a family member or neighbor. This means that if a business had just one dissatisfied customer a day, the word about their dissatisfaction could spread to 3,650 people in one year (GRM Business Solutions, LLC, 2008).

In any health care setting, the level of customer service can significantly influence the success or failure of a program or organization. This influence includes the ability to meet marketing and financial goals, relationship-building, delivery of care, and sustainability of the organization. Today, health care costs are skyrocketing and the health care market is highly competitive. The ability to attract and retain customers has greatly affected the financial status of most health care organizations. Providing a consistently high level of customer service leads to name recognition and repeat visits or sales.

Companies with noted quality service include Marriott, Nordstroms, and the Disney Corporation. Health care organizations are not often included in such a list. However, provision of health care is a business and is subject to the same principles of customer service. In leading the revolution, today's consumers begin to buy goods and services at a younger age. They are consumers for a longer period and are much more sophisticated than the consumers of the past. They are empowered to declare their dissatisfaction with service, which influences the profits of providers and organizations. In order to be competitive, health care services have recognized the importance of satisfied consumers and have made providing quality customer service a major initiative.

A consumer-centric organization is one that approaches its processes from the viewpoint of the consumer or customer. Particularly in health care, this is a very different approach. Most health care processes are still derived from a procedural model that is convenient for and centered on the provider. A few organizations are now changing the relationship dynamics between the health care consumer and health care provider.

An organization can promote a customer service focus, but it is the customer's expectation and perception of the experience with the staff that is most important. By being one of the initial contact points for the organization, the telehealth professional has a unique opportunity to develop the relationship between the organization and its customers. The nurse's mannerisms and attitude with customers are important and powerful influences on marketing, customer satisfaction, and patient retention. Additionally, the nurse's mannerisms and attitude contribute to the reputation and success of the organization. The nurse has the ability and opportunity to develop a positive and trustful relationship with the customer and to serve as a bridge between the patient and provider.

Customers are often reluctant to discuss their dissatisfaction with their health care providers due to the personal nature of the situation, or customers may fear that their future needs will not be met if they

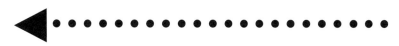

complain. Caregivers should view the feedback from dissatisfied consumers as an opportunity to improve processes. The telehealth professional can be an objective and empathetic discoverer of a person's satisfaction or dissatisfaction in the health care organization. Many health systems are utilizing their telehealth staff for assistance to better understand consumers' needs. To obtain information about customer service from the majority of consumers who never verbalize their opinions, organizations use customer satisfaction surveys collected anonymously.

CUSTOMER DISSATISFIERS

Some common areas of dissatisfaction identified by health care consumers that pertain to the telehealth nursing practice are:

Not being called back in a timely fashion. Telehealth personnel may use a call-back scenario for non-emergent calls. Delay of Care case law is increasing. Appropriate response times need to be identified and clearly communicated to the caller. If the response requires contacting a provider, it will generally result in a longer response time. Contract with the caller a time parameter in which to expect a response and be prepared to renegotiate when necessary.

Being placed on hold for an extended time. Be proactive by thanking the patient for holding and express appreciation for their time on hold. If the caller is left on hold longer than expected, take the time to go back on the line and question whether the caller is willing to continue holding or would prefer to be called back within a specified time frame. The telephone technology needs to be designed to deliver an inquisitive (not frustrated) customer. Understand your systems and make them user-friendly.

Being put on hold without permission. Ask permission before placing a caller on hold. Be sure to wait for the response. Some valid reasons that a caller may not be able to hold are:

❖ The situation is emergent.
❖ The caller's cell phone connection or battery is weak.
❖ The caller may have a limited amount of time to hold. For example, the caller may be on a work break or calling between classes.

Inadequate technical equipment. Technology that inadequately supports the telehealth program can be greatly dissatisfying to callers. Issues include receiving busy signals because of overloaded trunk lines, extended hold times in queue, and telephone announcements that are confusing, too long, or too repetitive.

The telephone technology needs to be designed to deliver an inquisitive (not frustrated) customer. Understand your systems and make them user-friendly.

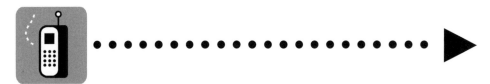

Being transferred from person to person. "Bouncing" is very frustrating for the caller for multiple reasons. There is always the risk that the call may be accidentally disconnected. Before transferring a call, be sure to give the caller the extension of the intended recipient of the transfer. Although expeditious, blind transfers should never be a regular occurrence. Do not hang up until the recipient acknowledges the transferred call. Many calls are personal in nature, and most callers do not like to repeat their private information to multiple people. It is important to transfer to the correct person the first time. If the nurse is unsure who this may be, it is best to explain to the caller the situation while volunteering to research the appropriate placement of the call. Ask permission to call back with the requested information within a short period.

Broken commitments. Credibility is lost when a commitment made by the nurse to a caller is not kept. If unable to fulfill a commitment such as returning a collaborative call within an hour, the caller should be notified and a new period established.

Being treated rudely and without compassion. When callers are ill, they want to be treated with kindness and compassion. In fact, all people should be treated in a professional manner, similar to how we would like to be treated in the same situation.

CUSTOMER SATISFIERS

Presentation and Relationship-Building

Presenting a positive attitude that is reflected in voice, choice of words, and actions can go a long way in meeting customer expectations. Communicating respect, empathy, and politeness are very important customer satisfiers that cost nothing. In today's marketplace, it is not enough to just meet customer expectations. To be a leader in customer service, exceeding customer expectations will result in "delighted" customers.

Customer Delight

Finding ways to delight the caller is the new standard for customer service. Offering to take care of needs beyond the original reason for the call is one way to delight the customer. A telehealth example might be offering to set up future appointments as part of the call. Another opportunity is expanding the focus of the call beyond the immediate need by reviewing the patient's immunizations and preventative care services (mammograms, pap smears, etc.) with them. An additional service may be offered after an illness-related phone call. Follow-up calls may be placed to check on the condition of the patient and inquire if they need further medical services. Another idea is reaching out to those with chronic illnesses such as diabetes, heart disease, or asthma to see if there are any

When callers are ill, they want to be treated with kindness and compassion. In fact, all people should be treated in a professional manner, similar to how we would like to be treated in the same situation.

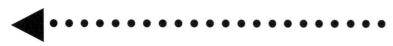

barriers to following their treatment plan. This can communicate caring and an interest in their well-being. It may also give those who may find it difficult to disclose socio-economic barriers the opportunity to open up and allow proactive problem-solving.

SUMMARY

While it is easy to state what not to do, identifying those behaviors that constitute exceptional service is really much more an integration of values and common sense. What does great telephone service feel like? It has been described as feeling as if you just talked to a dear friend who shared timely information, listened to your concerns, and truly cared about you and your family's well-being.

As demand for health care services from a successful customer-focused organization increases, nurses will see the organization's culture being transformed. A customer-focused organization differentiates itself from the competition and will achieve many successes. Organizations must recruit and retain competent personnel who will assist in building respect and loyalty with all types of customers and within the community. A survey by Solucient, LLC (2003) showed that good telehealth services in call centers will support patient loyalty, attract customers from premium target groups, increase satisfaction with their health care provider, and can augment revenues downstream from the initial contacts. Nurses will achieve higher personal and professional satisfaction when they are able to provide quality service that meets patients' needs.

The telehealth practice nurse has an important role in providing high-quality customer-focused service. By doing so, the nurse has the unique opportunity to have positive interactions with the customer, build a trusting relationship, and seek to have the organization viewed as a caring and supportive health care delivery system. It is all about relationship-building and the art of patient care.

A customer-focused organization differentiates itself from the competition and will achieve many successes.

TIPS & PEARLS

☎ The primary consumer driving force is customer satisfaction, which occurs when expectations are met or exceeded.

☎ Telehealth customers include patients, patients' family and/or friends, as well as members of the health care team (e.g., health care providers, health plans, etc.).

☎ The telehealth nurse has a unique opportunity in developing a positive relationship between his/her organization and its customers.

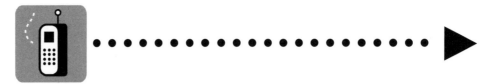

References

GRM Business Solutions, LLC. (2008). *Effective customer service management for Internet businesses.* Retrieved September 14, 2008, from http://www.effectivecustomerservicemanagement.com/

Solucient, LLC. (2003). *The call center as a marketing channel: A report from Solucient.* Evanston, IL: Author.

Zemke, R. (2003). *Delivering knock your socks off service* (3rd ed.). New York, NY: AMACOM Publishing.

Answer/Evaluation Form
Continuing Nursing Education Activity
Telehealth Nursing Practice Essentials
Chapter 3: Customer Service

AMBP9c02

This activity provides 1.0 contact hour of continuing nursing education (CNE) credit in nursing.
(Contact hours calculated using a 60-minute contact hour.)

This test may be copied for use by others.

COMPLETE THE FOLLOWING:

Name: _____

Address: _____

City: _____ State: _____ Zip: _____

Telephone number: (Home)_____ (Work)_____

Email address:_____

AAACN Member Number and Expiration Date: _____

Processing fee:　AAACN Member:　$12.00
　　　　　　　　Nonmember:　$20.00

Answer Form: (Please attach a separate sheet of paper if necessary.)
1.　What did you value most about this activity?

_____
_____
_____
_____

2.　If you could imagine that you have fully integrated your learning into practice, what would be different about your present practice?

_____
_____
_____
_____
_____

Evaluation	Strongly disagree				Strongly agree
3.　The offering met the stated objectives.					
a. Describe the impact of customer service as it relates to health care.	1	2	3	4	5
b. Explain how the telehealth practice nurse provides high-quality customer service.	1	2	3	4	5
c. Offer key customer service interventions to quickly improve customer satisfaction.	1	2	3	4	5
4.　The content was current and relevant.	1	2	3	4	5
5.　The content was presented clearly.	1	2	3	4	5
6.　The content was covered adequately.	1	2	3	4	5

7.　How would you rate your ability to apply your learning to practice following this activity? (Check one)

☐ Diminished ability　☐ No change　☐ Enhanced ability

8.　Time required to complete reading assignment and answer form: ___ minutes
Comments _____
_____

I verify that I have completed this activity:

_____
Signature

Objectives
This educational activity is designed for nurses and other health care professionals who provide telehealth care for patients. This evaluation is designed to test your achievement of the following educational activities.
1.　Describe the impact of customer service as it relates to health care.
2.　Explain how the telehealth practice nurse provides high-quality customer service.
3.　Offer key customer service interventions to quickly improve customer satisfaction.

Evaluation Form Instructions
1. To receive continuing nursing education (CNE) credit for individual study after reading the indicated chapter(s), please complete the evaluation form (photocopies of the answer form are acceptable). Attach separate paper as necessary.
2. Detach (or photocopy) and send the answer form along with a check, money order, or credit card payable to *AAACN* East Holly Avenue/Box 56, Pitman, NJ 08071-0056. You may also send this form as an email attachment to ambp401@ajj.com.
3. Answer forms must be postmarked by December 31, 2011. Upon completion of the answer/evaluation form, a certificate for 1.0 contact hour will be awarded and sent to you.

Payment Options
☐ Check or money order enclosed (payable in U.S. funds to AAACN)

☐ MasterCard　☐ VISA　☐ American Express

Credit Card #:_____

Expiration Date: _____ Security Code:_____

Card Holder (Please print):

_____

Signature:

_____

This educational activity has been co-provided by the American Academy of Ambulatory Care Nursing (AAACN) and Anthony J. Jannetti, Inc. (AJJ).

AAACN is a provider approved by the California Board of Registered Nursing, Provider Number CEP 5336.

AJJ is accredited as a provider of continuing nursing education by the American Nurses Credentialing Center's Commission on Accreditation.

This book was reviewed and formatted for contact hour credit by Sally S. Russell, MN, CMSRN, AAACN Education Director, and Maureen Espensen, MBA, BSN, RN, Editor.

American Academy of Ambulatory Care Nursing
East Holly Avenue/Box 56, Pitman, NJ 08071-0056
Phone: 800-AMB-NURS; Fax: 856-589-7463
Web: www.aaacn.org; Email: aaacn@ajj.com

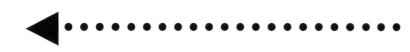

CHAPTER 4
Communication Principles

Objectives

1. Compare and contrast the conventional communication model with the Telehealth Nursing Communications (TNC) Model.
2. Identify the differences in which the patient and the nurse approach an encounter.
3. Describe influences which may affect the nurse-patient encounter.

Communication has multiple definitions. Merriam-Webster (2008) described the verb form of the word *communicate* as to:

- ❖ Share.
- ❖ Convey knowledge or information about; make known; to reveal by clear signs.
- ❖ Cause to pass from one to another.
- ❖ Transmit information, thought, or feeling so that it is satisfactorily received or understood.
- ❖ Open into each other.

Adler and Elmhorst (2006) described communication as the process that people use to exchange messages or information through various channels and respond through verbal and non-verbal feedback. The feedback can be interrupted or diminished by physical, physiological, or psychological noise from the sender or the receiver. Common to all definitions is that communication involves an exchange of information and that there are challenges in order to have a clear understanding of this exchange.

COMMUNICATION MODELS

Within telehealth nursing practice, clear and understandable communications become especially challenging because the nurse and the caller cannot observe non-verbal behaviors as a means to confirm the understanding or misunderstanding of the message. Auditory cues are used to clarify the communicated message (such as background noise, quality of speech, and voice energy, volume, and tone) when using the telephone. However, when interacting via Web-based technology, communication is based only on the written word.

Within telehealth nursing practice, clear and understandable communications become especially challenging because the nurse and the caller cannot observe non-verbal behaviors as a means to confirm the understanding or misunderstanding of the message.

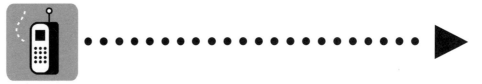

Traditional Communication Model

Telehealth nursing practice literature commonly presents a traditional model of communication. Figure 4-1 is a representation of a traditional communication approach.

Figure 4-1.

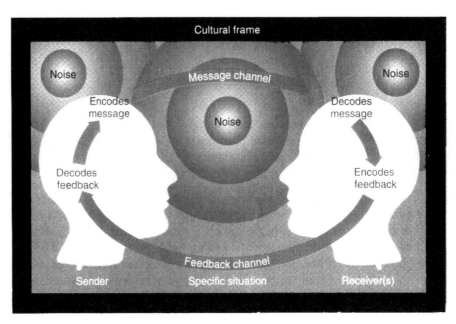

15. An early model of the communication model appears in Schramm, W. (1954). How communication works. In W. Schramm (Ed.), *The process and effects of mass communication* (pp. 3–10). Urbana: University of Illinois Press. Scholars in the ensuing decades have continued to refine the model.

The framework of culture surrounds this model and influences both the coding and decoding of the messages.

As represented in Figure 4-1, there is a sender and a receiver who participate in activities of encoding and decoding messages. A message channel is also present and for the purpose of telehealth nursing practice, the message channel is usually the telephone, but can also be via Web-based technology. In this model, the sender is the patient contacting the nurse. The patient encodes or chooses the message to send to the receiver, who is the nurse. As the receiver of information, the nurse decodes the message in order to understand the information being shared. The nurse then offers feedback to the patient to clarify the specific information being shared. The framework of culture surrounds this model and influences both the coding and decoding of the messages (Schramm, 1954).

Telehealth Nursing Communications (TNC) Model

As telehealth nursing roles expand beyond the initial triage roles, the need for a new communication model is evident. Traditionally, the patient initiates

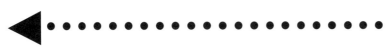

the nurse-patient encounter. Even though this is still a large part of the telehealth nursing role, it is now expected that the nurse also initiates outbound contact to the patient for consultation, follow-up care, and surveillance.

The Telehealth Nursing Communication (TNC) Model represents the nurse, the patient and family, and the exchange of information during the encounter. The contact may be initiated by either the nurse or the patient. The patient-initiated encounter to the nurse is usually to seek health information or advice, but it may also be a call for assistance with an appointment, prescription refill, or general information. The nurse-initiated encounter may be a consultation, a follow-up, or involve surveillance (monitoring).

The patient-initiated encounter to the nurse is usually to seek health information or advice, but it may also be a call for assistance with an appointment, prescription refill, or general information.

Figure 4-2.

Telehealth Nursing Communication Model

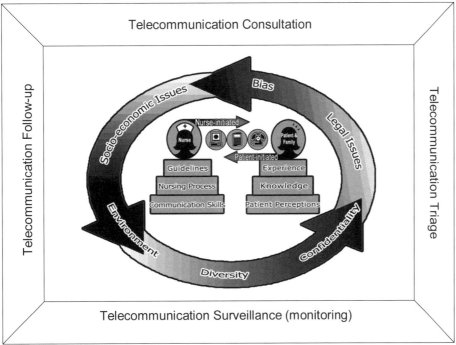

Copyright © 2009
American Academy of Ambulatory Care Nursing

In Figure 4-2, both the nurse and the patient approach the encounter from different perspectives. The nurse is supported by the nursing process, communication skills, and guidelines used during the progression of the encounter. The care provided is supported by the nursing process (assessing,

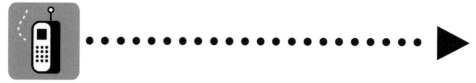

planning, implementing, and evaluating the problem or concern of the patient). The nurse's ability to provide care is also supported by communication skills and proficiency in handling various types of encounters (see Chapter 5, "Communication Techniques"). In addition, the nurse provides care through the use of decision support tools that have been approved by the management of the work setting. The guidelines include policies and procedures for documentation, risk management, use of equipment, and other factors.

As represented in Figure 4-2, the patient enters the process of information exchange with expectations of care supported by knowledge, perceptions, and past experiences. The patient may have a limited or vast knowledge of the problem or concern. The patient has a perception of what the nurse can do to be of assistance. Additionally, the patient may have had a positive or negative experience with the health care system.

The exchange of information is a process in which internal and external influences may distort the transmission for both the patient and the nurse, such as bias, socioeconomic factors, environment, diversity, legal issues, and patient confidentiality. These influences can alter how the nurse and the patient exchange information.

> *The exchange of information is a process in which internal and external influences may distort the transmission for both the patient and the nurse.*

As an example of bias, the nurse may assume all members of a certain group process health advice in a specific manner and therefore omit pertinent information when communicating. The patient may, due to socioeconomic factors, have limited access to health care, and the nurse must have full knowledge of potential social service support resources. The environment can influence the nurse's ability to communicate effectively. For example, if the working area is crowded and the noise level is high, the ability to process the encounter in a confident and professional manner may be hindered. Diversity can affect the exchange of information. The telehealth nurse must deliver nursing care that reflects the cultural, spiritual, psychosocial, and intellectual/educational differences of individual patients, families, or communities, and that preserves patient autonomy, dignity, and rights (AAACN, 2007).

Another influence that affects the information exchange is patient confidentiality. The conversation must be held in an area where information can be exchanged privately. Also, the nurse needs to be sensitive to the patient's issues when discussing personal information. Examples include family members present during the conversation or calling back at the patient's work site. Additionally, the nurse must be aware of organizational policies and legal ramifications affecting telehealth nursing. As a professional health care member, the nurse must be sensitive to negative influences and seek ways to minimize their affect on the exchange of information. The nurse is responsible for building a trustful, working relationship with the patient and seeking ways to meet their health care needs.

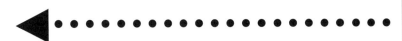

Framing the TNC Model, four types of telehealth roles are depicted. These are consultation, triage, surveillance (monitoring), and follow-up.

Consultation is the exchange of information, offering advice, health education, and symptom management. Either the nurse or patient initiates the encounter. *Triage* is the process of identifying the patient's health problem or concern, deciding on the level of acuity, and facilitating the appropriate disposition. The patient generally initiates the encounter. *Surveillance (monitoring)* is described as a nursing intervention utilized when working with patients on specific equipment related to home care (for example, a cardiac monitor that can transmit readings over the telephone line). The nurse is responsible for gathering and interpreting data from the equipment to assist the patient and their caregivers in administering care. *Follow-up* is the management of patient symptoms, determining compliance, or addressing knowledge deficits; the nurse usually initiates the follow-up.

The TNC Model incorporates the expanded roles associated with telehealth nursing practice. This model illustrates the information exchange, the multiple roles of the patient and the nurse, as well as the support underlying and surrounding the importance of communication in telehealth nursing practice.

Framing the TNC Model, four types of telehealth roles are depicted. These are consultation, triage, surveillance (monitoring), and follow-up.

SUMMARY

Telehealth nursing practice has expanded to include four main interventions: consultation, triage, surveillance, and follow-up. Communication can be influenced by various factors. Both the nurse and the patient have expectations regarding the process of telehealth communications. The nurse is a provider of care and is supported by the nursing process, communication skills, and guidelines. Knowledge, perceptions and experiences support the patient's expectations. Applying relevant communication techniques utilizing telecommunication devices to interact with and educate patients is a core dimension fundamental to telehealth nursing practice (Becker & Haynes, 2006).

TIPS & PEARLS

☎ The Telehealth Nursing Communication Model represents the nurse, the patient and family, and the exchange of information during an encounter.

☎ The information exchange can be affected by influences, such as socioeconomic factors, patient confidentiality, bias, environment, diversity, and legal issues.

☎ Telehealth nursing practice roles include triage, consultation, follow-up, and surveillance.

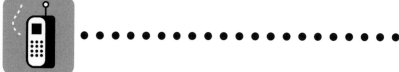

References

Adler, R.B., & Elmhorst, J.M. (2006). *Communicating at work – Principles and practices for business and the professions* (8th ed.). New York: McGraw-Hill.

American Academy of Ambulatory Care Nursing (AAACN). (2007). *Telehealth nursing practice administration and practice standards* (4th ed.). Pitman, NJ: Author.

Becker, C.A., & Haynes, T.S. (2006). Telehealth nursing practice. In C. Baker Laughlin (Ed.), *Core curriculum for ambulatory care nursing* (pp. 137-148). Pitman, NJ: American Academy of Ambulatory Care Nursing.

Merriam-Webster. (2008). *Communicate: Definition from the Merriam-Webster online dictionary.* Retrieved March 1, 2008, from http://www.merriam-webster.com/dictionary/communicate

Schramm, W. (Ed.) (1954). The process and effects of mass communication. In *How communication works* (pp. 3-10). Urbana: University of Illinois Press.

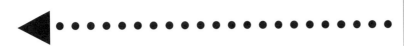

CHAPTER 5
Communication Techniques

Objectives

1. Propose ways to project a positive telecommunication personality and effective voice quality.
2. Describe effective telehealth communication techniques.
3. Explain necessary telecommunication mechanical competencies.
4. Understand basic information about motivational interviewing.
5. Summarize strategies to reduce communication barriers and to manage challenging communication situations.

The ability to communicate with others is paramount. In telehealth nursing practice, the nurse's use of communication skills can ultimately affect the health and lives of patients being served. Effective communication skills are essential in providing the basis for which the nursing process can be adapted for telehealth practice.

Telecommunications is the use of the telephone, Internet, interactive video, remote sensory devices, or robotics to transmit information from one site to another (American Academy of Ambulatory Care Nursing [AAACN], 2007). Telecommunications eliminates or reduces use of the senses of sight and touch because nursing care and services are delivered across distances. Patient assessment skills are challenged as most nurses are more confident when completing data collection using visual and tactile sensations. The nurse must remain aware of the crucial role data collection and assessment play throughout the nursing process. This requires a focus on maximizing communication techniques and strategies with benefits, which include:

> *Effective communication skills are essential in providing the basis for which the nursing process can be adapted for telehealth practice.*

- ❖ Development and maintenance of supportive and trusting relationships.
- ❖ Provision of the most appropriate level of care.
- ❖ Improved patient compliance.
- ❖ Increased satisfaction for both patient and nurse.

AAACN's *Guide to Ambulatory Care Nursing Orientation and Competency Assessment* (2005) competency statement for telehealth nursing practice/interpersonal skills/communication skills states: "Uses effective interpersonal communication skills to engage in, develop, and disengage in a therapeutic encounter" (p. 81). With effective communication, the nurse can be more confident in the ability to obtain a

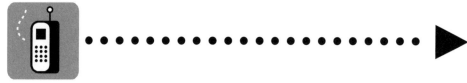

complete history and assessment, thereby assisting the patient to receive the most appropriate care.

TELECOMMUNICATION PERSONALITY

The first 10 to 20 seconds of a telephone encounter significantly affect the patient's perception of the nurse and the ability and desire of the nurse to meet the patient's needs.

With the telephone being the most common mode of telecommunication encounters, the nurse can begin by asking a few self-assessment questions to examine his/her current telephone personality. The patient will immediately identify with the nurse's personality and determine if the nurse is trustworthy enough to provide health care advice and support. When communicating face-to-face, individuals often draw upon body language and other visual cues to develop perceptions of one another. The telephone encounter limits the time and methods to project personality and intentions. The first 10 to 20 seconds of a telephone encounter significantly affect the patient's perception of the nurse and the ability and desire of the nurse to meet the patient's needs. *Who* the nurse is, whether right or wrong, has been established in that patient's mind.

As noted by Wheeler and Windt (1993), "the first words of the greeting to the way (the nurse) listens, responds, and questions will demonstrate the warmth, caring, and trustworthiness that is charisma" (p. 45). For this reason, the nurse needs to focus on call initiation. The simple technique of pausing and taking a breath before each encounter will help maintain the freshness of the nurse's voice quality.

Similar techniques apply to Internet-based encounters (nurse/patient emails or chats). A momentary pause and deep breath will help the nurse focus on the task at hand. Carefully worded statements will convey empathy and concern, as well as a desire to meet the patient's needs. Proper spelling and grammar is essential in conveying professionalism.

The patient's perception of the nurse's attitude often serves to define the potential for a trusting, positive relationship. The nurse must expand development of communication beyond being merely skill-based. Adopting certain attitudes that bring a more human quality to each encounter can enhance much of the nurse's "charisma." The nurse's attitude allows the creation of an understanding atmosphere that neither patronizes the patient, nor belittles the problem (Wheeler & Windt, 1993).

A caring attitude toward patients is the focus of positive communication. Although realistically caring for all patients may be challenging, it is crucial that the nurse be considerate to all. Nothing else defines care and consideration like the *Golden Rule*: treat each patient in a manner the nurse would like to be treated. One technique often used is keeping a mirror on your desk and looking at the reflection during a patient encounter. The reflection represents that the person could be you at the other end of the encounter. This applies to all types of telecommunication encounters. Other ways to portray care and consideration in the nurse's communication style include:

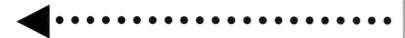

- ❖ Avoiding assumptions or stereotypes.
- ❖ Envisioning the patient as someone the nurse knows personally, such as a parent or friend.
- ❖ Empathizing with the patient's circumstances, no matter how different from one's own.
- ❖ Using reflective speech or verbal utterances to project interest and active listening.
- ❖ Addressing the patient by name throughout the encounter. Initially use more formal titles, such as "Mr." or "Ms.," unless the patient gives the nurse permission to use another form of their name. Under no circumstances should terms of endearment, such as "Honey" or "Sweetie," be used; these are often viewed as demeaning.

Effective communication is further supported by the nurse's commitment to meeting the individual needs of each patient while respecting the diversity of all individuals. In some circumstances, the nurse will need to take extra time or effort to meet the patient's needs and must know when to think "outside the box." In addition, a committed attitude toward quality telehealth nursing practice will allow the nurse to naturally project confidence and compassion. This, in turn, will positively influence the work environment, serving to decrease stress and minimize burnout. Observing peers who exhibit a committed attitude during patient encounters is one way to refine the nurse's skills.

Ongoing changes in the world, including health care, emphasize the importance of flexibility and creativity. The nurse must look for new ways to solve problems and meet the needs of patients. This can include maintaining a thorough resource listing and participating in ongoing education affecting practice. The nurse should also remain up-to-date with the organization's administrative directives related to specific circumstances.

The attitude of consistency can apply to various aspects of telehealth nursing practice guideline development, documentation standards, and communication techniques. In this chapter, consistency refers to the nurse treating each encounter as the first contact of the day. Most encounters are the patient's first contact with the nurse on any given day. Yet, consistency combined with control may be difficult attitudes to maintain, particularly when dealing with challenging patients. In these situations, the nurse should not personalize the situation. Generally, the patient's emotions are a result of a previous difficult encounter in which resolution was not reached.

Finally, self-confidence can affect the nurse's communication efforts. Lack of confidence will be communicated to the patient. The nurse can gain confidence by participating in mock telecommunication scenarios. The nurse's confidence is also supported by knowledge of the technical

Ongoing changes in the world, including health care, emphasize the importance of flexibility and creativity. The nurse must look for new ways to solve problems and meet the needs of patients.

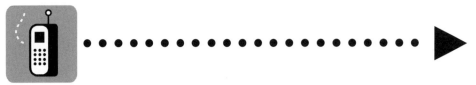

and interpersonal aspects of the job. Simple actions such as having the basic day-to-day tools (e.g., pens, paper, and phone numbers) readily available allow the nurse to focus on the important task of developing a trusting relationship with the patient. In addition, the nurse should be knowledgeable of role expectations and be clear on what resources are available to expedite the appropriate access to care.

Recognizing the internal affect of attitudes on the nurse's communication skills is important when projecting an appropriate telecommunications personality. Blending these attitudes with ongoing skill development will further enhance the nurse's overall communication excellence.

VOICE QUALITY

Both the nurse's and patient's sensory input is limited to the auditory sense when providing or receiving care over the telephone. A primary influence on effective care, advice, and intervention is perception. Voice qualities, including tone, volume, clarity, and speed, generally serve as a foundation for these perceptions. Each auditory characteristic has an impact on the personality and sincerity projected. Ultimately, voice quality affects overall spoken communication.

Tone

Tone of voice portrays various shades of meaning. The nurse can sound abrupt, disinterested, or unfriendly, or perhaps merely monotonous and emotionless. Instead, the nurse needs to use a tone of voice that has vitality. For example, by fluctuating voice pitch, the nurse may be more successful in engaging the patient. Use of a pleasant, natural tone of voice further conveys a sense of friendliness and willingness to help. This is particularly important at the initiation of an encounter. Smiling when speaking will naturally raise the pitch of the voice; how the nurse is feeling is reflected in facial expression and then translated through tone of voice. Having a mirror on the desk will help to serve as a reminder to smile. In turn, patients' emotions can also be expressed in their tone of voice. The nurse should take note of these auditory cues in assessment of the patient.

Volume

Throughout the encounter, the nurse needs to remain aware of voice volume. Variations in volume can add emphasis to these encounters. By attempting to speak in a soft, quiet tone, the nurse may seek to project consistency even when attempting to diffuse a tense situation. However, there is the potential for further inflaming the patient if they view this approach as minimizing his/her concern. On occasion, it may be necessary to match the patient's voice volume in response to anxious or angry

By fluctuating voice pitch, the nurse may be more successful in engaging the patient. Use of a pleasant, natural tone of voice further conveys a sense of friendliness and willingness to help.

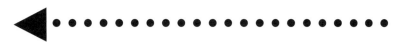

behavior. The key is *temporarily* meeting the volume, and then quickly returning to a calmer level. This technique serves to bring the nurse's volume to the patient's attention.

On a more basic level, some people speak loudly, while others can barely be heard. If the patient's volume level is the concern, the nurse can bring the problem to their attention. A nurse who is prone to either characteristic can make a conscientious effort to speak more softly or loudly. By manually adjusting the volume control of the telephone and being aware of the position of the headset mouthpiece or handset, the nurse can control the volume of the call. Placing the receiver on the chin or below the mouth can result in a muffled, quieter exchange. The nurse can ask a co-worker for input on voice volume or record a tape of normal speaking voice to perform a self-assessment.

Clarity and Speed

Clarity and speed are two voice qualities that are closely connected. The combination of careful enunciation and pace moderation will support positive communication techniques. The most effective speaking rate is within the range of 125-160 words per minute (Adler & Elmhorst, 2006). The nurse can easily keep within this range by speaking rapidly enough to avoid a boring drone, yet slowly enough to be clearly understood. Variation in rate of speech can be used to reflect mood changes and to emphasize points. The nurse must listen to the patient for direction based on the patient's ability to respond to questions. The nurse may need to vary the pace when speaking to someone who has communication impairment or whose primary language is not English. In this case, it is important not to sound condescending or remedial. Finally, the nurse may improve clarity by avoiding the use of medical or technical terms unless the nurse is validating the patient's use of such terms. A patient's use of medical terms does not necessarily indicate accurate knowledge.

The nurse will need to train his/her voice to excel in all the above-mentioned qualities. Audiotaping can improve the nurse's awareness of voice qualities.

The most effective speaking rate is within the range of 125-160 words per minute. The nurse can easily keep within this range by speaking rapidly enough to avoid a boring drone, yet slowly enough to be clearly understood.

CORE COMMUNICATION TECHNIQUES

Most nurses should be able to easily identify ineffective communication techniques. It is the nurse's responsibility to identify and remove such barriers between the nurse and the patient. Some examples of barriers are:

❖ Being abrupt or sounding busy (this can be conveyed through writing too).

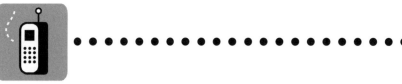

- ❖ Using inappropriate slang or expletives.
- ❖ Arguing with or intimidating the patient.
- ❖ Judging or blaming the patient or other health care providers.
- ❖ Being authoritarian by lecturing the patient or minimizing the patient's concerns.
- ❖ Rushing through the encounter.
- ❖ Losing professional perspectives.
- ❖ Having something in the mouth (such as food, gum, or a pen) when conversing with a patient.
- ❖ Speaking too loudly or softly.
- ❖ Carrying on more than one encounter at a time.
- ❖ Not having a quiet, secure area to conduct the encounter.
- ❖ Being unprepared to respond to the patient's need.

Listening Skills

As previously mentioned, telehealth nursing practice relies upon thorough assessment, much of which can be obtained through listening. Listening is more than merely hearing. Hearing is primarily a physiological process, while listening is a psychological process. Real listening means the nurse pays closer attention and understands that there is meaning beyond just the words the patient uses. The nurse must consider the literal meaning of the words and think about what is being said. To fully understand what is being heard, the nurse should consider the patient's emotions or "the message behind the message." As an attentive listener, the nurse will pick up various clues, providing a sharper picture of the patient's needs and motivations. This concept applies to other forms of telecommunication encounters. By being attentive to what is being said or written, the nurse can also determine if there is an underlying message.

Listening has a natural barrier in misunderstandings. During an average conversation, only 25-50% of the interpretations are accurate (Adler & Elmhorst, 2006). For this reason, the nurse will want to concentrate on the development of patient-centered listening skills. That is, the nurse takes an approach to listening that does not inhibit but encourages the patient to talk. Through a mixture of silence and prompts, the patient is invited to continue speaking. Skilled listening is not a natural talent, so the nurse will need to practice this skill. The nurse can recognize various causes for poor listening and address each one by asking the following questions.

- ❖ **Is the nurse really concentrating?** It is easy to give in to physical and mental distractions, allowing thoughts to wander rather than concentrate on what is being communicated.

Listening has a natural barrier in misunderstandings. During an average conversation, only 25-50% of the interpretations are accurate.

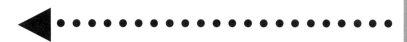

  o **Solution** – The nurse must force the focus if distracted, making a conscious effort to listen/read more carefully to what the patient is communicating.
- ❖ **Is the nurse listening too closely?** The nurse may become so engrossed in the details that the facts or main points may become confused.
  o **Solution** – The nurse mentally reviews what the patient has already communicated and makes sure it is understood.
- ❖ **Is the nurse jumping to conclusions?** By failing to listen to the patient and prematurely anticipating his/her needs, the nurse may erect a barrier. This might result in finishing the patient's thought or perhaps prematurely concluding that the patient is boring, misguided, or rambling. Each of these situations can result in misdirected or inappropriate delivery of care.
  o **Solution** – Do not anticipate the response from the patient. Listen/read carefully, giving the conversation full attention. Plan the response after hearing/reading the entire statement. Restating what the patient has said/written can also assist in clarity.

Finally, the nurse should become familiar with auditory cues such as noises or sounds that may accompany speech. Vocal sounds provide vital cues of emotion that can be a powerful conveyor of information. If the patient's verbal cues do not match what is being said, the nurse should suspect that something is wrong. For example, a patient may say they are in extreme pain but talks effortlessly and laughs during the conversation. Listening for auditory cues will aid in the assessment process.

Vocal sounds provide vital cues of emotion that can be a powerful conveyor of information. If the patient's verbal cues do not match what is being said, the nurse should suspect that something is wrong.

INTERVIEWING STRATEGIES

Since assessment is the key element to successfully directing a patient to the appropriate level of care, the nurse also needs to be skilled in interviewing techniques. These include the use of questions and statements that are worded to elicit specific types of answers.

Questioning Techniques
One of the most successful questioning strategies is the use of open-ended questions. The intent of this type of interviewing strategy is to illicit greater amounts of information, since it eliminates only "yes" or "no" responses. Additionally, this strategy reinforces the patient's trust in the nurse due to the perceived value that the nurse now places on the patient's input and involvement in care delivery. The encounter becomes more interactive and personal. Use of summarizing statements by the nurse such as, "These seem to be your concerns," will help establish a basis for further discussion. In addition, by using reflective statements such as,

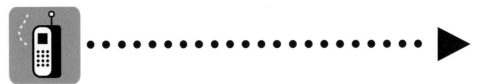

"You seem rushed," the nurse conveys observations and attention to more than just the verbal/written exchange. The nurse's perceptions of the patient's emotional state may also be acknowledged using reflection such as, "You seem very angry."

Various types of questions will encourage the patient to continue to share such as, "Please tell me more about..." Encouraging statements can reinforce the nurse's interest in the patient. Affirming statements are important in relationship-building as they acknowledge the efforts already made. For example, "What you have done to reduce your child's temperature is what I would have asked you to do..." Initially, it is not desirable to ask leading questions; however, at a later point in the encounter, the nurse may need to be more focused with the patient, especially if the patient tends to ramble or is a poor historian.

By using clarification, the nurse may get a clearer understanding of the patient's response, particularly if the patient is very anxious or symptoms need to be quantified. These could include such questions as, "When did you take the medicine?" or "How many times did you vomit?" Restating can demonstrate that the nurse is paying attention and understanding what the patient is communicating (for example, "So you would say you feel worse today?"). Other forms of clarification include asking the patient to repeat what they understood the nurse to say. Throughout the assessment, the nurse should use validation statements. These will continue to acknowledge the worthiness and abilities of the patient. For example, "You have taken the right actions so far. I appreciate the concerns that prompted your contacting us." If possible, avoid leading questions such as, "Is the bleeding bright red?" The patient may be cued to give the nurse a perceived desirable response that may be inaccurate.

Rephrasing

Each patient has a specific motivation for contacting the nurse. By choosing to construct statements and questions in a positive manner, the nurse will motivate cooperation. The intent is to rephrase statements in a way to more positively encourage a response or a more thorough answer. The following are examples of the rephrasing technique.

The first statements should appeal to the patient's sense of autonomy. Most people do not like to be told what to do. The nurse should instead appeal to the patient's desire to feel needed. Consider some alternative statements.

Instead of communicating:	*Say or write:*
"You have to..."	"I need you to..."
"You should..."	"It would be helpful if you would..."

Each patient has a specific motivation for contacting the nurse. By choosing to construct statements and questions in a positive manner, the nurse will motivate cooperation.

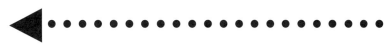

Sometimes the nurse needs to clarify or be more definite about what has or is being communicated. The following phrases support this technique:

Instead of communicating:	Say or write:
"I'll try to do it..."	"I will do it..." (Only commit to this promise if you will truly complete the action)
"I'll have Dr. Smith contact you..."	"I'll ask Dr. Smith to contact you..." (The nurse cannot guarantee that Dr. Smith will contact the patient. The responsibility is placed on Dr. Smith, not the nurse).
"I'll contact you as soon as possible."	"I will contact you between 9 a.m. and 11 a.m." (Identify the timeframe and be sure to contact the patient, even if the situation is not yet resolved, to provide an update.)

When communicating in writing such as by email, the above statements may need to be adjusted slightly. The focus still should be on collaborative communication instead of being overly direct in telling the patient what to do.

Even if the patient is difficult or requesting "unreasonable" demands, the nurse always has some options. Consider what can be done rather than the focusing on perceived barriers. This positive attitude demonstrates flexibility, creativity, and collaboration.

Instead of communicating:	Say or write:
"That's impossible and it cannot be done!"	"Instead, this is what can be done."
"I don't know."	"I do not know, but I will find out."

Closure of the Encounter

Closure is a critical component of each encounter. If appropriate time is spent reaching closure, miscommunications can be decreased and compliance increased. The nurse should use the skill of summarizing in an effort to review progress and pull important facts together. The nurse asks whether the patient has the resources or ability to carry out the instructions given. Then the nurse reiterates instructions so that the patient clearly understands their responsibilities by using "I will/you will" statements. For example, "You will check your child's temperature again in 30

Closure is a critical component of each encounter. If appropriate time is spent reaching closure, miscommunications can be decreased and compliance increased.

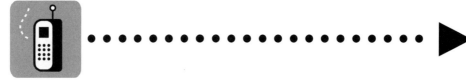

minutes. If the temperature does not decrease to 101 degrees Fahrenheit, you will need to contact me."

The nurse should instruct the patient to follow-up if symptoms persist, worsen, or change. The nurse should confirm the patient's compliance with the agreed upon actions. For example, the nurse may communicate, "I will call the pharmacy with the prescription the doctor has authorized. Does this meet your needs?" Next, the nurse clarifies the instructions and proceeds to end the encounter. Throughout the encounter, the nurse and patient have worked to establish a plan of care that includes follow-up.

Although first impressions have great impact on the success of the encounter, last impressions are equally important. The nurse should continue to pay attention to tone of voice, rate of speech; or what is put into writing and personalize the closure by again using the patient's name. Finally, the nurse should allow the patient to end the encounter first. This allows an opportunity for the patient to ask additional questions if desired.

Motivational Interviewing

Motivational interviewing (MI) is a patient-centered therapeutic technique designed to help individuals develop a commitment to changing problematic behaviors. Telling or instructing the patient to change behavior or what has been done in the past is ineffective in many cases. MI has proven effective when a patient is ambivalent by facilitating recognition of the situation and building a case for positive change. The health care provider no longer "tells" the patient to change their habits, but rather works with the patient to verbalize their own reasons, arguments, or desire to change behavior. In doing so, the patient/person becomes more committed to making the change. It is crucial to form an equal, assertive, and positive partnership with the patient and encourage "change talk."

While MI was originally described in 1983 to address problem drinkers, the theory and practice has been applied to a variety of health behaviors, such as smoking cessation, dietary change, medication adherence, treatment compliance, disease management, etc., as well as to diverse patient populations. The practice can be applied, in whole or part, to all clinical encounters based on the nurse's style and patient needs.

The foundation of MI is patient-nurse communication. Using open-ended questions, affirmations, reflective listening, and summaries (OARS), will encourage a collaborative spirit and build a solid relationship (Borrelli, 2006).

Four basic interventions are used by the nurse: expressing empathy, developing discrepancy, rolling with resistance, and supporting self-efficacy.

The nurse should instruct the patient to follow-up if symptoms persist, worsen, or change. The nurse should confirm the patient's compliance with the agreed upon actions.

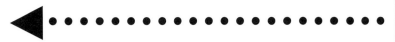

❖ *Expressing empathy* requires that the nurse accurately reflect what the patient is communicating. This requires the nurse to employ active listening skills. For instance, "What is the message?"

❖ *Developing discrepancy* involves eliciting from the patient that which is important and at odds with the behavior needing to be changed.

❖ *Rolling with patient resistance* necessitates utilizing reflection in an effort to decrease resistance, rather than confrontation.

❖ *Supporting self-efficacy* includes focusing on the patient's strengths, based on the abilities and resources they possess. It is essential for the nurse to elicit self-motivational communication from the patient.

The nurse must be cognizant in matching the interventions to the patient's level, emphasizing the patient's personal choice, recognizing that ambivalence and resistance are a normal part of the change process, and that goals are collaboratively set (Squires & Moyers, 2008).

A very simplistic example is a parent calling about his/her child who has asthma. After assessing the child's needs and determining the disposition to be one in which patient education or home care instructions are provided (e.g., not an emergent disposition), the nurse may learn that the parent smokes in the child's presence. The parent may state he/she has tried to quit many times. The nurse's response could be, "It sounds like you have been persistent. This change must be very important to you." Asking the parent to identify options to smoke away from the child may be the next step. This would be a positive change for both the child and the parent. It removes the child from the irritant and results in a changed behavior for the parent; this could progress into further attempts at quitting.

Motivational interviewing can be used in telehealth encounters, especially when the nurse has ongoing contact with the patient. The nurse can set goals with the patient, reinforce these goals, and provide ongoing support and motivation to being successful in achieving the desired health care change.

TELECOMMUNICATIONS MECHANICS AND ETIQUETTE

Communication techniques such as listening and interviewing are fundamental to professional interpersonal competency. However, for a telehealth nurse, basic telecommunication mechanics and etiquette are also crucial. The nurse should become as proficient with telecommunications hardware as with a stethoscope. Successfully executing the options of hold, transfer, and conference calling with the telephone and forwarding, replying, and attaching files for Web-based technology will affect the patient's/recipient's confidence in the nurse's abilities. If the nurse loses a

The nurse must be cognizant in matching the interventions to the patient's level, emphasizing the patient's personal choice, recognizing that ambivalence and resistance are a normal part of the change process, and that goals are collaboratively set.

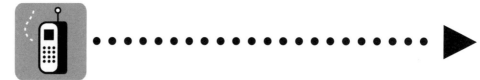

telephonic patient in an attempt to transfer or place on hold, it may undermine the patient's confidence in the nurse's ability to provide care. The nurse should engage in periodic practice of various telecommunication mechanics. Techniques and procedures can change as telecommunication equipment is updated. The proper use of equipment not only includes manual skills, but etiquette as well. For instance, it is essential to know how to answer incoming calls, but it is equally important to understand the need to answer any type of call promptly. Prompt answering supports the patient's perception of the nurse's access and willingness to provide for their needs. The nurse should answer a telephone call using name and title to make the encounter more personal and enhance the patient's confidence.

Hold Option

Placing patients on hold is sometimes a necessity. However, some patients will not be willing or able to hold for a variety of reasons, such as long distance charges, location of telephone, cellular phone limitation, or time constraints. If the patient must be placed on hold, the nurse should follow these guidelines:

- ❖ Before actually placing a patient on hold, ask permission *and* wait for a response before proceeding.
- ❖ When returning to the encounter, thank the patient for holding. It is not necessary to say, "Sorry you had to hold," if indeed the nurse asked permission and then returned to the call in a timely manner.
- ❖ Limit hold time to 60 seconds or less. If the situation cannot be resolved within a minute, return to the patient and offer one of the following options:
  - o "Do you wish to remain on hold while I continue to work on this?"
  - o "May I take some information and call you back?"

Transfer of Encounter

On occasion, it is necessary to transfer an encounter to another location. To maintain the patient's confidence, the nurse must know how to properly complete the transfer in one attempt. The goal of transferring is "the right place, the first time." The following techniques are useful to successfully complete a transfer:

- ❖ Collect as much information from the patient as possible, including the reason for the encounter.
- ❖ Before initiating the actual transfer, provide the patient with the following information:
  - o Why the patient is being transferred.

On occasion, it is necessary to transfer an encounter to another location. The goal of transferring is "the right place, the first time."

Telehealth Nursing Practice Essentials © American Academy of Ambulatory Care Nursing, 2009

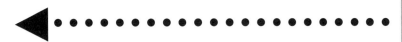

 o To whom (person and/or department) the encounter is being transferred.
 o The telephone number of the receiving person.

Each of these pieces of information helps assure the patient that the call is being sent to the appropriate place. The patient's impression of the nurse will affect their confidence in the health care organization as well as the nurse's abilities to meet future needs. To complete the transfer cycle, the nurse should announce the transfer by providing the receiving party with the following information:

- ❖ The nurse's name and location.
- ❖ The patient's name (and other identifiers).
- ❖ Reason for the transfer.

If the line is busy or the transfer will not go through, the nurse should return to the patient. The nurse must avoid completing transfers into voice mail or on-hold lines without the express permission of the patient. When appropriate, the nurse can offer the correct phone number or offer to take a message.

The nurse must avoid completing transfers into voice mail or on-hold lines without the express permission of the patient. When appropriate, the nurse can offer the correct phone number or offer to take a message.

Conference Calls

The use of conference calling can enhance the efficiency of a single encounter. The nurse initiating the conference call needs to include each step delineated in the above section on transferring calls. The etiquette of collecting information and announcing calls is vital to maintaining confidence and comfort with the nurse's delivery of care. Each new person being included in the encounter should be provided with the following information:

- ❖ The names of those already on the encounter.
- ❖ The purpose of the encounter.
- ❖ The option to join the encounter. If the new person chooses to join, their presence is announced to the other attendees.

Web-Based Encounters

Verbal encounters have traditionally been the mechanism for communicating health information. However, with advancing technology, Web-based applications are becoming another viable avenue for communication exchange of health information. Email messages can provide or link to educational materials as well as other resources. Considerations to email communications include issues of privacy, confidentiality, and security, as well as a delay in which the email response occurs by one or both parties.

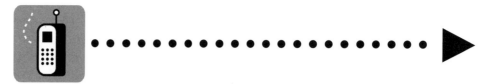

The American Medical Association (AMA) has published communication and medico-legal and administrative guidelines for email communication (2008). It is important to make certain there is a disclaimer or standard block of text explaining anticipated turnaround time, reminders about security, and the importance of not using this form of communication for urgent or emergent situations. Other guidelines include establishing types of transactions to be handled via email, type of concise information the patient should provide, permission agreement, policies for writing and electronic form, and a means to archive and/or retrieve communications (AMA, 2008).

Instant messaging is real-time and should also have guidelines established by the organization regarding security, types of encounters to be managed, documenting the information exchange on the patient's permanent record, etc. This form of telecommunication can undoubtedly increase efficiencies, but policies and processes must be clearly defined and enforced. No matter what form of transaction is utilized, it is essential to maintain professionalism, use correct spelling and grammar, and convey a willingness to help the patient with whatever his/her reason for contact might be.

CARE DELIVERY BARRIERS

> *When communicating with the patient, the nurse can anticipate that barriers may be present. By knowing where the barriers exist, the nurse can then begin to overcome the communications barriers, regardless of whether they originate with the patient or the nurse.*

When communicating with the patient, the nurse can anticipate that barriers may be present. Some barriers cannot be removed but can be avoided or addressed. By knowing where the barriers exist, the nurse can then begin to overcome the communications barriers, regardless of whether they originate with the patient or the nurse.

Patient Barriers

The telehealth practice nurse can be challenged by a variety of factors, including the patient's unique personality. These personalities comprise various characteristics and beliefs, including patient expectations, socioeconomic issues, diversity, physical or environmental limitations, and education or level of understanding.

Patient Expectations: Some patients who are not familiar with using telecommunication devices to access care may be resistant to the process, where others may expect to get an appointment without discussion or recommendations for home care. Some patients do not wish to speak with anyone other than the provider. In these circumstances, the patient's needs are met first. Then the nurse may engage the provider in educating the patient about the role of the telehealth practice nurse. The nurse will need to be flexible during the encounter and may spend extra time building the nurse-patient relationship through skill-based communication techniques. This can be enhanced by empathetic awareness of feelings and the nurse's telecommunication personality in demonstrating warmth through voice

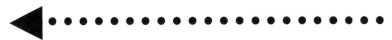

and choice of words. The nurse should be willing to educate the patient about the benefits of receiving health care in this manner. The nurse can collaborate with the health care team to be prepared to meet the patient's demands, such as speaking directly with an individual provider.

Socioeconomic Issues: A key element in preparing to care for a population is being aware of various socioeconomic factors. As an integral part of the health care team, the telehealth nurse should work with the organization to complete a thorough population assessment to identify the composition of its service area. The nurse's ability to care for patients is impeded without assessment and evaluation of social and economic resources, including awareness of fluctuations in the service area's economy, socioeconomic makeup, and various available resources.

Diversity: Important to any population assessment is an awareness of the various cultural and ethnic groupings within a service area. Readily apparent evidence of ethnic diversity is language differences. Even though the nurse may be unable to communicate in the patient's language, it is extremely important that the language barrier not impede care. The following can help in this area:

- ❖ The nurse must not change voice volume or speak slower than his/her usual rate of speech. Often, the nurse is inclined to speak louder and slower when trying to overcome language differences.
- ❖ The nurse should build and utilize a network of on-call translators.
- ❖ The nurse can assess and consider the use of a family member or friend of the patient to serve as an immediate translator solution. A translator from within the organization is a more appropriate solution.
- ❖ The organization may contract with a telecommunication foreign language translation service (such as the AT&T Language Line) for phone or document translation. Web-based technology translation is available in some languages.
- ❖ If the demand for specific fluency in a particular foreign language increases, the organization should consider adding this as a job skill for nurses, and providing educational opportunities for existing staff to increase their skill set.

Diversity differences within a service population may include more than cultural, racial, or language differences. For example, the difference may also include a redefinition of the term *family,* as it has indeed become much different from past traditional assumptions. In developing communication techniques and interviewing skills, the nurse needs to consider and address the possibility of blended families, custodial vs. non-custodial care of a minor, single parent homes, elderly adult caregivers, and same-sex partners.

As an integral part of the health care team, the telehealth nurse should work with the organization to complete a thorough population assessment to identify the composition of its service area. The nurse's ability to care for patients is impeded without assessment and evaluation of social and economic resources.

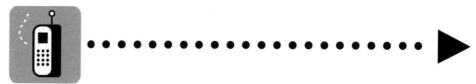

Physical and Environmental Limitations: The mere use of the telephone implies that both the patient and nurse can hear and verbally exchange information. However, this can be both physically and environmentally challenging. The nurse's organization must provide for the needs of deaf patients. As with foreign language speakers, translation services may be helpful, or nurses can be prepared and skilled in the use of Telecommunication Devices for the Deaf (TDD). Such encounters may take longer than usual because of the need for additional keyboard exchanges and lack of verbal cueing. If the patient's only communication avenue is by sign language, TDD services will not be useful. In this case, the patient should be assessed in person or via Web-based technology, if available and appropriate.

Environmental considerations may also exist, such as distracting background noise, lack of privacy, and quality of line connections for both telephone and Web-based applications. The nurse must be prepared with alternatives, such as offering to call the patient back, offering other telecommunication services, and/or using interviewing techniques that include closed-ended statements to minimize the need for intimate or revealing responses.

Education and/or Level of Understanding: The inability to visually confirm that the patient understands instructions or education supports the need for a longer communication exchange. To begin to meet these communications challenges, the nurse must consider interpretation, ambiguity, and retention.

Various words, directions, and terms can be interpreted differently, especially without visual assistance. A variety of words may have different meanings to the nurse and patient. It is crucial that the patient clearly understands the nurse's questions. If not, the patient's responses to the questions may be inaccurate. The nurse must verify that the patient understands by asking them to repeat what they understood the nurse to say or by rephrasing the patient's response.

The nurse must also be aware of ambiguous terms, such as *often*, *sometimes*, or *usually*. The patient and nurse may use these terms to quantify such things as health habits, body fluids, or symptoms. Various patient responses could be more accurate if instead the nurse's question includes use of a percentage or specific number.

Environmental considerations may also exist, such as distracting background noise, lack of privacy, and quality of line connections for both telephone and Web-based applications.

Initial question:	Less ambiguous question:
Have you been vomiting a lot?	"How many times have you vomited in the last 24 hours?"
Is there much blood?	"When you changed the last bandage, how big was the area of blood on the bandage?"
Are you changing the bandages all the time?	"How many bandages and what size have you used today?"

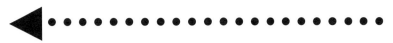

Do you sometimes have headaches in the morning?	"Out of 7 days in a week, how many mornings do you have a headache?"

How much a patient truly understands and retains can be difficult to accurately assess. A person with more education is not necessarily better able to understand questions or instructions during a telehealth encounter. For this reason, the nurse needs to frequently clarify and confirm information with the patient. The nurse can have the patient repeat the instructions or elicit the patient's degree of comfort with the encounter by asking, "How does that sound to you?" Finally, the nurse should be prepared to reinforce teachings with mailings or follow-up encounters.

If the nurse confirms that a patient has a learning disability, care must still be provided. In these situations, the nurse will want to apply all the same techniques, but increase the frequency of clarifying and asking the patient to repeat back statements. In addition, the nurse should have the patient write down instructions or speak to a support person who may be available to that patient.

Nurse Barriers

Some barriers the nurse brings that may interfere with effective communication are *knowledge gaps*, *willingness*, and *bias*. If present, the nurse is responsible for decreasing or eliminating these personal barriers.

Knowledge Gaps: With the rapid change in health care knowledge, the growing learning needs of the nurse must be addressed. Gaps in knowledge can be partially closed by using decision support tools, but these needs are more successfully managed by commitment to lifelong learning. This commitment becomes increasingly challenging as patients become more and more skilled at acquiring health information via media and Internet access.

Willingness: The nurse must be willing to ask for help when needed. Telehealth nursing practice requires autonomy; however, like any type of nursing, telehealth nursing practice benefits from teamwork. If the nurse is unwilling to capitalize on teamwork, both the patient and nurse will suffer. By working with others as part of a team, the nurse is given broader resources, expertise, decision-making, and emotional support, which will benefit the nurse and ultimately the patient.

Bias: The ability to maintain objectivity and avoid bias is central to nursing practice. The reality for many nurses is to meet the challenge of not allowing bias to influence care. When working "blindly" over a telecommunication device, the nurse may be apt to make certain assumptions based on the patient's speech patterns or communication styles. For example, if a patient's speech is slurred, the nurse may assume that the patient's intelligence is low or perhaps that the patient is intoxicated. The reality may be that the patient has experienced a stroke and has difficulty speaking. Another example is if a patient's written

A person with more education is not necessarily better able to understand questions or instructions during a telehealth encounter. For this reason, the nurse needs to frequently clarify and confirm information with the patient.

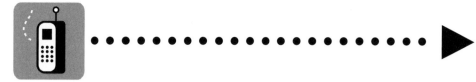

communication has many misspelled words, the nurse may think the person illiterate, when they are simply using a coded language similar to that which is used in text messaging.

In addition, the pitch of a person's voice tends to imply gender. The nurse must not make assumptions, but instead it is important to use skilled interviewing techniques to secure conclusive data.

Biases only serve to interfere with the nurse's ability to provide safe and appropriate care. The nurse is a central access point for care and is obligated to provide quality care to all people, regardless of bias or prejudice.

CHALLENGING COMMUNICATION SITUATIONS

Communication is often challenging. In telehealth nursing, that challenge is heightened. Like most practices, there are situations or patients that test the nurse's abilities to maintain professionalism. The following sections on difficult patients, emergency situations, refusal to follow advice, and obscene encounters will consider critical attitudes and techniques to facilitate care in less-than-optimal situations.

Difficult Patients

The "difficult" patient describes a variety of people and problems. It may be an irate patient demanding an appointment in one hour for a cough, or the sobbing new parent sure that her newborn has a severe illness because the infant will not burp. In either example, the problem is real to the patient. Though it may seem so on a trying day, most difficult encounters are not the result of someone waking up and deciding to contact the nurse for the sole purpose of making his/her day miserable. Instead, the stress of an unforeseen illness, its inconvenience, or perhaps lack of health care knowledge can affect a patient's ability to effectively deal with the situation. By feeling a loss of control or frustration with the situation, the patient has a compromised ability to communicate with the nurse. This is important for the nurse to remember when encountering difficult patient. Regardless of the level of difficulty, the nurse's goal should remain to assist the patient to find a means to regain or maintain health and well-being. To do this, the nurse must deal with two separate areas: the patient's actual feelings and then the problem itself.

Most difficult encounters are not the result of someone waking up and deciding to contact the nurse for the sole purpose of making his/her day miserable. Instead, the stress of an unforeseen illness, its inconvenience, or perhaps lack of health care knowledge can affect a patient's ability to effectively deal with the situation.

- ❖ To properly identify and address the patient's emotion and to be able to address it, the nurse should take a systematic approach.
- ❖ The nurse must look beyond the obvious and avoid prematurely reacting to a perception of the patient's emotions.
- ❖ The nurse should work to heighten the ability to empathize with patients.

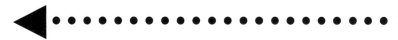

- ❖ The nurse should listen to understand, although not necessarily with agreement. This technique will help to cultivate a trusting relationship. Trust and objectivity can lead to a more positive outcome.
- ❖ The nurse should avoid saying or writing, "I know how you feel," because the nurse really may not know.
- ❖ The nurse should try to remain calm and non-confrontational.
- ❖ The nurse should allow the patient to ventilate emotions by hearing them out, not just listening for an immediate solution.
- ❖ The nurse can use reflective statements to clarify the patient's feelings.
- ❖ The nurse must know organizational policy for when and how to terminate an encounter.

After dealing with the patient's emotion, the nurse can attempt to focus on the real problem and find out what the patient *really* wants by asking questions, sharing information, and verifying understanding. The nurse can ask, "What can I do for you today?" The nurse may suggest alternatives in attempting to find a positive solution whenever possible by emphasizing collaboration as part of the situation. The nurse should thank the patient at the closure of the encounter and be sure to follow-up on and perform any agreed-upon actions.

In addition, the perception of what is a difficult patient may vary. One co-worker may truly enjoy a type of encounter that another nurse considers difficult. This includes dealing with various conditions or age groups. The elderly patient with multiple chronic concerns may be "difficult" if the nurse's expertise is in pediatrics. The only way to address such difficulties is education and reliance on other resources.

The nurse must be cautious in dealing with the patient that frequently contacts the organization. This person may be viewed as difficult strictly based on the amount of time spent responding to non-urgent needs. If the nurse becomes too complacent or familiar with these patients, the nurse might miss legitimate, urgent needs. This can be countered if the nurse strives to maintain a fresh approach and treat each encounter as the first of the day or the first from that patient.

Emergency Situations

Any form of emergency can strain the ability of the patient to communicate. Rational, logical thought is replaced with frustration and loss of control. It is the nurse's role to ensure a safe and effective disposition of the crisis. To do so in the presence of communication barriers, the nurse needs to use expert communication to solicit a thorough assessment by focusing on techniques and attitudes necessary to building and sustaining trust with the patient. During an emergency, the nurse should focus on a systematic approach in communication efforts.

During an emergency, the nurse should focus on a systematic approach in communication efforts.

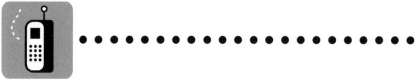

❖ ***Reassure and engage the patient.*** The patient in crisis may need ongoing reassurance that can be communicated with statements. Some examples include:

  o "I want to help you."
  o "Let's figure out what we can do to improve this."
  o "You have contacted the right place."
  o "You may say whatever you need to."
  o "I'm listening, please continue."

❖ ***Provide calm and specific advice.*** The tone of the nurse's voice is paramount, along with the accurate support of decision support tools for the particular crisis. By providing specific actions, the nurse assists the patient to feel more in control of the situation.

Refusal to Follow Advice

As a nurse, it is easy to assume that if someone is contacting you, that person wants assistance. However, seeking help may not assure the patient's willingness to follow the nurse's actual advice. When the patient refuses to follow advice, two foci for the nurse's communication repertoire that address this issue are prevention and consequence.

As noted throughout this chapter, building a trusting relationship is crucial to enhancing the type of care the nurse can provide. To help in preventing the patient's refusal, the nurse should strive to build a relationship with each patient. When determining the most appropriate access to care, the nurse must collaborate with the patient. This serves to restore some control to the patient. When the nurse performs an ongoing evaluation of the patient's acceptance with statements such as "Do you feel comfortable with this suggestion?" or "Are there other things we should consider?" the patient feels more ownership. Hopefully, this ownership and collaboration will prevent later refusal.

If the patient chooses to not follow the advice given, the nurse should clearly state and document the consequence of that action. By answering the phone or responding via Web-based technology, the nurse is legally placed in a responsible relationship with that patient. The nurse must ask the patient, "Do you understand what could occur if you do not follow this advice?" If the patient still refuses to follow the advice given, another question that can be asked is "What would you prefer to do?" If the outcome is not positive, the nurse should document the exchange noting the patient's response to each question. Later, the nurse might consider following-up by contacting the patient.

Obscene Encounters

On occasion, the nurse may receive threatening or obscene contacts. This type of contact can be particularly upsetting because the tone tends to feel more personal. The nurse should first consider whether the patient's use of foul language is an intentional affront or normal vocabulary for that

If the patient chooses to not follow the advice given, the nurse should clearly state and document the consequence of that action. By answering the phone or responding via Web-based technology, the nurse is legally placed in a responsible relationship with that patient.

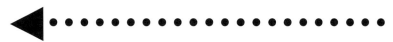

person. The nurse should focus on getting to the root of the problem by attempting to calm the patient with a quiet tone of voice, the use of nonverbal utterances, and/or carefully worded responses. Periodically, the nurse can use reflective statements to emphasize active listening. Whenever possible, it is best for the nurse to try not to match the patient's frustration level and/or obscene language. The nurse can attempt to clarify both the patient and nurse's expectations of the encounter. Ultimately, if the abusive or obscene language continues, the nurse must follow organizational policy. This may include telling the patient that if the language continues, the encounter will be concluded. The nurse must be aware of legal consequences of terminating encounters. In these situations, the criteria for terminating an encounter as well as an offer for alternative care must be followed per policy. Otherwise concluding the encounter may be considered abandonment. If an encounter is ended in this fashion, the nurse should follow policy regarding notification, and thoroughly and objectively document the exchange.

SUMMARY

The ability to effectively communicate is the foundation of telehealth nursing practice. Communication is the platform for creating an atmosphere in which the patient and nurse can work together to achieve mutually desired outcomes. Communication techniques used effectively will allow the nurse to obtain a more complete history and assessment to reduce communication barriers and manage challenging communication situations. The nurse must be aware of anticipated barriers and understand how to effectively overcome those barriers. Facilitating a positive exchange with the individual serves to support and maintain trusting relationships with the nurse and the organization.

Communication techniques used effectively will allow the nurse to obtain a more complete history and assessment to reduce communication barriers and manage challenging communication situations.

TIPS & PEARLS

☎ Examine your own telecommunication "personality."
☎ Practice actively listening.
☎ Spend adequate time reaching closure with the call/encounter.
☎ Be aware of patient and nurse communication barriers.
☎ Be prepared to handle difficult situations.
☎ Recognize that communications extend beyond the telephone and that appropriate techniques must be used when communicating by email, TDD, and other devices.

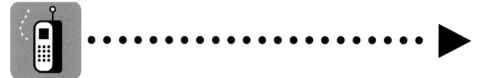

References

Adler, R.B., & J.M. Elmhorst. (2006). *Communicating at work – Principles and practices for business and the professions* (8th ed.). New York: McGraw-Hill.

American Academy of Ambulatory Care Nursing (AAACN). (2005). *A guide to ambulatory care nursing orientation and competency assessment.* Pitman, NJ: Author.

American Academy of Ambulatory Care Nursing (AAACN). (2007). *Telehealth nursing practice administration and practice standards* (4th ed.). Pitman, NJ: Author.

American Medical Association (AMA). (2008). *Guidelines for physician-patient electronic communications.* Retrieved on March 7, 2008, from http://www.ama-assn.org/ama/pub/category/print/2386.html

Borelli, B. (2006). *Using motivational interviewing to promote patient behavior change and enhance health.* Retrieved on February 23, 2008, from http://www.medscape.com/viewprogram/5757_pnt

Squires, D.D., & Moyers, T.B. (2008). *Motivational interviewing: A guideline developed for the Behavioral Health Recovery Management project.* Retrieved on February 23, 2008, from http://www.bhrm.org/guidelines/motiveint.pdf

Wheeler, S., & Windt, J. (1993). *Telephone triage theory, practice & protocol development.* Albany, NY: Delmar Publishers, Inc.

Answer/Evaluation Form
Continuing Nursing Education Activity

AMBP9c03

Telehealth Nursing Practice Essentials
Chapter 4: Communication Principles and Chapter 5: Communication Techniques

This activity provides 1.3 contact hours of continuing nursing education (CNE) credit in nursing.
(Contact hours calculated using a 60-minute contact hour.)

This test may be copied for use by others.

COMPLETE THE FOLLOWING:

Name: _____

Address: _____

City: _____ State: _____ Zip: _____

Telephone number: (Home)_____ (Work)_____

Email address:_____

AAACN Member Number and Expiration Date: _____

Processing fee: AAACN Member: $12.00
                  Nonmember: $20.00

Answer Form: (Please attach a separate sheet of paper if necessary.)
1. What did you value most about this activity?

_____
_____

2. If you could imagine that you have fully integrated your learning into practice, what would be different about your present practice?

_____
_____

Evaluation	Strongly disagree				Strongly agree
3. The offering met the stated objectives.					
a. Compare and contrast the conventional communication model with the Telehealth Nursing Communications (TNC) Model.	1	2	3	4	5
b. Identify the differences in which the patient and the nurse approach an encounter.	1	2	3	4	5
c. Describe influences which may affect the nurse-patient encounter.	1	2	3	4	5
d. Propose ways to project a positive telecommunication personality and effective voice quality.	1	2	3	4	5
e. Describe effective telehealth communication techniques.	1	2	3	4	5
f. Explain necessary telecommunication mechanical competencies.	1	2	3	4	5
g. Understand basic information about motivational interviewing.	1	2	3	4	5
h. Summarize strategies to reduce communication barriers and to manage challenging communication situations.	1	2	3	4	5
4. The content was current and relevant.	1	2	3	4	5
5. The content was presented clearly.	1	2	3	4	5
6. The content was covered adequately.	1	2	3	4	5

7. How would you rate your ability to apply your learning to practice following this activity? (Check one)

☐ Diminished ability   ☐ No change   ☐ Enhanced ability

8. Time required to complete reading assignment and answer form: ___ minutes
Comments _____

_____

I verify that I have completed this activity:

_____
Signature

Objectives

This educational activity is designed for nurses and other health care professionals who provide telehealth care for patients. This evaluation is designed to test your achievement of the following educational activities.
1. Compare and contrast the conventional communication model with the Telehealth Nursing Communications (TNC) Model.
2. Identify the differences in which the patient and the nurse approach an encounter.
3. Describe influences which may affect the nurse-patient encounter.
4. Propose ways to project a positive telecommunication personality and effective voice quality.
5. Describe effective telehealth communication techniques.
6. Explain necessary telecommunication mechanical competencies.
7. Understand basic information about motivational interviewing.
8. Summarize strategies to reduce communication barriers and to manage challenging communication situations.

Evaluation Form Instructions

1. To receive continuing nursing education (CNE) credit for individual study after reading the indicated chapter(s), please complete the evaluation form (photocopies of the answer form are acceptable). Attach separate paper as necessary.
2. Detach (or photocopy) and send the answer form along with a check, money order, or credit card payable to *AAACN* East Holly Avenue/Box 56, Pitman, NJ 08071-0056. You may also send this form as an email attachment to ambp401@ajj.com.
3. Answer forms must be postmarked by December 31, 2011. Upon completion of the answer/evaluation form, a certificate for 1.3 contact hours will be awarded and sent to you.

Payment Options
☐ Check or money order enclosed (payable in U.S. funds to AAACN)

☐ MasterCard   ☐ VISA   ☐ American Express

Credit Card #:_____

Expiration Date: _____ Security Code:_____

Card Holder (Please print):

_____

Signature:

_____

This educational activity has been co-provided by the American Academy of Ambulatory Care Nursing (AAACN) and Anthony J. Jannetti, Inc. (AJJ).
AAACN is a provider approved by the California Board of Registered Nursing, Provider Number CEP 5336.
AJJ is accredited as a provider of continuing nursing education by the American Nurses Credentialing Center's Commission on Accreditation.
This book was reviewed and formatted for contact hour credit by Sally S. Russell, MN, CMSRN, AAACN Education Director, and Maureen Espensen, MBA, BSN, RN, Editor.

American Academy of Ambulatory Care Nursing
East Holly Avenue/Box 56, Pitman, NJ 08071-0056
Phone: 800-AMB-NURS; Fax: 856-589-7463
Web: www.aaacn.org; Email: aaacn@ajj.com

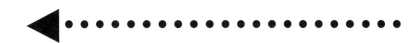

CHAPTER 6
Legal Aspects of Telehealth Nursing

Objectives

1. Define the unique legal issues that affect telehealth nurses.
2. Review practices that can be used to manage risk.
3. Discuss developments in licensure, laws, and practices that may affect telehealth nursing in the future.

CREATING A LEGAL RELATIONSHIP

Every time a telehealth nurse is in contact with a patient, a relationship is created with that patient. This relationship is fraught with risk from a legal standpoint for at least three reasons.

First, the telehealth nurse is expected to maintain the level of care provided in face-to-face nursing while operating at a distance from the patient. This situation creates unique challenges for the telehealth nurse. The telehealth nurse assesses symptoms and offers advice without ever viewing the patient. The nurse often has little or no access to a patient chart or medical history, and may have limited access to reference materials or other resources. The telehealth nurse must rely on the patient or family member's cooperation in order to provide care and monitor compliance.

The nurse often has little or no access to a patient chart or medical history, and may have limited access to reference materials or other resources.

Second, telehealth nurses practice in different settings with their employers having varied levels of awareness of professional standards. In some situations, it may mean that the telehealth nurse is forced to become the advocate for acquiring and maintaining the resources and materials required to meet professional standards. In addition, the telehealth nurse may be forced to serve as his/her own risk manager, educating the employer about current standards, legal risks, and new developments in telehealth nursing practice, along with laws and licensure.

Third, the telehealth nurse works in a setting where legal standards continue to evolve and licensure issues are being evaluated at both the state and national level. Consequently, the telehealth nurse must continually monitor developments to ensure appropriate practice within the state Nurse Practice Act and national standards, such as the American Academy of Ambulatory Care Nursing (AAACN) *Telehealth Nursing Practice Administration and Practice Standards* (2007).

Fortunately, for the telehealth nurse, these risks can be managed. The challenge for telehealth nurses is to minimize exposure to risk, while providing high-quality care for patients.

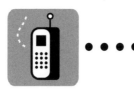

UNDERSTANDING LIABILITY

Liability is the term used to describe the assignment of responsibility of duties that an individual or organization is legally bound to fulfill. Thus, nurses or organizations that are found negligent in performing their duties can be held responsible – or *liable* – for the outcome of their actions. Almost all negligence cases involving telehealth nurses will take place in a civil courtroom, rather than a criminal proceeding.

There are four elements to negligence cases involving nurses. They include:

1. The nurse had a ***duty*** to provide care to the patient by following an accepted standard of care.
2. The nurse ***failed*** to adhere to this standard of care.
3. The nurse's failure to adhere to the standard of care was the ***cause*** of the patient's injuries.
4. The patient suffered ***damages*** – some type of ***hurt*** or ***injury*** – that were an ***effect*** of the nurse's negligent actions.

Another way to sum up the concept of negligence is to ask these four questions:

- ❖ Did the nurse have a duty to care for the patient?
- ❖ Did the nurse fail to fulfill that duty?
- ❖ Was there a "cause and effect" relationship between the nurse's actions and the outcome for the patient?
- ❖ Did the patient suffer damages (also described as hurt or injury) as a result?

Although the law of telehealth nursing is still evolving, it is clear that juries are willing to hold both telehealth nurses and their employers responsible for poor outcomes in cases involving telehealth nurse information, assessment, or advice. Telehealth nurses can be named as part of a lawsuit involving an employer, or they may be the sole defendant in a lawsuit. In addition, telehealth nurses may face disciplinary action for violating standards in state Nurse Practice Act.

A telehealth nurse must always consider the legal implications of telehealth encounters. For example, upon picking up the telephone, the nurse hears heavy breathing on the other end of the call. The nurse must listen carefully and decide if the "heavy breathing" is from a semi-conscious patient or is because someone fell asleep while waiting for his/her call to be answered. Alternatively, is the call is from someone playing a prank? There is an inherent risk whenever a nurse picks up the telephone and as much of a risk when choosing to hang up. The nurse must make a judgment on how to handle the situation. What if the nurse

A telehealth nurse must always consider the legal implications of telehealth encounters.

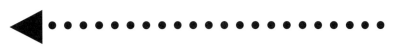

thinks it is a prank call and hangs up, only to learn later that it was actually a semi-comatose patient? In this case, in a court of law, hanging up the telephone may be considered "abandonment of care."

THE NURSE'S DUTY

The telehealth nurse has an implied agreement to provide care upon responding to a telehealth request. In other words, once the nurse answers a call, responds to an email, or begins a telemonitoring encounter, the nurse has accepted a duty to provide care for the patient.

There are five areas where failure to fulfill this duty creates liability for telehealth nurses:

- ❖ *Failure to ensure patient safety.* For example, if the nurse fails to:
  - o Assess and triage the patient appropriately.
  - o Follow clinical guidelines as written.
  - o Report situations where a child or elderly person is at risk.
  - o Follow-up with patients to ensure that instructions were understood and appropriate care was sought.
- ❖ *Failure to communicate.* The most essential skill in telehealth nursing is communication. This includes active, participatory listening. Failure to communicate adequately (either written or verbally) during the encounter may result in misperceptions, jumping to conclusions, or leading the caller. The nurse must:
  - o Listen to the patient's concerns.
  - o Convey written and verbal information in a manner that the patient and family can readily understand.
  - o Carefully clarify information to ensure that the patient fully understands.
  - o Document the encounter to make it possible to reconstruct the call in the future and for others.

  Additionally, lawyers advise that nurses have a responsibility to inform callers of the seriousness or life-threatening nature of their decision when the patient does want to be compliant with the recommended care advice. This process ensures that patients understand the risk and dangers associated with non-compliance.
- ❖ *Failure to follow policies and procedures.* The nurse must clearly understand policies and specific call handling procedures. Policies must be updated on a regular basis to match current practices and reflect current standards. If the nurse ignores policies and procedures, both the nurse and the employer are at risk.
- ❖ *Failure to act on professional judgment.* The nurse's ability to apply professional judgment is a core reason why the nurse is an irreplaceable part of the telehealth service. Without professional judgment, a computer could dispense decision support tools and

The telehealth nurse has an implied agreement to provide care upon responding to a telehealth request. In other words, once the nurse answers a call, responds to an email, or begins a telemonitoring encounter, the nurse has accepted a duty to provide care for the patient.

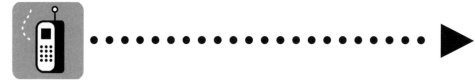

perform the job. However, the clinical knowledge and decision-making skills of a registered nurse are needed to interpret and correlate data in order to render appropriate professional judgment. In court, abandoning professional judgment in favor of just following physician orders or the decision support tools will be an inadequate defense. The nurse must be able to show that professional judgment was used during every patient contact.

❖ *Failure to document.* The nurse must demonstrate careful, clear documentation to recreate the encounter for medical and legal reasons.

Based on these five failures, it is possible to develop a checklist in order to fulfill the duty to the patient. Did the nurse and/or contact center…

❑ Monitor the patient and situation?
❑ Assess the situation using professional judgment?
❑ Provide information and education to the patient?
❑ Maintain a safe environment for the encounter by controlling noise, workspace, and workload?
❑ Guard confidentiality by preventing telephone calls and conversations with patients from being overheard?
❑ Protect the encounter records by not allowing all office personnel access to the documentation?
❑ Assign appropriate types of staff and adequate staffing levels to handle patient encounters?
❑ Perform quality improvement measurements on encounter handling, documentation, and clinical outcome analysis?
❑ Develop and follow policies and procedures?
❑ Document the encounters according to policy?
❑ Understand and implement standards of practice?
❑ Practice within the state Nurse Practice Act (the appropriate scope of practice)?

STANDARDS OF CARE

In essence, standards determine the expectations for nursing performance in patient care and system operations.

Standards are defined as "statements enunciated and promulgated by the profession by which the quality of practice, service, or education can be judged" (AAACN, 2007). In essence, standards determine the expectations for nursing performance in patient care and system operations. At the same time, standards define the type of nursing care that is expected, as well as provide a means of controlling barriers that could impair that care. Standards should be reflected in every telehealth delivery model. This includes one-person physician offices, mid-size clinics, and community nurse lines, as well as more than 100-seat contact centers.

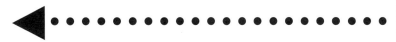

Standards are found in a variety of formats including policies and procedures, job descriptions, performance standards or other goals, decisions support tools, and written standards of care developed specifically for each telehealth center.

Six types of standards that affect telehealth nurses should be taken into account when developing telehealth nursing materials. Applicable standards of care include:

1. *Personal standards* include actions and decisions of a reasonable ordinary person who is a model citizen if under similar circumstances. These standards are developed based on community beliefs, morality, and ethics.

2. *Legal standards* include applicable state and federal laws. Each state has requirements for nursing care defining the nurse's scope of practice. In addition, telehealth nurses handling patient encounters (emails and telephone calls) from other states may be required to meet the license requirements of the state in which the patient resides. The telehealth nurse must also be aware of new state or federal laws that address emerging concerns about telehealth nursing.

3. *Professional standards* are obtained from professional organizations, especially those focusing on telephone triage, telehealth nursing, and telemedicine. Organizations that have issued statements addressing telephone triage include the American Academy of Ambulatory Care Nursing (AAACN), the American Association of Office Nurses (AAON), and the Emergency Nurses Association (ENA). In some cases, these standards may overlap or even contradict each other. For example, the American College of Emergency Physicians issued a policy statement in July 2000 recommending that emergency departments not attempt medical assessment or management by telephone. It is important for telehealth nurses working in specialized contact centers (such as for oncology patients) to be aware of standards specifically written for their area of specialty (oncology) and understand how the specialty standards apply in telehealth practice.

4. *Regulatory standards* are developed by agencies and organizations charged with reviewing and maintaining the health care system. These standards are created by local and state health departments, the Joint Commission, the Occupational Safety and Hazards Administration (OSHA), the Food and Drug Administration (FDA), the Americans with Disabilities Act (ADA), and the National Committee for Quality Association (NCQA), among others. Many of the standards written by each of the organizations are applicable to telehealth nursing even when it is not directly stated. It is important to recognize that although telehealth nurses

Each state has requirements for nursing care defining the nurse's scope of practice. In addition, telehealth nurses handling patient encounters (emails and telephone calls) from other states may be required to meet the license requirements of the state in which the patient resides.

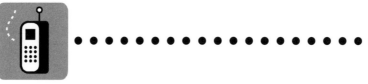

provide care to patients remotely through telecommunication devices, The Joint Commission and other accreditation bodies can certainly survey them. Currently, the American Accreditation HealthCare Commission, Inc. (otherwise known as URAC) is the only accrediting body that specifically reviews and certifies health contact centers.

5. ***Structural standards*** reflect the conditions, equipment, and materials needed to reliably operate a nursing contact center or telehealth program. Typically written in the format of policies, these standards may spell out the means that will be used to handle long wait times or calls waiting in a queue. Once these policies are created, the contact center has an obligation to provide the equipment and materials needed to fulfill them.

6. ***Process standards*** define how the telehealth nurse will provide care, as well as the type or quality of care that the nurse be expected to provide. The standards will outline requirements for the nurse's actions, knowledge, skills, and behavior.

SCOPE OF PRACTICE

The nurse's scope of practice is determined by each state's Nurse Practice Act, as well as the State Medical Board and other professional organizations that provide guidelines for appropriate roles of physicians and nurses.

The nurse's scope of practice is determined by each state's Nurse Practice Act, as well as the State Medical Board and other professional organizations that provide guidelines for appropriate roles of physicians and nurses. In applying these guidelines, the telehealth nurse typically faces three types of challenges.

Interstate Licensure

First, variations in state nurse practice acts continue to create challenges for telehealth nurses. These acts can vary significantly from state to state in the level of independence granted to the nurse for assessment, triaging, and scope of practice. The National Council of State Boards of Nursing (NCSBN) developed the Nurse Licensure Compact to resolve the issues created by services that function across state lines. States that approve the compact agree to allow a nurse to hold one license in the state where the nurse resides. The nurse can then practice in other states covered by the compact using either physical or electronic methods as long as he/she acknowledges that the nurse is subject to each state's practice laws and discipline. Nurses must meet the home state's qualifications for licensure and comply with all current laws. Twenty-three states had adopted the compact as of March 2008, and many others states were considering participation. The NCSBN provides updates on state compact bill status at its Web site (www.ncsbn.org).

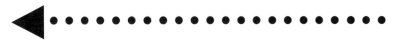

Scope of Care

Second, the telehealth nurse must clearly understand the scope of care the nurse is allowed to provide under the requirements of the home state's nurse practice act. There are some issues, however, that apply to all nurses, regardless of location. Wherever the nurse resides, the nurse must scrupulously avoid practicing medicine by medically diagnosing patients or prescribing treatment. In other words, the nurse's role must be limited to assessing symptoms and offering information related to those symptoms. The nurse must never cross into the territory of the physician by attempting to diagnose conditions. The nurse must also be careful to follow policies, procedures, and professional standards in determining when the physician or another provider must be brought in to assist in handling the call or responding to the caller's concerns. The telehealth nurse's role includes:

❖ *Assessment.* Appropriately assessing, prioritizing, and initiating the encounter including performing complex interviewing.

❖ *Planning.* Choosing appropriate decision support tools, using them correctly, collaborating with the patient and other health care providers, and referencing resources.

❖ *Implementation.* Effectively solving problems, applying intervention techniques, activating the disposition of care including teaching and counseling, educating, coordinating resources, and facilitating follow-up care.

❖ *Evaluation.* Documenting, communicating with others, and analyzing outcomes.

Wherever the nurse resides, the nurse must scrupulously avoid practicing medicine by medically diagnosing patients or prescribing treatment. In other words, the nurse's role must be limited to assessing symptoms and offering information related to those symptoms.

Employment of Others

Third, the registered nurse must be aware that his/her license may be used to justify the employment of licensed practical nurses (LPNs) or unlicensed assistive personnel (UAP) to perform duties that may be legally restricted to RNs. These practices should particularly concern nurses who oversee LPNs or UAPs as part of their role as nurse manager. The use of LPNs and UAPs can be particularly troublesome in physician offices or contact centers. UAPs often have years of experience in obtaining medical information from patients or dispensing medical advice on the physician's behalf. Consequently, they accept this role as a customary part of their position and may even expect to perform these duties. However, if an RN serving in a supervisory role appears to allow this practice, a court may be able to assume that the UAP acted under the nurse's license. In most states, RNs violate the practice act if they delegate telephone advice to UAPs, such as medical assistants. RNs should also be wary of situations when physicians ask them to exceed the limits of the state Nurse Practice Act by independently providing treatment information. Such information

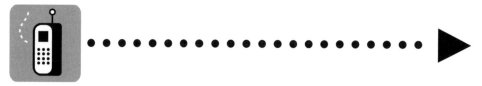

should only be dispensed under the specific direction of a physician using approved guidelines.

To control these risks, nurses should ensure that job descriptions clearly outline the roles of RNs, LPNs, and UAPs. Policies and procedures should reinforce the job description by outlining appropriate roles for all staff members. URAC (2007) standards allow for the use of non-clinical personnel in the telehealth practice arena. However, they are very specific in outlining that:

To control risks, nurses should ensure that job descriptions clearly outline the roles of RNs, LPNs, and UAPs. Policies and procedures should reinforce the job description by outlining appropriate roles for all staff members.

Non-clinical staff:

- ❖ Do not perform clinical activities;
- ❖ Are qualified and trained to perform screening, as defined by the organization, of service requests;
- ❖ Are supported by policies and procedures on the collection of non-clinical data;
- ❖ Are trained in the principles and procedures of screening callers, collection and transfer of service requests, maintenance of confidentiality of individually identifiable information and provider-specific information, and the URAC *Health Call Center Standards* (2007);
- ❖ Through an established process, promptly transfers a telephone call or other communication requiring clinical intervention to a licensed clinical staff person; and
- ❖ Have clinical monitoring, oversight, and immediate availability of a licensed clinical staff person for clinical issues (URAC, 2007).

Furthermore, URAC standards state that the organization restricts performance of clinical triage and health information services to:

- ❖ Registered nurses possessing a current, unrestricted license issued by a state or jurisdiction within the United States to practice nursing (or if the license is restricted, have a process to ensure practice is within the scope of licensure as outlined by the state board).

RN Scope of Practice Summary
(Note: Please review individual state nurse practice acts for specific information.)

The scope of practice for a registered nurse does not include medically diagnosing or prescribing. The scope of practice for a registered nurse includes:

1. Independent assessment and triaging.
2. Developing a nursing diagnosis.
3. Independent clinical judgment and decision-making.
4. Independent education of patients.

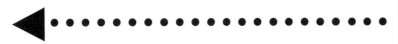

5. Analyzing outcomes.
6. Coordinating care.

LPN/LVN Scope of Practice
(Note: Scope of practice varies from state to state.)
1. Cannot independently assess and triage.
2. Can gather general information about the patient.
3. Can present data to the RN or physician for analysis and triaging.
4. Cannot independently educate patients, but can provide general information as directed by the RN or physician.

Non-Licensed Personnel
(For example: Nurse's aides, medical assistants, and receptionists.)
1. Can gather basic information from the patient.
2. Can screen service requests (URAC, 2007).
3. Cannot assess, triage, or make independent decisions on the care or disposition of a patient.

Examples of Practice Issues
The following examples illustrate scope of practice issues. It is recommended that telehealth nurses discuss these examples with their administration and legal counsel.

❖ It is a frequent practice for long-term care facilities (such as nursing homes) to contact the physician's office to report patient falls. Frequently, the provider's secretary handles the telephone call and gathers the information from the nursing home registered nurse. In some states, this may be a breach in the chain of duty because the registered nurse provided the information to a secretary. Perhaps the communication needs to be from the registered nurse in the long-term care facility to the registered nurse in the physician's office.

❖ A registered nurse in a centralized triage service assesses and triages patients by telephone and offers first-time appointments to patients. The triage nurse contacts a physician's office for an appointment and is told that there is not an appointment available until 5 days later. However, the triage disposition recommends that the patient be seen within the next 1-2 days. The patient states that he can wait for the appointment in 5 days. The nurse agrees and overrides the triage decision by downgrading the triage disposition. What is the nurse's liability because of downgrading the patient's disposition?

❖ The office secretary routinely answers all incoming calls. The secretary decides which calls are handled first and which patients should be seen in the earliest period. What are the issues in

It is a frequent practice for long-term care facilities (such as nursing homes) to contact the physician's office to report patient falls.

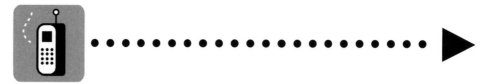

allowing a secretary to use independent decision-making and choose which patients have the most urgent needs?

STRATEGIES TO MINIMIZE LIABILITY

Strategies to minimize the liability of telehealth nursing involve the nurse, the employer, and the health care provider. The following strategies address risk management for telehealth nurses by considering optimum practice for both individual nurses and their employers. The strategies are divided into two groups – before the encounter and after the encounter.

1) **Strategies to develop BEFORE the nurse responds to an encounter:**
   ❖ *Identify the telehealth functions, purpose, and goals.* Statements should also include the limits of telehealth nursing services, as well as specific objectives that telehealth nurses should seek to meet.
   ❖ *Create job descriptions that accurately reflect the scope of telehealth nursing.* The job description should include detailed information about the scope of the telehealth nurse's responsibilities and minimum qualifications (a minimum of 3 years of RN experience in an applicable clinical area prior to telehealth nursing is the industry standard) (Espensen, 2001). The job description should detail accountability for outcomes. The document should be reviewed and updated on an annual basis to ensure it reflects current responsibilities.
   ❖ *Create and update policies and procedures that reflect current standards.* Inevitably, new medical discoveries will affect clinical care, referral information will change, providers will merge, and new health issues will emerge. Policies and procedures must be updated as these changes occur. In addition, all policies and procedures should be reviewed on at least an annual basis to ensure that the written policies match actual practice, with the date of the last review noted as part of the policy. Policies should be reasonable and obtainable. Lawyers warn that writing "pie in the sky" policies that are unattainable can expose the telehealth nurse to additional risk. Some examples of policies that could be unattainable are "every call must be answered within 20 seconds," and "every patient must be seen within 12 hours." Instead of having these service standards as policies, they can be implemented as service goals to use as guidance for practice. A department goal or guideline to answer calls within 20 seconds is just that. However, if written as a policy, the department may not be able to answer calls within this timeframe, and this causes a policy violation.

Inevitably, new medical discoveries will affect clinical care, referral information will change, providers will merge, and new health issues will emerge. Policies and procedures must be updated as these changes occur.

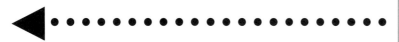

❖ *Provide formal telehealth nurse orientation and continuing education.* A formal orientation strengthens telehealth service and assists nurses in understanding their role and responsibilities. Orientation should include learning the unique aspects of assessing a patient without face-to-face contact, triaging with clinical guidelines, performing adequate telecommunication skills, and supporting patient advocacy. Accreditation bodies such as URAC expect that the orientation process is documented specifically for each nurse. The industry average for telehealth orientation is 2-4 weeks. Additionally, URAC and others expect documentation of ongoing continuing education. Education should include clinical information, issues identified through quality assurance, and broader issues related to job performance and nursing care.

❖ *Identify physicians to oversee the decision support tools.* Physicians are ultimately responsible for the care of their patients. Because of this responsibility, a physician needs to oversee the clinical assessment and triage system used by the telehealth nurses. Generally, the physician consultant is a family practice, emergency department, or internal medicine physician. Other physicians are utilized for reviewing system-specific clinical guidelines, such as an obstetrician for the obstetrical and gynecology guidelines. Although physicians oversee the clinical guidelines system, it is important that the decision support tools be developed for the RN to use as non-diagnostic tools. The assessment guidelines need to be symptomatic and not written as a medical diagnosis.

❖ *Identify patient care standards especially for emergent situations.* In emergent situations, courts have ruled that nurses have an obligation to send patients to the nearest emergency facility. Telehealth nurses also have an obligation to access emergency services such as 911 when appropriate. Some telehealth services expect the nurse to stay on the line with the patient until the ambulance arrives, while other telehealth services do not. Patient abandonment is a concern if the nurse does not continue "caring" for the patient until help arrives. The telehealth nurse needs to investigate how and when to transfer calls to 911 and the expectations of administration. In addition to emergency situations, the telehealth nurse must know how to respond and direct patients when emergency calls are received from patients outside their 911 service area or network.

❖ *Identify encounters that must be referred immediately to emergency services or providers.* The telehealth service should have clear guidelines on calls that must be linked to emergency services, immediately referred to a provider, or otherwise handled according to a procedure that acknowledges the urgency of the

Although physicians oversee the clinical guidelines system, it is important that the decision support tools be developed for the RN to use as non-diagnostic tools. The assessment guidelines need to be symptomatic and not written as a medical diagnosis.

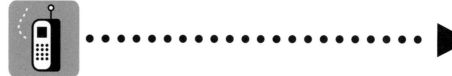

call. If these guidelines and/or policies are not followed, there is an increased medical legal risk of "delay in care."

❖ ***Select, maintain, and use an appropriate decision support tool system.*** Some "informal" telehealth services in physician offices continue to rely on case-by-case assessment responses based solely on the nurse's knowledge and personal experience. If this information is challenged in court, the nurse may find it difficult to accurately re-create the situation decision. In fact, it is difficult to defend the fact that information was given "off the top of the head," and that this was an appropriate resource for providing quality care. Because standards of practice have been written for telehealth nursing, a court of law will find it unacceptable that the nurse gave spontaneous information. Instead, telehealth nurses should rely on a formal decision support tool system of guidelines, protocols, or algorithms, which may be developed in-house or purchased. If purchased, the tools should be adapted to respond to provider practices, state laws governing emergencies, and community practices. Whenever decision support tools are implemented or changes are made, the tool should be reviewed and approved by appropriate physicians. Finally, when the nurse uses a care guideline, it is extremely important to document which specific guideline was used as the source of information. The nurse should read the information directly to the caller, rather than relying on memory.

❖ ***Monitor encounter volumes and staff appropriately.*** The telehealth staff should demonstrate their awareness of peak call or email times and respond appropriately with adequate staffing levels. Additionally, procedures need to be put in place so that requests are not left until the next day, especially assessment calls (symptom-based calls). This would be considered abandonment of care.

❖ ***Notify patients if there is a wait to be in contact with the nurse.*** The message should advise the patient to seek immediate help from emergency services if there is an emergency. The message should give clear, direct instructions: "If this is an emergency, hang up and call 911 or your local emergency response unit."

❖ ***Monitor the nurse's interactions with patients to improve performance.*** Quality programs should include goals for improving individual and department-wide performance, including skill validations in assessment, triaging, communication, and documentation. This can be accomplished via competency testing or call auditing and monitoring.

❖ ***Develop new procedures in response to special issues.*** As the field of telehealth nursing continues to evolve, new issues are certain to arise, such as handling requests by email or fax. In addition, a

When the nurse uses a care guideline, it is extremely important to document which specific guideline was used as the source of information. The nurse should read the information directly to the caller, rather than relying on memory.

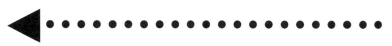

community may have specific demands that require a specific response. For example, an *E. coli* outbreak caused by contaminated drinking water can prompt a flood of calls about how to determine whether drinking water is safe. The savvy contact center will quickly create health education statements to specifically respond to these inquiries.

❖ *Protect patient confidentiality on all outbound calls, faxes, and electronic transmissions, which include patient identifiable information (including email).* Although patient confidentiality falls under HIPAA regulations, state laws may be more stringent. It is important to know which law supersedes in each patient's state. The nurse has a duty to protect the patient's identity. A frequent confidentiality conflict occurs when placing outbound calls or follow-up calls to patients. Caller identification systems (Caller I.D.) and answering machines provide an opportunity for the non-caller to learn that someone contacted a telehealth nurse. To avoid these problems, the telehealth nurse should dial the caller identification block on outgoing calls. In addition, a policy should be developed about leaving messages on answering machines or voice mail systems. Emails and patient data transmissions should be sent as encrypted or by a HIPAA privacy secure system.

❖ *Consider whether taping calls is a benefit or a risk.* Some services tape patient calls as a means of protecting the nurse. The taped call provides a recording of the exact conversation when there is a question of what the nurse said versus what the patient recalled. Taping also protects the institution because the taped nurse tends to "stay within boundaries" of appropriate communication and scope of practice. In other words, taped nurses avoid sharing their own opinions with callers. Taping calls can be beneficial for telehealth programs. In informal settings with limited experience or poorly defined professional standards however, taped calls can become a liability by revealing the shortcomings of the nurse and/or the nurse's employer. When taping is used, the caller must be notified that the call will be taped before they begin interacting with the nurse. Typically, this message is provided as part of the standard greeting before the call is transferred to the telehealth nurse.

❖ *Provide an appropriate environment and equipment for telehealth nursing.* The setting should be controlled in order to reduce noise. The nurse needs a quiet environment to concentrate. The patient needs to hear a quiet environment in order to trust the nurse. Although, noise-canceling headsets are beneficial to decrease background noise, they do not guarantee that office conversations will not be overheard by the caller. Co-workers may need to be reminded to keep their conversations at a low level

Although patient confidentiality falls under HIPAA regulations, state laws may be more stringent. It is important to know which law supersedes in each patient's state.

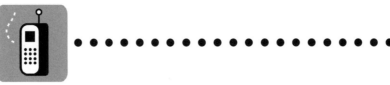

when others are handling patient calls. Appropriate equipment is essential, including telephone systems and computers. When these systems fail, the telehealth nursing program must have a back-up plan available to continue providing services. The implications of providing telehealth nursing services from remote sites, such as home, also need to be considered. Back-up systems (phone, computer, etc.) are needed when telecommuting from home or other locations.

❖ *Provide the appropriate resources necessary for telehealth nursing.* In addition to decision support tools. the nurse should be provided with:

   o Telephone equipment for transferring calls and placing calls on hold. Additionally, it is important to have a phone with a 3-way call feature to interact with emergency services and the patient.

   o Reference material (approved resources, books, and Web sites for providing general health information).

   o Equipment manuals and online resources as applicable.

   o Poison control center access or appropriate information.

   o Directory of approved community resources and hotline phone numbers.

   o Standards of practice, such as from AAACN.

❖ *Monitor laws, licensure requirements, and court actions that may affect telehealth nursing.* The passage of the nurse licensure compact, changes in laws governing telehealth and telemedicine services, managed care steerage issues, federal regulations (such as HIPAA, Stark, and Safe Harbor acts), and court cases all affect telehealth nursing. Programs that ignore developments in these areas are placing themselves at risk for legal action.

❖ *Avoid making false promises in marketing materials.* Marketing materials should accurately describe the limits of services provided by telehealth nursing programs. Physician practice and telehealth service brochures should not give promises or create false expectations, such as, "We always return calls within 2 hours." It is less risky to state, "We generally return phone calls within 2 hours."

2) **Strategies DURING and AFTER the call:**

❖ *Document calls to recreate the situation.* The documentation should indicate which decision support tools were used, detailed information that was given to the patient, any resources used, any referrals given, and confirmation that the patient demonstrated an understanding of the information (typically by repeating the information back to the nurse). Brief telephone notes or message notes will not provide enough detail to recreate the call. Instead, a standardized form should be used to aid in documentation and

Brief notes will not provide enough detail to recreate the call. A standardized form should be used to aid in documentation and ensure that all the appropriate information is captured.

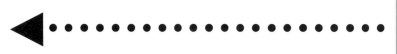

ensure that all the appropriate information is captured. Notes should be taken throughout the call, and documentation should be completed immediately following the conclusion of the call. Often, using checkboxes for specific phrases can strengthen documentation, particularly when these phrases document routine actions that the nurse might ignore or miss documenting in an abbreviated form. Suggested checkbox phrases include:

- ❏ "Care instructions explained and questions answered."
- ❏ "Encouraged to ask questions."
- ❏ "Instructed to call back if symptoms worsen."
- ❏ "Advised to watch for new or urgent symptoms and seek medical care."
- ❏ "Warned regarding the need for urgent treatment and the need to take action."
- ❏ "Numbers and resources given to the patient."
- ❏ "Asked to repeat instructions."

❖ *Inform patients about the telehealth service limitations.* The nurse should inform the patient that he/she is a registered nurse and that the patient must see a doctor to be diagnosed or to obtain a physician opinion. The nurse should also communicate with the patient in a manner that emphasizes assessment, information, and treatment options, rather than telling the patient what to do, or giving information that might be mistaken for diagnosis or treatment. The patient should always be made aware that the patient/caller holds final responsibility for pursuing care and acting upon the options presented by the telehealth nurse.

❖ *Provide patient instructions on when and how to obtain additional care.* The nurse should document that the patient was provided with information on when and how to seek care (such as referrals to specialists, community agencies, social service, or walk-in clinics) and that the patient understands the reason for the referral. The nurse should also discuss and document the contingency plan if the patient or nurse are unable to secure services. By discussing and documenting the contingency plan, the next health professional assisting the patient will have this information readily available and have a broader understanding of the patient treatment plan.

❖ *Provide precise, non-judgmental information.* When the patient misunderstands the information provided by the nurse, the results can be disastrous. The nurse should avoid making ambiguous statements that could be interpreted in different ways. When providing information to difficult callers or callers who have already spoken with the nurse about the same complaint, avoid remarks that might imply that the nurse is judging the caller's

The nurse should inform the patient that he/she is a registered nurse and that the patient must see a doctor to be diagnosed or to obtain a physician opinion.

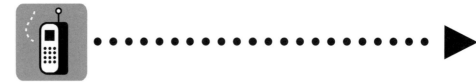

behavior or compliance with earlier recommendations. Instead, the nurse should concentrate on evaluating the health problem.

❖ **Provide appropriate services for the population served.** The telehealth service needs to provide access to a foreign language line as well as services for hearing impaired callers, either with a Telephone Device for the Deaf (TDD) or a relay service.

❖ **Never deny patient contact with a provider.** The telehealth service (especially an *after hours* service for physicians) should not be developed to protect physicians from receiving calls. If a patient insists on speaking to a provider, he/she should not be denied this contact.

❖ **Avoid making promises.** Nurses are advised against using any language that infers promises that a certain action will occur, either in individual interactions with callers or when representing its program or employer at public events. Hollow reassurances (such as telling callers that "everything will be alright") are likely to worsen the situation if things go wrong.

❖ **Initiate follow-up calls.** Information obtained during follow-up calls may be used for quality improvement, to check the status of callers with serious conditions, or to monitor patient compliance. Some telehealth programs prioritize follow-up encounters based on the severity of the symptoms reported by the caller. Others rely on decision support tools that specify which cases should receive follow-up calls. In severe cases, these calls can help minimize liability by revealing significant changes in symptoms, clarifying information provided by the nurse to the caller, or referring the caller to additional resources.

❖ **Protect patient confidentiality in the office.** The nurse must ensure that communications regarding patients not be overheard by others in the office. The nurse should handle calls or speak to patients in a private area away from other patient rooms, the waiting room or a hallway. Documentation should also be protected because it is a medical record. This means not having telephone notes in an area that others may read. Guarding documentation also includes locking files at night and not keeping charts out on the desk where cleaning staff and others may have access.

❖ **Adhere to the same standard of care.** Some telehealth nurses enjoy speaking or conversing with their "special" patients and end up spending more time with those patients. However, if patients are treated differently, there is inconsistency in the standard of care provided to patients. Likewise, sometimes the staff picks and chooses the callbacks to make to patients based on their concern. This favoritism is a legal risk because the nurse is providing a differentiated "level of service" to only certain patients.

Information obtained during follow-up calls may be used for quality improvement, to check the status of callers with serious conditions, or to monitor patient compliance.

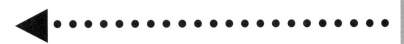

❖ *Have a plan when a patient refuses to provide his/her medical history.* When the patient refuses to provide his/her medical history (such as when contacting a community nurse triage line), the nurse does not have enough information to make an informed triage decision. The organization needs to decide how the triage nurse will proceed when the patient refuses to provide any medical history. The nurse will not be able to fully complete an assessment because of not knowing if the patient has chronic conditions, is on medications, or a recent medical history. The organization should provide scripting on interacting with these patients. If the nurse is still unable to obtain the history, the nurse should ensure documentation reflects the patient unwillingness to disclose their medical information. The nurse should not provide suggestion for over-the-counter medication use; care advice will be given and a disclaimer should be read that care advice is minimal based on not knowing the patient's medical history and contraindications for certain care techniques.

When the patient refuses to provide his/her medical history (such as when contacting a community nurse triage line), the nurse does not have enough information to make an informed triage decision.

RISK MANAGEMENT POLICIES

Policies can help telehealth nurses manage risk by anticipating problems and detailing procedures. Depending on the setting, policies should be developed to manage risk in the following areas:

❖ Communication with minors.
❖ Non-compliant patients.
❖ Angry or obscene callers.
❖ Inability to contact the patient or caller.
❖ Anonymous callers.
❖ Third party callers (baby-sitters, neighbors, or others calling on behalf of the patient, with or without the patient's permission).
❖ Family member calls (such as a minor calling for a parent who does not speak English or partners calling on behalf of his/her spouse).
❖ Calls from caregivers.
❖ Refusals from patients to provide a medical history.
❖ Language barriers (may be combined with hearing-impaired callers).
❖ Hearing-impaired callers (may be combined with language barriers).
❖ Back-up technology systems (computers crashing, loss of telephone lines).
❖ Access to emergency medical services (911, ambulance, and fire).

- ❖ Referrals to providers and services (the policy should include providers' inclusion criteria in the physician referral service or referrals to community agencies).
- ❖ Confidentiality of the actual call and the documentation.
- ❖ Nursing boundaries for call handling.
- ❖ Out-of-state calls.
- ❖ Prioritizing calls by call type (triage or general question) and severity of call.
- ❖ Types of calls to handle (triage, prescription refills).
- ❖ Callers who are not patients of your clinic or your providers.
- ❖ Medical and prescription benefit-related calls
- ❖ Repeat callers within a certain time frame (for example, the organization may set a policy that a person calling more than 3 times in 24 hours requires an automatic trigger to be seen and evaluated).

TRIAGE POLICIES

Policies that guide the triage process for telehealth nurses can also manage risk. Depending on the practice setting, telehealth nurse programs should consider creating policies to address the following conditions:

- ❖ Multiple symptom calls and clinical guidelines to use.
- ❖ Overriding guidelines.
- ❖ "No-protocol" calls when the symptoms do not "fit" any protocol.
- ❖ Providing over-the-counter medication dosages.
- ❖ New prescriptions and refills.
- ❖ Laboratory test ordering and disclosing results.
- ❖ Child abuse and neglect.
- ❖ Elderly abuse and neglect.
- ❖ Ingestions and poisonings.
- ❖ Sexual assault calls.
- ❖ Suicide or psychiatric calls.
- ❖ Chronic callers.
- ❖ Birth control and abortion calls. The nurse should follow a policy instead of his/her opinion and personal beliefs.

SPECIAL POPULATIONS

Some populations have inherent barriers that the nurse must overcome to communicate effectively. Court cases have established that it is the nurse's responsibility to overcome these barriers by communicating in a manner that the patient can understand. This means telehealth nurses must be prepared to communicate with patients regardless of age, mental

Some populations have inherent barriers that the nurse must overcome to communicate effectively. Court cases have established that it is the nurse's responsibility to overcome these barriers by communicating in a manner that the patient can understand.

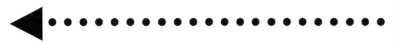

disability, language barriers, domestic disturbances, or lack of access to an adult.

Minor patients pose a special challenge because they may have special needs related to communication and consent. Minors may contact the telehealth nurse by phone or email for several reasons. They may be calling about their own symptoms and do not want to involve an adult. Teens may be emailing on behalf of a peer. Minors may also be put in a situation where they must act as the family spokesperson and translate for an adult who does not speak English.

Legal definitions of *minor* may vary from state-to-state. In some states, married minors older than age 15 are considered adults for health care purposes. Most states recognize emancipated minors and also consider a minor emancipated if the minor is a parent of a child. For minors, each state varies in their parental notification requirements for birth control counseling, abortion, tattooing, and other special conditions. Telehealth nurses should verify state laws and regulations that affect telehealth information to minors and develop policies accordingly. Additionally, administrative policies need to define what types of calls are accepted from minors and the information that can be provided.

Language barriers can also hamper telehealth nurses. The telehealth staff should be prepared to assist patients with no English or only limited English skills. In many cases, this means having a translator available or using a language translation service, such as a Language Line. When the community includes a large ethnic population, the contact center may need to have bilingual nurses on staff. To reduce legal risks of misinterpretation, the contact center should verify that the translator or translation service understands medical terminology and can accurately translate these terms into the second language. In addition, telehealth nurses must be trained in how and when to use the interpreter service. When there are common requests for interpreters for a specific language, such as Spanish, the nurse should learn the necessary Spanish phrase to ask the caller to hold for a translator. Using family members and/or other personnel to help with language interpretation may restrict the information that is shared by the patient. Additionally, it is a patient's right to have direct access to a neutral third party for language interpretation services.

Cultural and socioeconomic differences can create problems that may be further magnified by language barriers. In some populations, social taboos may prevent discussion of some types of health problems or even bar direct communication with certain family members, such as when only the husband speaks for the wife. When patients with poor vocabulary skills or cultural taboos are encountered and the patient has difficulties communicating (especially about bodily functions), the nurse must have some communication strategies readily available. Other issues include being aware of and making unique arrangements for patients with limited access to a telephone, transportation, and/or health care.

When the community includes a large ethnic population, the contact center may need to have bilingual nurses on staff. To reduce legal risks of misinterpretation, the contact center should verify that the translator or translation service understands medical terminology and can accurately translate these terms into the second language.

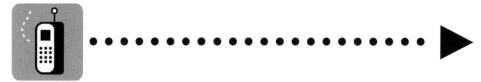

Access for people with hearing impairment. The telehealth nurse must have access to hearing-impaired callers by providing a TDD, training the staff in TDD operations, and publicizing the TDD telephone number. If having a TDD is not possible, all staff members should know how to access the state relay telephone service for the hearing impaired and communicate with a hearing-impaired caller via the relay center.

SPECIAL ISSUES

The same technology (telephones and computers) that makes it possible to provide telehealth assessment and information is likely to lead to additional issues in health information delivery. Emerging issues that create special legal concerns for telehealth nursing include Internet communications, email, texting, and standing orders for physicians.

Some telehealth nursing programs continuously or intermittently use the Internet to communicate with patients and providers. Special concerns include maintaining technology connections with patients, managing patients outside the provider's service area (state practice act), and protecting the patient's confidentiality. Because information sent online can be intercepted, telehealth nurses must take special measures to protect patient confidentiality. Nurses should still rely on the telephone when patients seeking information online want to discuss in-depth personal health conditions. Email delivered via the Internet should be used only with an agreement from the patient and only for general, non-specific information. In all cases, the nurse should remember that Internet-based email is similar to sending information through the United States Postal Service using a postcard that can be viewed by anyone who handles it. Unless encryption technology is available so that the consumer's email has the same security as a sealed first-class letter, telehealth nurses should continue relying on the telephone.

Because information sent online can be intercepted, telehealth nurses must take special measures to protect patient confidentiality.

The field of telehealth nursing is expanding roles and responsibilities. One example is the use of standing orders by some after-hours programs. These standing orders allow the telehealth nurse to issue prescriptions for callers with specific conditions based on guidelines approved by the caller's physicians. Issues that must be addressed before using standing orders include regulations contained in the nurse and pharmaceutical practice acts of the applicable states, determination of appropriate conditions, development of physician guidelines, and telehealth nursing education.

SPECIFIC CALLS TO 'HANDLE WITH CARE'

Strategies that minimize liability by providing high-quality patient care are essential, particularly in the area of sound nursing practices and call documentation. Yet, the telehealth nurse can provide another layer of

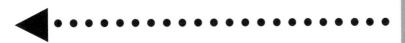

protection by consciously recognizing calls that must be handled with special care. In essence, this means recognizing high-risk situations and implementing strategies to limit risk. In addition to the calls and issues mentioned earlier in this chapter, there are numerous callers and conditions requiring special care by the nurse. In all of the situations listed below, the nurse should always err on the side of caution.

Providing advice when off duty. When a friend or neighbor contacts telehealth nurse at home during non-working hours, the temptation to provide medical "advice" may be hard to resist. Yet even in informal situations, the telehealth nurse must adhere to policies and protocols or accept exposure to legal risk. The "friendly neighbor" who called for your advice will not be so friendly in a court of law if given the wrong information. When outside of work, the nurse should limit medical legal risks by encouraging friends, neighbors, and family members to contact their health care provider for medical or health care advice.

Caregivers or third party calls. The nurse faces special challenges any time a third party is used to relay information. In some cases, the patient may not be able to communicate directly with the nurse due to injury, illness, language issues, or cultural taboos. This forces the nurse to rely on perceptions of a caregiver who is "assessing" the patient.

Patients with chronic disease. Chronic conditions are complex problems that often require specialized information. Specific clinical guidelines need to be developed if the nurse is handling calls for chronic illnesses, such as diabetes or congestive heart failure, or for patients undergoing chemotherapy.

Pregnant patients. Calls dealing with pregnancy should be handled with care, especially when the patient has a condition that labels her as "high risk." Many contact centers are no longer handling pregnancy calls but instead direct patients to contact their obstetrician, perinatologist, or mid-wife.

Infants under 2 months of age. Because infants under 2 months of age have an under-developed immune system and other special considerations, a general rule is that patients in this age group with symptoms need to be seen instead of being "assessed and treated" via technology.

Parents of ill children. Parents of chronically ill children may become overly anxious about minor ailments or they may be relatively unconcerned by potentially dangerous conditions. Either attitude can lead to miscommunication. Nurses must be particularly careful to provide clear, straightforward guidelines to parents without judging their inaction or belittling their pro-active approach.

Elderly callers. Elderly callers are more susceptible to a host of conditions. At the same time, they may be reluctant to share information or seek help due to a desire to protect their ability to live independently.

Calls dealing with pregnancy should be handled with care. Many contact centers are no longer handling pregnancy calls but instead direct patients to contact their obstetrician, perinatologist, or mid-wife.

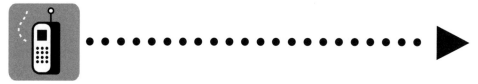

The nurse must triage cautiously, and when in doubt, request that the patient be seen by a provider.

Frequent, chronic, or repeat callers. Callers who repeatedly contact the telehealth program may be ignored on the one occasion when they truly have a complaint, or the nurse may miss the progression of complaints due to familiarity with the caller.

Patients with recent surgery. Any patient who has undergone surgery in the last 4-8 weeks and is having symptoms should be referred to the surgeon or primary care provider. The old adage to "err on the side of caution" always takes priority over not contacting physicians during their off hours.

Calls that take less than 3 minutes or more than 10 minutes. If the assessment portion of a call takes more than 10 minutes, it's likely that the patient needs to be seen. If an assessment takes less than 3 minutes, the nurse and caller have not shared enough information to adequately assess symptoms and triage appropriately. By handling calls in this manner, nurses put themselves at risk (Espensen, 2000).

If the assessment portion of a call takes more than 10 minutes, it's likely that the patient needs to be seen. If an assessment takes less than 3 minutes, the nurse and caller have not shared enough information to adequately assess symptoms and triage appropriately.

TIPS & PEARLS

☎ The telehealth nurse is expected to maintain the same standard of care provided in face-to-face nursing while operating at a distance from the patient.

☎ The telehealth nurse must monitor developments to ensure appropriate scope of practice within the state(s) Nurse Practice Act, from which they are interacting with patients and national standards such as AAACN's *Telehealth Nursing Practice Administration and Practice Standards.*

☎ Telehealth nurses must understand their liability. They can be named in a lawsuit involving an employer, or they may be the sole defendant in a lawsuit. Additionally, they may face disciplinary action for violating standards in state Nurse Practice Acts.

☎ The telehealth nurse has an implied agreement to provide care upon responding to a telehealth request (e.g., answering a call, responding to an email, or a taking part in a telemonitoring encounter).

☎ Develop and follow strategies to minimize liability before, during, and after an encounter.

☎ Develop and follow policies and procedures to manage risk.

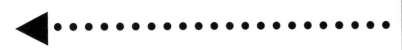

References

American Academy of Ambulatory Care Nursing (AAACN). (2007). *Telehealth nursing practice administration and practice standards* (4th ed.). Pitman, NJ: Author.

American Accreditation HealthCare Commission, Inc. (URAC). (2007). *Health call center (HCC) standards.* Retrieved February 11, 2009, from http://www.urac.org

Espensen, M. (2001). Telehealth nursing practice. In Robinson, J. (Ed.), *Core curriculum for ambulatory care nursing.* St. Louis, MO: Harcourt Health Services.

Special Acknowledgement

Physician Referral & Telephone Triage Times. National monthly publication for telephone nursing professionals; HMR Publications Group, Inc., 3180 Presidential Drive, Suite K, Atlanta, GA 30340; (770) 457-6106.

Suggested Readings (taken from AAACN, 2007)

RISK MANAGEMENT (CURRENT)

$841,500 verdict: Nurse mishandles postoperative patient's calls. (2003). *OB-GYN Malpractice Prevention, 10*(3), 21-22.

Castledine, G. (2003). Triage nurse who did not follow the protocols and forged her references. *British Journal of Nursing, 12*(10), 589.

Houge, E.E. (2005). Telemedicine and telehealth articles risk management in home telehealth. *Telehealth Practice Report, 9*(6), 1, 9-10.

McLean, P. (2003). Professional liability risks and risk management for nurses in telehealth. *Medicine and Law, 22*(4), 683-692.

Reese, P., & Huff, K. (2003). Defending the negligent credentialing claim. *Journal of Legal Nurse Consulting, 14*(3), 3-7.

Waters, R.J. (2005). Telehome care – Legal advice for telehealth pioneers. *Caring, 24*(5), 32-38.

RISK MANAGEMENT (ARCHIVED)

Hickson, G., & Federspiel, C. (2002). Patient complaints and malpractice risk. *JAMA, 287*(22), 2951–2957.

Hyde, J. (2002). Managed care and its effect on the healthcare system: Is it just an accident waiting to happen or will it improve patient outcomes? *Journal of Legal Nurse Consulting, 13*(2), 26-29.

Kinsella, A. (2002). Home telehealthcare: Good idea, but with safety concerns. *Medical Malpractice Law & Strategy, XIX*(7), 5-8.

Landry, H., & Landry, M. (2002). Nursing ethics and legal issues. *Journal of Nursing Education, 41*(8), 363-364.

Meaney, M. (2002). Exercise ethical leadership in case management. *Total Case Management, 12*(6), 34.

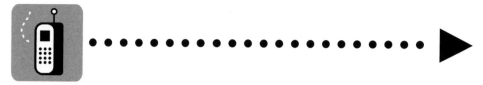

COURT CASES INVOLVING AMBULATORY CARE – TRIAGE LITIGATION (ARCHIVED)

HMO – Breach of contract and wrongful death. Thornton v. Shah MD. 333 Ill.App.3d, 777 N.E.2d 396 (1st Dist., 2002).

HMO telephone triage: Court sees no legal duty to preserve nurses' logs. (2002). *Legal Eagle Eye Newsletter for the Nursing Profession 10*(9), 4.

Medical assistant in violation of Nurse Practice Act. People of the State of Illinois v. Stults. 291 Ill.App.3d 71, 683 N.E.2d 521 (2nd Dist, 1997).

Answer/Evaluation Form
AMBP9c04
Continuing Nursing Education Activity
Telehealth Nursing Practice Essentials
Chapter 6: Legal Aspects of Telehealth Nursing

This activity provides 1.2 contact hours of continuing nursing education (CNE) credit in nursing.
(Contact hours calculated using a 60-minute contact hour.)

This test may be copied for use by others.

COMPLETE THE FOLLOWING:

Name: _____

Address: _____

City: _____ State: _____ Zip: _____

Telephone number: (Home)_____ (Work)_____

Email address:_____

AAACN Member Number and Expiration Date: _____

Processing fee: AAACN Member: $12.00
              Nonmember: $20.00

Answer Form: (Please attach a separate sheet of paper if necessary.)
1.   What did you value most about this activity?

_____
_____
_____
_____

2.   If you could imagine that you have fully integrated your learning into practice, what would be different about your present practice?

_____
_____
_____
_____

Evaluation	Strongly disagree				Strongly agree
3. The offering met the stated objectives.					
a. Define the unique legal issues that affect telehealth nurses.	1	2	3	4	5
b. Review practices that can be used to manage risk.	1	2	3	4	5
c. Discuss developments in licensure, laws, and practices that may affect telehealth nursing in the future.	1	2	3	4	5
4. The content was current and relevant.	1	2	3	4	5
5. The content was presented clearly.	1	2	3	4	5
6. The content was covered adequately.	1	2	3	4	5

7. How would you rate your ability to apply your learning to practice following this activity? (Check one)

☐ Diminished ability ☐ No change ☐ Enhanced ability

8. Time required to complete reading assignment and answer form: ___ minutes
Comments _____
_____

I verify that I have completed this activity:

_____
Signature

Objectives
This educational activity is designed for nurses and other health care professionals who provide telehealth care for patients. This evaluation is designed to test your achievement of the following educational activities.
1.   Define the unique legal issues that affect telehealth nurses.
2.   Review practices that can be used to manage risk.
3.   Discuss developments in licensure, laws, and practices that may affect telehealth nursing in the future.

Evaluation Form Instructions
1. To receive continuing nursing education (CNE) credit for individual study after reading the indicated chapter(s), please complete the evaluation form (photocopies of the answer form are acceptable). Attach separate paper as necessary.
2. Detach (or photocopy) and send the answer form along with a check, money order, or credit card payable to *AAACN* East Holly Avenue/Box 56, Pitman, NJ 08071-0056. You may also send this form as an email attachment to ambp401@ajj.com.
3. Answer forms must be postmarked by December 31, 2011. Upon completion of the answer/evaluation form, a certificate for 1.2 contact hours will be awarded and sent to you.

Payment Options
☐ Check or money order enclosed (payable in U.S. funds to AAACN)

☐ MasterCard ☐ VISA ☐ American Express

Credit Card #:_____

Expiration Date: _____ Security Code:_____

Card Holder (Please print):

Signature:

This educational activity has been co-provided by the American Academy of Ambulatory Care Nursing (AAACN) and Anthony J. Jannetti, Inc. (AJJ).
AAACN is a provider approved by the California Board of Registered Nursing, Provider Number CEP 5336.
AJJ is accredited as a provider of continuing nursing education by the American Nurses Credentialing Center's Commission on Accreditation.
This book was reviewed and formatted for contact hour credit by Sally S. Russell, MN, CMSRN, AAACN Education Director, and Maureen Espensen, MBA, BSN, RN, Editor.

American Academy of Ambulatory Care Nursing
East Holly Avenue/Box 56, Pitman, NJ 08071-0056
Phone: 800-AMB-NURS; Fax: 856-589-7463
Web: www.aaacn.org; Email: aaacn@ajj.com

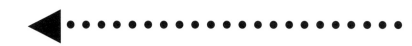

CHAPTER 7
Decision Support Tools

Objectives

1. Compare and contrast the types of decision support tools used in TNP.
2. Describe the benefits associated with the use of decision support tools.
3. Identify the essential components of decision support tools adequate for TNP.
4. Describe common challenges with using decision support tools.
5. Describe a framework that can be used to evaluate decision support tools.

Nurses rely on support tools to make sound decisions, direct their actions and complete thorough assessments of patients. Telehealth nursing is based on using decision support tools for effective and safe practice. Without decision support tools, telehealth nursing practice is undefined and unprofessional. By using clinical decision support tools, the nurse can effectively manage patients and decrease inappropriate use of health care resources by properly directing the patient to an appropriate level of care. Decision support tools provide an avenue by which nurses can use their nursing judgment to effectively guide the patient through the health care system while using standardized information. The goal of this chapter is to increase understanding of the components and benefits of using decision support tools in the practice of nursing telehealth advice.

Telehealth nursing is based on using decision support tools for effective and safe practice. Without decision support tools, telehealth nursing practice is undefined and unprofessional.

DEFINITIONS AND TYPES OF DECISION SUPPORT TOOLS

The term *decision support tool* is used to comprehensively describe guidelines, protocols, and algorithms used for making sound clinical decisions. Guidelines are more general, steering the course of action that a nurse should take. Protocols and algorithms provide more specific information than guidelines in directing nursing practice.

Guidelines

A *guideline* is defined as a line by which one is guided or an outline of policy or conduct (Merriam-Webster, 2008). A guideline for nursing practice is a vehicle that directs the nurse to individualize a plan of care to meet the needs of the patient. Guidelines provide flexibility by allowing modification of nursing practice to tailor advice to patients' needs while maintaining specific standards of care. Guidelines can be used as a framework for the interaction between the nurse and the caller. For example, the nurse utilizes

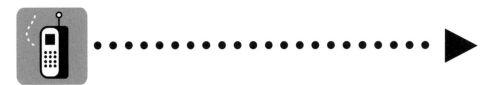

the "back pain" guideline or decision support tool while assessing a caller and determines the appropriate disposition is home care. Because the nurse is using a decision support tool, the home care advice within can be tailored to meet the needs of the patient. If the patient lives by himself and there is no one to help at home, the nurse can make the decision not to discuss the advice related to having someone massage the area of pain, even though this is part of home care advice. All other home care advice related to back pain is relayed to the patient. The nurse has stayed within the standard of care by appropriately determining the disposition by the assessment criteria, yet has made a judgment within the nursing practice portion of the guideline to best meet the patient's needs.

Well-written decision support tools should utilize the nursing process, be symptom-based, have well-defined assessment steps (including consistent disposition criteria), and contain appropriate interim care advice with both education and counseling text to support nurses during patient encounters. There is a need to establish guidelines that will hold providers and call centers accountable for providing timely access to care in an appropriate setting without compromising quality and more importantly, patient safety(American Academy of Pediatrics, 1998).

Protocols

A *protocol* is defined as "a plan for carrying out a scientific study or a patient's treatment regimen" (Merriam-Webster, 2008). Protocols are intended to be followed as written without deviation. This interpretation does not provide flexibility for the nurse to exercise nursing judgment while using protocols. If protocols are used, the process by which a nurse may deviate from a protocol should be completely stipulated by organizational policy, and the nurse must fully understand the ramifications of any deviations.

Because protocol use implies they are followed without attempting interpretation, protocols may seem to be the perfect answer for inexperienced nurses, medical assistants, or medical receptionists. However, protocols rely on the provider's ability to appropriately gather assessment data, make a determination based upon the patient's responses to the questions, and assess the patient's ability to follow the instructions given. An inexperienced nurse or unlicensed person generally lacks these critical thinking skills that are developed through experience, expertise, and education. Inexperienced nurses may follow the protocol standard without overlooking a critical aspect of care, but will lack the personalized variation and nursing judgment that comes with the interpersonal, intellectual, technical, and moral/ethical competence of the experienced nurse.

Algorithms

Merriam-Webster (2008) defines *algorithms* as "a set of rules for solving a problem in a finite number of steps, as for finding the greatest common

Well-written decision support tools should utilize the nursing process, be symptom-based, have well-defined assessment steps (including consistent disposition criteria), and contain appropriate interim care advice with both education and counseling text to support nurses during patient encounters.

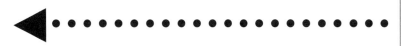

divisor." The development of an algorithm for nursing practice uses a flow chart format to put clinical questions and written decision-making processes into logical, step-by-step sequences. Along the way, decision points should be included within algorithms so that the nurse can decide upon options after receiving input from the patient.

For assessment situations that are straightforward, algorithms serve a very worthwhile purpose. For example, clinical management of children experiencing shock and/or respiratory failure is outlined utilizing algorithms in the *Pediatric Advanced Life Support (PALS) Provider Manual* (American Heart Association, 2006). The steps in the algorithm to manage a child who presents with bradycardia are logical, easy to follow, and based upon sound clinical practice. Virtually anyone can follow the steps in the algorithm. However, effective use of the algorithm assumes that the user initially has made the correct assessment of bradycardia and then knows when to stop the algorithm.

Like protocols, algorithms are used effectively in certain clinical situations. However, within telehealth nursing practice, they are of limited use because the nurse does not have the flexibility to customize the flow chart elements to the needs of a specific patient.

BENEFITS OF DECISION SUPPORT TOOLS

Standardization

Decision support tools provide structure for nursing telehealth assessment and advice by insuring consistency, accuracy, completeness, and quality of practice regardless of individual nurses' backgrounds, education, and experiences (American Academy of Ambulatory Care Nursing [AAACN], 2007). This benefit lends credibility to the practice because the patient receives the same disposition and similar advice regardless of which nurse answers the call.

Decision Support

Using decision support tools results in more appropriate triage decisions by providing decision support because guidelines assist the nurse in analyzing and classifying symptoms. Decision support tools make decision-making choices easier by assisting in organizing large amounts of significant information and helping to show the interrelationship of data. Decision support tool use improves the efficiency of the nurse because not only decisions are easier, but also because the nurse saves time by not having to consult with a provider since most encounters will fall within parameters of the written guidelines. Decision support tools are not intended to be used by the inexperienced or untrained nurse. Instead, they are a tool for the skilled, experienced nurse who must employ critical thinking skills as well as nursing judgment. Nursing judgment is largely based on thinking, reasoning, and

Like protocols, algorithms are used effectively in certain clinical situations. However, within telehealth nursing practice, they are of limited use because the nurse does not have the flexibility to customize the flow chart elements to the needs of a specific patient.

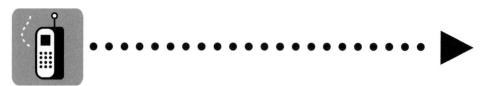

experience that differentiates the expert nurse from the less experienced nurse. Due to their experiential background, expert nurses can utilize nursing judgment to quickly and efficiently identify root problems instead of focusing on unnecessary considerations. Nurses at different levels of expertise utilize expert systems, like decision support tools, for different aspects of decision-making. For instance, a novice nurse may utilize a decision support tool as a knowledge base to formulate decisions while the expert nurse utilizes the knowledge base primarily to consider alternatives.

Although a nurse may be extremely familiar with a particular symptom-based guideline to use while assessing a patient, the guideline should be opened, visualized, and followed with each applicable call. The open guideline serves as a continual reminder of important facets of care that should be considered and evaluated. Working from an opened guideline helps the nurse stay focused even if physically or emotionally fatigued.

Occasionally, the nurse may decide to override the disposition indicated by a decision support tool due to the needs expressed by the patient or family. The nurse may recommend a more acute disposition than recommended by the guideline. This should be done with caution, and organizational policy should define how and when an override should occur. If a disposition is over-ridden, thorough documentation of the situation must be completed. At times, a nurse may disagree with the care recommendation and may want to recommend a lesser care disposition for the patient. The nurse should never downgrade a patient's disposition unless approved by the provider.

A guiding principle of nursing telehealth assessment and advice is that when in doubt, "err on the side of caution" for the patient. Nurses should utilize the strength of decision support tools and providers if unsure of the most appropriate patient disposition.

Using decision support tools including guidelines, protocols, and algorithms is not "cook book" medicine. Nurses providing telehealth assessment and advice should focus on the *three Rs*: the *right* care, with the *right* provider, at the *right* time. By focusing on the *three Rs,* all other benefits of TNP will naturally follow, such as quality patient care, satisfied customers, and cost benefits for the organization and the caller.

Legal Protection

Decision support tools offer some legal protection to nurses. Effective risk management is enhanced by the presence of well-defined standards and their consistent application. The standard of practice for telehealth nurses is the same as for any RN practicing in any other setting. As stated in the AAACN *Telehealth Nursing Practice Standards* (2007), telehealth nursing practice must be consistent with recognized professional standards of nursing and must comply with standards mandated by regulatory agencies. In an effort to perform a comprehensive encounter, telehealth practice nurses should ensure that each of the following components is addressed.

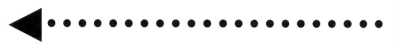

❖ Collection of appropriate, complete data from the patient.
❖ Appropriate assessment of the situation/problem.
❖ Appropriate decision support tool(s) selection.
❖ Adherence to organization-approved telehealth practice policies and standards of practice.
❖ Verification that the patient understands the advice/information, and the ability of the patient to comply with the advice.
❖ Complete and accurate documentation of the telehealth interaction.

In order to provide legal protection for nurses, the written decision support tool must reflect the *standard of practice*. An organization should select decision support tools after ensuring that they are evidenced-based and written by a collaborative team of nurses and physicians. Once decision support tools are selected for use by an organization, it is a requirement by regulatory bodies (such as The Joint Commission) that the decision support tools be reviewed and revised on a regular basis. Many organizations have annual reviews and updates. This review includes approval by both nursing and medical leadership who have responsibility for supervising and managing the telehealth practice nurses.

An organization should select decision support tools after ensuring that they are evidenced-based and written by a collaborative team of nurses and physicians.

Documentation Ease

Most organizations providing telehealth nursing organize documentation formats similar to the flow of their guidelines. This enables the nurse to easily document the telephone encounter while collecting data and providing the intervention.

COMPONENTS OF DECISION SUPPORT TOOLS

According to AAACN (2007), the components of decision support tools should define the ongoing care or management of a broad problem or issue in six areas:

❖ Assessment/data collection/caller interview process.
❖ Classification/determination of acuity.
❖ Nature/type/degree of advice/intervention/direction to the caller.
❖ Information/education of caller.
❖ Validation of patient understanding/verbal contracting.
❖ Evaluation/follow-up/effectiveness of advice or intervention.

These six areas encompass the nursing process essential to TNP. If any of these components are missing from the decision support tools, the nursing process is incomplete, thereby possibly allowing a potential gap in the quality of care. Many decision support tools do not specifically include the steps to

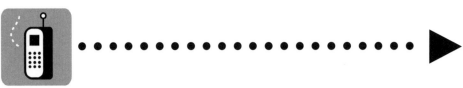

validate the patient's understanding or to evaluate the follow-up/effectiveness of advice or intervention given. Validation is an important part of the nursing process and should be part of the telehealth encounter.

No matter how decision support tools are defined, they serve as an essential tool in TNP. Well-written guidelines provide standardization, decision support, legal protection, and documentation ease to the nurse.

> **No matter how decision support tools are defined, they serve as an essential tool in TNP. Well-written guidelines provide standardization, decision support, legal protection, and documentation ease to the nurse.**

Essential Components

Essential components of decision support tools should:

❖ **Follow a logical thought process.** Good decision support tools are written so that nurses can competently and safely provide appropriate care, even without expertise in a particular field. A user-friendly format that is orderly and enables the nurse to elicit information by asking open-ended questions is beneficial to obtain information from the patient.

❖ **Trigger assessment questions.** Whatever type of decision support tool the organization is using (algorithm, protocol, or clinical guidelines), the tool should include assessment questions. Assessment questions should rule out emergent symptoms first and then move to less serious symptoms. It is important that assessment questions are asked in lay language. Communication with a general audience in the United States should be at a 6th-8th grade reading level (Association of Medical Directors of Information Systems and The Improve-IT Institute, 2008). There is a risk of collecting incorrect data if medical terminology or jargon is used, because patients may not understand the questions and may not request clarification.

❖ **Classify or determine acuity.** Acuity is usually determined within decision support tools by defining a period for receiving care and appropriate place for care. For example, for a patient who calls with symptoms of possible dehydration, the acuity level is determined to be *emergent.* The options for receiving emergent care may be referral to the emergency room, the primary care site, or the *urgent care* site. There are also situations requiring additional care, such as from Poison Control or a Rape Crisis Center.

❖ **Demonstrate consistency** for symptom definition and symptom disposition whenever possible. For example, the disposition for *severe difficulty breathing* should be "call 911 now" in all guidelines where severe difficulty breathing is assessed. The disposition for respiratory arrest should not be different in the *Asthma* guideline than it is in the *Chest Pain* guideline. Additionally, symptoms of dehydration should not be defined differently in the *Diarrhea* guideline than it is in the *Vomiting* guideline. This consistency of dispositions will only occur if the decision support tools dispositions

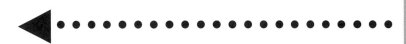

are concretely defined and consistently applied. For example, a patient calls at 4:55 PM and the office is scheduled to close at 5:00 PM. Does consistency require the office remain open for the patient to come in, or can the patient be seen early the next morning? If there is a clear definition of the disposition *same day care,* which means an appointment within 2-18 hours, the nurse can utilize nursing judgment on the appropriateness of having the patient come in early in the morning or having the patient go to an urgent care site or emergency room.

❖ **Identify high-risk patients or concerns.** High-risk patients or concerns should be included in the guidelines. For example, elderly, diabetic, immunosuppresed, recent surgical patients, or cardiac patients are at a much higher risk for serious complications from a wound or a fever than a healthy adult.

❖ **Include appropriate and accurate information and education for patients.** Nurses should provide information and education to patients during most telehealth encounters. The information may be explaining to the patient why a provider appointment is necessary. It may be giving interim care advice. Whatever information or education is given to the patient, it is essential that it be given in terms understood by the caller. It is also important for home care advice to be safe and practical. Lastly, it is crucial to verify that the information relayed to the caller/patient is understood.

Nurses should provide information and education to patients during most telehealth encounters.

❖ **Describe criteria to help patients evaluate their symptoms.** Evaluation of a patient's condition differs when giving nursing telehealth advice rather than "hands-on" patient care. When the patient is available for face-to-face patient care, the nurse can perform an objective and subjective assessment. Via the telehealth device, the nurse is limited by the patient's clues. Hence, there is a need to educate patients on how to evaluate the problem themselves. For example, when nurses evaluate post-surgical wounds in the hospital setting, the wound can be visualized for redness, odor, heat, and healing progress. Via the telephone, nurses must teach patients how to evaluate their own wounds with appropriate assessment questions in the decision support tool.

❖ **Prompt the nurse to use disclaimers.** A common disclaimer is, "If anything new develops, if anything gets worse, or if you are increasingly concerned for any reason, either call us back or proceed immediately to an ER or seek urgent care." Other common disclaimers are warnings about medicine usage with certain medical conditions or increasing fluid intake with certain medical conditions. Some telehealth services close the encounter with a statement such as, "This telehealth information was provided free of charge and does not replace your health care provider's advice. Contact your provider to discuss your personal medical condition." The telehealth nurse should be aware of and follow all disclaimers required by the organization.

❖ **Prompt the nurse when patient evaluation or follow-up is necessary.** The purpose of patient follow-up is:
  o To avoid potential serious outcomes.
  o Customer service.
  o Evaluation for the nurse giving the advice or directing the intervention.

If the tool does not specify the circumstances requiring follow-up, the organizational policy should define when follow-up is necessary. For example, follow-up may be required for all high-risk patients (those with diabetes, who are immunosuppressed, or who are HIV positive), infants less than a certain age, or elderly patients. Some organizations require 100% follow-up on all symptom-based calls, and others require follow-up only on specific dispositions or symptoms.

ADDITIONAL HELPFUL COMPONENTS OF DECISION SUPPORT TOOLS

Potential Medical Diagnosis

Although most decision support tools are symptom-based, some display potential medical diagnoses for particular symptoms. The purpose is not to have the nurse make a medical diagnosis, but to alert the nurse to potential outcomes. It is important not to disclose the possible medical diagnosis to the caller, but rather to be cognizant of the potential diagnosis. By being aware of the potential diagnosis, it may assist the nurse with additional assessment questions.

Resources

Community, regional, and national resource numbers should be readily available to the nurse. Whether this is part of the guideline book or a separate list, the nurse must have access to crisis line telephone numbers, self-help groups' telephone numbers, community resources, and additional educational materials for specific disease (see Chapter 12, "Clinical Knowledge – Special Situations").

Patients frequently ask for additional information not included in the guidelines. Each organization must identify the approved resources to assist the nurse with these questions.

Patients frequently ask for additional information not included in the guidelines. Each organization must identify the approved resources to assist the nurse with these questions. Perhaps the organization uses specific reference books or employs an audio library with textbook-type discussion about medical topics such as chicken pox, multiple sclerosis, eczema, etc. Frequently, pertinent written information is also mailed to the patient. When providing information to the caller from an approved resource, it is advisable to cite the source being used both verbally to the patient and in the written record. This practice provides credibility and ensures accuracy.

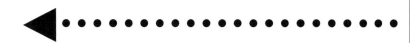

SELECTION OF DECISION SUPPORT TOOLS

The nursing process is the backbone of TNP. Every step of the nursing process is brought into play when determining the appropriate tool (guideline, protocol, algorithm) to select. Evaluation, the last step of the nursing process, is continually being utilized for every step of the process. There are a number of challenges that make choosing the right decision support tools difficult.

Multiple Symptoms or Complaints

Patients frequently contact the nurse with multiple symptom complaints, making it difficult for the nurse to know which guideline to use. The nurse must first always rule out emergent criteria. If a patient complains of emergent symptoms such as respiratory distress, cardiac symptoms, or a recent change in mental status, then the nurse should first use the most acute tool. When using the tool, the symptom with the most serious potential outcome is selected first, and then a disposition is determined by using further decision points in the tool. For example, a patient contacts the nurse complaining of chest pain. Due to the potential emergent nature of that symptom, the nurse initially uses the guideline that screens for myocardial infarct. If upon further assessment, the patient states his chest only hurts with coughing and the cough has been present for several days, the guideline selection then changes. The next decision support tool may be *cough and/or chest congestion*.

The nurse must first always rule out emergent criteria. If a patient complains of emergent symptoms such as respiratory distress, cardiac symptoms, or a recent change in mental status, then the nurse should first use the most acute tool.

If the patient is not complaining of an obvious emergent symptom, the nurse determines the chief complaint from the collected data. If the nurse has difficulty determining the chief complaint, it may be helpful to ask the patient, "What symptom is causing you the most concern today?" Even after a chief complaint has been identified, it is not uncommon for nurses to work with two or three tools at the same time. Frequently, the nurse discovers another, more serious patient symptom as the assessment data is collected. For example, a patient complains of a pulled muscle in his left arm. As the nurse questions the patient more thoroughly, the patient discloses the pain began while mowing the lawn and mentions some vague pain in the sternal area. At this point, the nurse would immediately use the *chest pain* guideline. If the nurse determines a more critical symptom than the one currently being assessed, it is imperative to switch to the more appropriate decision support tool. When utilizing more than one guideline, the nurse considers the guideline with the safest and most effective care for the patient. The guiding rule is to "err on the side of caution" in favor of the patient.

The Patient Is a Poor Historian

Appropriate decision support tools selection may also be difficult if the patient is a poor historian. For example, the patient is unable to describe the location of the pain or adequately quantify the pain. Another example would

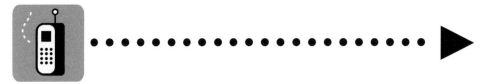

be if a child or an older adult calls for assistance. People who may be poor historians are:

- ❖ Alzheimer's or dementia patients.
- ❖ Head-injured or mentally handicapped patients.
- ❖ Patients with a language or communication barrier.
- ❖ Patients seeking drugs (narcotics).
- ❖ Frequent callers who just seem to be lonely most of the time.
- ❖ Patients embarrassed by their problem (such as contracting a sexually transmitted disease).

Having access to the patient's medical records is extremely helpful in many of these situations. If medical records are not accessible, the nurse may need to consult with the patient's primary care provider. For some of the above situations, the nurse may need to request contact with a spouse, daughter/son, or caretaker while being compliant to HIPAA. If the nurse is unable to collect adequate data via the telehealth device and the situation is not urgent or emergent, the patient should be given the option of making an appointment with the primary care provider.

If the nurse is unable to collect adequate data via the telehealth device and the situation is not urgent or emergent, the patient should be given the option of making an appointment with the primary care provider.

Patients with a Complex History

Chronically ill patients or patients with multi-system problems frequently have complex histories. Again, having access to the patient's medical records or the patient's primary care provider is very helpful. An adequate assessment cannot be completed without knowing the patient's past medical history, current medications, and allergies to medications.

Symptoms Are Not Described In a Decision Support Tool

Organizational policy should direct the nurse's action if a patient has a symptom or complaint for which there is no decision support tool. The policy should dictate the appropriate action for the nurse to take. There are usually three choices:

1. Instruct the patient to come in for a provider appointment.
2. Collaborate with a provider in determining next steps.
3. Instruct the patient to re-contact the nurse if any new or worse symptoms develop.

For example, an elderly man calls complaining, "I'm just not feeling well today." The nurse rules out any possibility of emergent/urgent symptoms. The man cannot describe any specific symptoms other than that he "just does not feel well today." There is no tool named *Just Does Not Feel Well*. At this point, the nurse would most likely instruct the patient to make an appointment with his provider in the next 24 hours, adding the caution to call

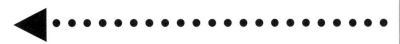

the nurse back at any time. Some decision support tools have a designated "no listed guideline" tool that is selected when none of the guidelines are suitable.

The Insistent Patient

Organizational policy should determine what process a nurse should follow when home care advice is adequate and the patient still insists on a provider appointment. Most organizations will support the nurse in allowing the patient to be seen by a provider. This decision is due to medical legal risk as well as the desire to provide excellent patient care and customer service. A "patient first" philosophy is often the mission of many organizations. Customer service experts know that one dissatisfied customer can influence a number of friends, family members, neighbors, and co-workers to not use an organization's services. Hopefully when the patient is seen, the provider will take the time to educate the patient about the benefits of TNP.

DECISON SUPPORT TOOL EVALUATION AND REVIEW

Purpose of Review

Although the process of evaluating decision support tools can be a long and tedious process, it is essential for maintaining quality of the tools used in practice. The purpose of the review is to ensure the timeliness of the information contained within the guidelines and to reflect changes in practice. Trends in practice and changes in medical and nursing standards, such as national disease-specific practice guidelines, influence the delivery of health care and the necessity to review the decision support tools. Additionally, whether the decision support tools were written by the nurse's organization or were purchased, the review process must verify the guidelines are pertinent and specific to the organization. Considerations before starting the review include:

- ❖ Identifying the appropriate personnel to review the tools.
- ❖ Assessing how frequently the specific tool is used.
- ❖ Identifying how often the tools should be reviewed.
- ❖ Analyzing which aspects of the tool to review.

Although the process of evaluating decision support tools can be a long and tedious process, it is essential for maintaining quality of the tools used in practice. The purpose of the review is to ensure the timeliness of the information contained within the guidelines and to reflect changes in practice.

Identifying Reviewers

Nurses and providers who use the decision support tools should not only be familiar with the decision support tools content, but are also responsible in verifying the content meets practice standards and is within the philosophy of the organization. Therefore the ownership of the decision support tools' review belongs to the users: the nurses and providers.

For the review to be accurate, both input from providers and nurses is required. Generally nurses should review all decision support tools and

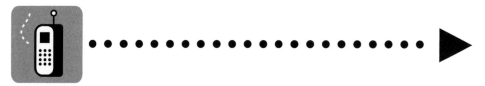

providers should review the decision support tools that encompass their area of practice.

Sub-specialists should review the decision support tools specific for the specialty. For instance, cardiologists should review the decision support tools related to chest pain and emergency providers should review the decision support tools related to trauma and injuries. This lends much more credibility to the decision support tools and helps ensure consistency of practice.

After the nurses and providers have made their changes, the appropriate administrative forum must approve the decision support tools for medical and nursing staff. This may be the medical practice board, nursing senior leaders, medical and nursing directors of a call center, or other leadership forums within an organization. Administration is ultimately held responsible for the entire process of TNP and must be an integral part of the review and approval process.

Frequency

In considering how frequently decision support tools should be reviewed, there are many constraints imposed upon organizations that influence the period for review of policies and decision support tools. At the very least, standards by national accreditation bodies (such as The Joint Commission and the National Committee for Quality Assurance [NCQA]) that govern the organizations using the decision support tools set the minimum standard for review. Often these accreditation bodies leave the time frame for review up to the organization. Most organizations adopt a yearly time frame. This assures that information remains current and applicable to the population served. When changes are suggested or needed, a current, documented reference (within the last five years is preferred) is essential to ensure that evidence-based information is included.

The most frequently used decision support tools should undergo a stringent review process, both formally by being examined yearly and informally by virtue of their daily use.

The most frequently used decision support tools should undergo a stringent review process, both formally by being examined yearly and informally by virtue of their daily use. When each nurse on the service accesses the *pediatric fever* decision support tool six times a day, both positive and negative issues related to that tool become clearer. Most other decision support tools will not need such a stringent review within the one-year time period. These include the decision support tools that focus on developmental issues (thumb sucking, toilet training, etc.) instead of symptoms, and those at low-risk and are rarely used. If new information is published, or if there are issues related to the decision support tool, changes may need to be made more frequently.

Any information related to support groups and resources given to the patient must be updated at least yearly. Because this information changes frequently, it is crucial to verify support groups, phone numbers, and resources.

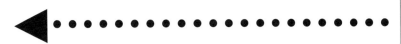

Aspects to Review

A thorough review should encompass all aspects of the decision support tool. Areas of alerts, red flags, and at-risk populations are just as crucial to evaluate as the emergent and urgent care criteria. The *interim care advice* section of the decision support tool may be the most time-consuming portion to review. This section may include proven remedies easily managed by the patient and should reflect current and accepted trends in health care. With the enormous amount of medical information readily accessible via many avenues, most patients insist upon and should receive the latest information available. The organization should consider including information on alternative medicine therapies and homeopathic remedies in the *interim care* or *home care* section.

QUALITY ASSURANCE AND IMPROVEMENT

Although the review process helps ensure content quality, it does not assure that the tools are being used appropriately and/or consistently. Having a mechanism in place to analyze that the nurses are selecting the appropriate decision support tool, that the presenting symptoms match the decision support tool that directs the disposition, and that the assessment triggers are up-to-date helps address this concern. For instance, a *quality assurance and improvement* (QA&I) audit may indicate that all patients presenting with a cough and a fever are referred for same-day appointments with their provider. The review team decides this is an inappropriate disposition for **all** patients with coughs and fevers, and only appropriate for some patients with coughs and fever. The recommendation goes to the decision support tool review team to add additional criteria to the tool for clarity. The team may decide to add criteria of fever of 100.5° for 3 days accompanied by a productive cough with brown sputum, which more clearly identifies the patients to be seen the same-day.

A well-coordinated and thoughtful QA&I process significantly affects the organization's care delivery system and should be an integral part of TNP. Ongoing quality assurance and quality improvement are one part of safe patient care; they assist in determining if the nurses are following the pre-determined process, and if the telehealth practice is beneficial to the organization.

Having a mechanism in place to analyze that the nurses are selecting the appropriate decision support tool, that the presenting symptoms match the decision support tool that directs the disposition, and that the assessment triggers are up-to-date helps address concern.

SUMMARY

Decision support tool use does not need be labor intensive, but should outline the information the nurse must obtain from the patient to dispense meaningful, safe advice (Wilkinson, Przestrzelski, & Duff, 2000). Decision support tools are to be used in conjunction with the nurse's experience and judgment. Appropriate decision support tool selection is essential to the

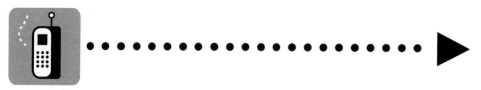

Appropriate decision support tool selection is essential to the success of nursing telehealth assessment and advice service. No matter how expert the nurses are that are employed by the service, they cannot make up for poorly written or developed decision support tools.

success of nursing telehealth assessment and advice service. No matter how expert the nurses are that are employed by the service, they cannot make up for poorly written or developed decision support tools. On the other hand, decision support tools are only as good as the nurses' abilities to use them. Nurses who have poor communication skills should not be employed in telehealth nursing practice, even with excellent decision support tools available for their use. Decision support tools adherence is basic to TNP and should be stressed in training and quality review.

TIPS & PEARLS

☎ Thorough education and preceptorship are a requirement for appropriate decision support tools usage. In-depth, working knowledge of the decision support tools' content is essential for expert practice.

☎ Decision support tools should be consistently reviewed and updated within an appropriate time by all appropriate parties, such as nurses who use the decision support tools, providers, and administrators.

☎ Decision support tools should always be referred to and followed, no matter how familiar the nurse is with the symptom or the decision support tool.

References

American Academy of Ambulatory Care Nursing (AAACN). (2007). *Telehealth nursing practice administration and practice standards* (4th ed.). Pitman, NJ: Author.

American Academy of Pediatrics. (1998). *Telehealth care.* Retrieved June 24, 2008, from http://www.aap.org/sections/telecare

American Heart Association. (2006). *Pediatric advanced life support (PALS) provider manual.* Retrieved on March 6, 2008, from http://www.americanheart.org

Association of Medical Directors of Information Systems and The Improve-IT Institute. (2008). *Informatics review* [e-journal]. Retrieved February 12, 2009, from http://www.informatics-review.com/

Merriam-Webster. (2008). *Merriam-Webster online dictionary.* Retrieved February 26, 2008, from http://www.merriam-webster.com/dictionary

Wilkinson, C., Przestrzelski, D., & Duff, I. (2000). Competency-based telephone triage curriculum. *Lippincott's Case Management: Managing the Process of Patient Care, 5*(4), 141-147.

Answer/Evaluation Form
Continuing Nursing Education Activity
Telehealth Nursing Practice Essentials
Chapter 7: Decision Support Tools

AMBP9c05

This activity provides 1.1 contact hours of continuing nursing education (CNE) credit in nursing.
(Contact hours calculated using a 60-minute contact hour.)

This test may be copied for use by others.

COMPLETE THE FOLLOWING:

Name: _____

Address: _____

City: _____ State: _____ Zip: _____

Telephone number: (Home)_____ (Work)_____

Email address:_____

AAACN Member Number and Expiration Date: _____

Processing fee: AAACN Member: $12.00
  Nonmember: $20.00

Answer Form: (Please attach a separate sheet of paper if necessary.)
1. What did you value most about this activity?

_____
_____
_____

2. If you could imagine that you have fully integrated your learning into practice, what would be different about your present practice?

_____
_____
_____

Evaluation	Strongly disagree				Strongly agree
3. The offering met the stated objectives.					
a. Compare and contrast the types of decision support tools used in TNP.	1	2	3	4	5
b. Describe the benefits associated with the use of decision support tools.	1	2	3	4	5
c. Identify the essential components of decision support tools adequate for TNP.	1	2	3	4	5
d. Describe common challenges with using decision support tools.	1	2	3	4	5
e. Describe a framework that can be used to evaluate decision support tools.	1	2	3	4	5
4. The content was current and relevant.	1	2	3	4	5
5. The content was presented clearly.	1	2	3	4	5
6. The content was covered adequately.	1	2	3	4	5

7. How would you rate your ability to apply your learning to practice following this activity? (Check one)
☐ Diminished ability ☐ No change ☐ Enhanced ability

8. Time required to complete reading assignment and answer form: ___ minutes
Comments _____

I verify that I have completed this activity:

_____
Signature

Objectives
This educational activity is designed for nurses and other health care professionals who provide telehealth care for patients. This evaluation is designed to test your achievement of the following educational activities.
1. Compare and contrast the types of decision support tools used in TNP.
2. Describe the benefits associated with the use of decision support tools.
3. Identify the essential components of decision support tools adequate for TNP.
4. Describe common challenges with using decision support tools.
5. Describe a framework that can be used to evaluate decision support tools.

Evaluation Form Instructions
1. To receive continuing nursing education (CNE) credit for individual study after reading the indicated chapter(s), please complete the evaluation form (photocopies of the answer form are acceptable). Attach separate paper as necessary.
2. Detach (or photocopy) and send the answer form along with a check, money order, or credit card payable to *AAACN* East Holly Avenue/Box 56, Pitman, NJ 08071-0056. You may also send this form as an email attachment to ambp401@ajj.com.
3. Answer forms must be postmarked by December 31, 2011. Upon completion of the answer/evaluation form, a certificate for 1.1 contact hours will be awarded and sent to you.

Payment Options
☐ Check or money order enclosed (payable in U.S. funds to AAACN)

☐ MasterCard ☐ VISA ☐ American Express

Credit Card #:_____

Expiration Date: _____ Security Code:_____

Card Holder (Please print):

Signature:

This educational activity has been co-provided by the American Academy of Ambulatory Care Nursing (AAACN) and Anthony J. Jannetti, Inc. (AJJ).
AAACN is a provider approved by the California Board of Registered Nursing, Provider Number CEP 5336.
AJJ is accredited as a provider of continuing nursing education by the American Nurses Credentialing Center's Commission on Accreditation.
This book was reviewed and formatted for contact hour credit by Sally S. Russell, MN, CMSRN, AAACN Education Director, and Maureen Espensen, MBA, BSN, RN, Editor.

American Academy of Ambulatory Care Nursing
East Holly Avenue/Box 56, Pitman, NJ 08071-0056
Phone: 800-AMB-NURS; Fax: 856-589-7463
Web: www.aaacn.org; Email: aaacn@ajj.com

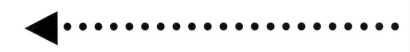

CHAPTER 8
Documentation of Telehealth Encounters

Objectives

1. Describe five reasons why documentation of telehealth encounters is essential to telehealth nursing practice.
2. Summarize the essential components of effective telehealth documentation.
3. Compare and contrast the various types of documentation tools and charting methods available for documenting various types of telehealth encounters.
4. Summarize procedures to maintain confidentiality of telehealth documentation.
5. Explain the effect of technology on telehealth documentation.

The practice of professional nursing includes communicating with the patient, family, and health care team through verbal and written interactions. Because of this, documentation is an integral part of delivering nursing care, and the documentation of telephone encounters is no exception. Good documentation describes the nursing process of assessment, nursing diagnosis and planning, implementing, and evaluating patient care.

Documentation of the telehealth encounter includes gathering data, analyzing the information through critical thinking skills, defining the plan of care, and translating this information into a permanent format as a summary of communications between the nurse and patient. Although these short verbal interactions may last only an average of 5-6 minutes, documentation provides evidence that the encounter has occurred. Documenting telephone encounters follows the same guiding principles as medical record documentation and is necessary to:

❖ Decrease legal risks.
❖ Demonstrate use of the nursing process.
❖ Demonstrate standards of care.
❖ Demonstrate quality and identify quality issues.
❖ Demonstrate the plan of care.

PURPOSE OF DOCUMENTATION

Decrease Legal Risks
A nurse may handle hundreds (and sometimes thousands) of telehealth encounters each year. In contrast, a patient may only have an encounter

> *Documentation of the telehealth encounter includes gathering data, analyzing the information through critical thinking skills, defining the plan of care, and translating this information into a permanent format as a summary of communications between the nurse and patient.*

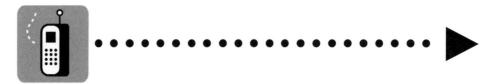

once or twice a year. As time passes, the patient is likely to be able to remember his/her one encounter compared to one of many by the nurse. In a court of law, a patient will certainly describe their encounter details more readily than the nurse. The patient's medical record has become the determining factor in 80-85% of all malpractice lawsuits involving patient care (Iyer & Camp, 2005).

Documentation of encounters can help protect the nurse from legal liability. Although a nurse may be an expert with assessment and communication skills, without thorough documentation, the nurse is not going to be able to protect herself/himself as well in a court of law.

As with other health care environments, the quality and completeness of the telehealth documentation is crucial when a malpractice claim goes to litigation. Concise and specific information that is neat, comprehensive, and understandable helps prevent misconstruing the meaning of a note. By applying principles and standards regarding what to document and basic guidelines on how to effectively document, the nurse increases the chance of defending professional judgment and actions if called upon in a court of law.

All telehealth practice settings should develop specific policies outlining telehealth documentation standards. Effective risk management is enhanced when these standards become a part of the nurse's core competencies for telehealth nursing practice. Whereas complete documentation of the telehealth encounter can be an effective defense for the nurse accused of negligence or malpractice, incomplete telehealth documentation increases the risk for malpractice. At the same time, too much documentation does not necessarily protect the nurse from legal action because it is the quality of documentation that determines its effectiveness, not the quantity.

Demonstrate the Use of the Nursing Process

Documentation should reflect that the nurse has applied the nursing process while handling an encounter. Documentation should include:

- ❖ **Assessment**
  - o Reason for the encounter or patient's chief complaint.
  - o History of symptoms and associated symptoms.
  - o Allergies and past medical history.
  - o Nurse's assessment.
- ❖ **Plan**
  - o Decision support tools used and triaged category.
  - o Recommendations for further care or disposition of the patient based on acuity (e.g., see provider, go to a walk-in clinic, need for teaching).

> *Documentation of encounters can help protect the nurse from legal liability. Although a nurse may be an expert with assessment and communication skills, without thorough documentation, the nurse is not going to be able to protect herself/himself as well in a court of law.*

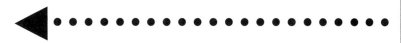

❖ **Intervention**
  ○ Nurse's intervention (e.g., transferred call to 911, set up an appointment).
  ○ Details about the information and education provided.
❖ **Evaluation**
  ○ Patient's acceptance and understanding of plan of care.
  ○ Follow-up actions and plans of nurse and patient.

Demonstrate Standards of Care

The primary focus of each encounter is to provide care of a consistently high standard. Standards of care that should be verified within the documentation include: assessment of symptoms, evaluation of the seriousness of those symptoms, determination of the appropriate triage level, and provision of health education. Documentation should reflect that the nurse is providing nursing care and making a nursing diagnosis, but is NOT providing a medical diagnosis.

The nurse should commit to using written decision support tools for assessing and triaging patients. By documenting that a decision support tool was used, the nurse validates that standards were followed and that information was not given "off the top of the head." Testimony that a decision support tool was used is insufficient evidence without the supporting documentation to prove that a reference was used for clinical decision-making.

Numerous organizations, including the American Academy of Ambulatory Care Nurses (AAACN) (2007), have written telehealth nursing practice standards. These standards should be reviewed on a regular basis and when new documentation procedures are implemented. Additionally, it is extremely important for the nurse to follow his/her employer's administrative and departmental policies. Nurses are responsible for knowing policies on appropriate documentation as well as the acceptable abbreviations and formats for documentation.

The Joint Commission for Accreditation of Healthcare Organizations (JCAHO) developed general standards on patient education and assessment. These standards need to be applied in the telehealth nursing practice setting. The standards state that patient education must be provided and documented (JCAHO, 2007). The Joint Commission also requires that all patients be assessed and that this assessment must be documented. In other words, when a patient makes a contact for general health information (such as, "How do I read a thermometer?"), the nurse should assess for symptoms and document the presence or absence of symptoms. In addition to The Joint Commission, the National Committee for Quality Assurance (NCQA) has defined documentation standards for the accreditation of health plan organizations as well as their affiliated providers for health care (NCQA, 2006).

Standards of care that should be verified within the documentation include: assessment of symptoms, evaluation of the seriousness of those symptoms, determination of the appropriate triage level, and provision of health education.

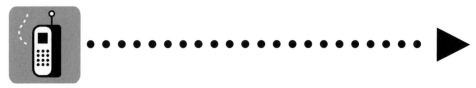

Demonstrate Quality and Analyze Quality Issues

Documentation can provide valuable information about the types of encounters (symptoms, referrals, lab results, prescription refills, patient education, and follow-up) handled in the telehealth setting.

Documentation can provide valuable information about the types of encounters (symptoms, referrals, lab results, prescription refills, patient education, and follow-up) handled in the telehealth setting. Documentation is one component of demonstrating quality practice and can also be used for analyzing quality issues. Documentation will provide information to the telehealth provider to aid in identifying why their population is making contact. By reviewing these encounters, improvements can be made in continuity, quality of care, and risk management issues. Additionally, the nursing staff can identify patient issues such as:

❖ Frequently occurring encounters, such as bee stings and chickenpox.
❖ Repetitive encounters, such as medication refills.
❖ At-risk encounters, such as pregnant patients experiencing possible labor.
❖ Clarifying encounters, such as the need for more instructions after being seen in the office.
❖ Educational encounters, such as requests for medication information.

Once encounters are analyzed and problems identified, an action plan to make quality improvements can be developed to improve services. For example, a practice setting with a high volume of medication requests and refills might decrease encounter volume by implementing proactive procedures to refill the medications during the office visit instead of later.

Documentation can be used to monitor the thoroughness of assessments and appropriateness of the disposition and plan of care. Quality measurements can analyze whether:

❖ Enough pertinent information was obtained.
❖ The appropriate decision support tool was used.
❖ The patient was triaged at the appropriate disposition level.

Documentation provides information on the volume and time distribution of encounters. This can help management to identify staffing requirements for peak hours and days. Additionally, analysis of the number of various types of telehealth encounters, assessments, consultations, and follow-ups can identify the staffing mix needed to handle these encounters.

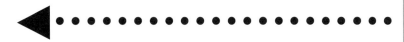

Demonstrate the Plan of Care

In addition to being used by health care providers, the nurse's documentation is used by the legal profession and regulatory agencies. The health care team uses the documentation as a comprehensive, ongoing record of the patient's episodic health care concerns. Care can be fragmented and duplicated, and excessive resources may be used unless there is a clear documentation and understanding of each encounter. A complete, well-documented record is essential to comprehensive, coordinated care.

Documentation provides a record that validates the need for a specific level of care or referral to health care services. Because most insurance companies cover the cost of care based upon the need for that care, documentation must demonstrate the need for care. The documentation must show that the patient was adequately assessed, referred to the most appropriate level of service, and in the most appropriate time frame. Using decision support tools with supporting documentation can prove that patients are being effectively managed. Telehealth nursing practice enables patients to manage their health care needs by safely guiding them to care and services compatible with their actual acuity and concerns. Telehealth may save the patient money and contribute to the overall lowering of health care costs.

Telehealth nursing practice enables patients to manage their health care needs by safely guiding them to care and services compatible with their actual acuity and concerns. Telehealth may save the patient money and contribute to the overall lowering of health care costs.

ESSENTIAL COMPONENTS OF TELEHEATLH DOCUMENTATION

Documentation Guidelines

Because documentation of the telehealth encounter becomes a permanent part of the patient's medical record, there are basic guidelines that should always be followed. These include:

- ❖ *Document each encounter.* Each time there is a point of contact between the nurse and the caller, that contact needs to be documented. The date and time of the contact should be recorded on the documentation tool. Follow-up encounters may occur on different dates but can be recorded on the same documentation form.
- ❖ *Document at the time of the encounter.* If documentation is delayed, the nurse may not accurately recall what was said. Documentation should be completed during or immediately after the encounter, before moving to next encounter. This prevents "mix-ups" by being able to clearly document the specifics about the current encounter before moving to the next one.
- ❖ *Focus on the facts.* A clear picture of the patient's situation can only be obtained through precise documentation of the patient's responses to assessment questions along with the nurse's

disposition, consultation, and/or follow-up. The nurse should avoid documentation language that implies assumptions, blames, is ambiguous, or is too generalized unless the language is a direct quote from the patient. Judgmental or opinionated words such as "appears," "seems to," and "sounds like" should also be avoided.

Documentation should reflect that collaborative communication took place. The nurse should use words such as "discussed" instead of "told to do." It is also important to document if the patient understood the information and if they agreed to the treatment recommendations.

During the encounter, the nurse should substantiate vague information with facts by using clarification techniques. "What do you mean when you say that your son is lethargic? Describe his behavior." Open-ended questions are the best. If the patient cannot explain what they mean, the generalization should be quoted.

It is particularly crucial to document by quotes if the patient threatens to sue, cause harm, or uses abusive language. The nurse should also document if a patient is planning to be non-compliant with the nurse's recommendations. To avoid an assumption of non-compliance, document the patient's stated reasons for his/her non-compliant behavior. The nurse's rebuttal to the non-compliance and the patient's response to the nurse's rebuttal should also be documented.

Clarity and Conciseness

Expansive and cluttered documentation does not always provide a complete and relevant record of the encounter, nor does it necessarily provide legal protection. Documenting irrelevant, unnecessary words by using formal complete sentences is time-consuming and does not add to the detail or quality of the note. Sentence fragments are acceptable. Some organizational policies do not allow charting only pertinent negatives, so it is important to learn about the documentation policies before handling encounters.

Documentation should not be wordy. For example:

> "The patient is complaining about chest pain on the left side of his chest. He has not experienced shortness of breath, diaphoresis, or radiation of pain to his arm or jaw. He describes the pain as aching and on a scale of 1-10, the intensity is an 8." This assessment could be re-written to be more clear, concise, and succinct: "c/o left sided aching chest pain. Intensity = 8 on a scale of 10. Denies SOB, diaphoresis, and radiating pain to arm, jaw."

The "wordy" documentation above contains all the elements necessary for good documentation. However, the excessive wordiness is caused by

Documenting irrelevant, unnecessary words by using formal complete sentences is time-consuming and does not add to the detail or quality of the note. Sentence fragments are acceptable.

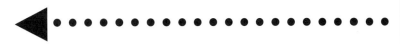

using complete sentences such as, "The patient is complaining about" instead of "c/o" (complains of).

Concise documentation should contain terms to qualify and quantify urgency and acuity, as well as to clarify the disposition, consultation, and follow-up. Descriptive terms assist in understanding the quality of symptoms. The patient should be asked to *qualify* (what is meant) symptoms regarding pain/discomfort, color, consistency, odor, alignment, activity level, and mood. *Quantifiable* (measurable) terms can be used to describe the quantity, amount, intensity, number of episodes, periods of time, frequency, duration, and onset. For example, during the assessment, the nurse asks:

❖ "What color was your vaginal bleeding?"
❖ "Any clots?"
❖ "How many pads did you use over a 2-hour period?"
❖ "What type of pad?"

The written documentation would be: *"Changed 4 mini pads q2h with bright red bleeding, no clots."*

Correct Spelling and Grammar

Spelling is very important, especially when documenting information about medication. Incorrect spelling can change the name of a medication and result in an adverse outcome.

The nurse should always ask the patient to spell the name of each medication. There are many medications with similar names and the telephone connection may make it difficult to hear the correct name. Additionally, the nurse may misinterpret the medication name because of the patient's accent or pronunciation of the medication. Examples of similar medication names include:

❖ Ceftin® and Cefotan®.
❖ Inderal® and Inderide®.
❖ Capoten® and Capozide®.
❖ Dimetane® and Dimetapp®.
❖ Zantac® and Xanax®.
❖ Zyprexia® and Zyrtec®.
❖ Clonidine® and Klonpin®.
❖ Celebrex® and Celexa®.

Spelling and grammar are a reflection of the nurse who is documenting the telehealth encounter. Prior to making the note part of the medical record, the nurse should proofread the documentation for clarity and correct language.

Spelling is very important, especially when documenting information about medication. Incorrect spelling can change the name of a medication and result in an adverse outcome.

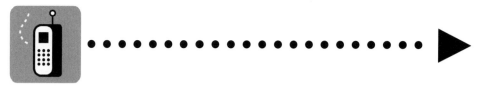

Symbols, Abbreviations, and Terminology

Most organizations and medical practices adopt a list of standardized symbols, abbreviations, and terminology. This facilitates communication as well as consistency and understanding among the health care writers and readers. However, the nurse's present place of employment may not use the same abbreviations and terminology that were approved by a previous employer. Some abbreviations are generic to the profession, while others are idiosyncratic to an organization. For example, in some facilities, the abbreviation "mx" is used for mammogram. This is not a standard abbreviation, nor is it widely used. Furthermore, "LOC" has several meanings depending on the area of specialty. It may mean, "level of consciousness," "loss of consciousness," or "laxative of choice." An incorrect abbreviation or symbol can alter the meaning of a word. The nurse should spell the word out if he/she is unsure of the approved abbreviation or meaning. A copy of the up-to-date and approved abbreviation list should be kept within reach for the telehealth staff.

Legibility

Illegible information may be misinterpreted, resulting in inappropriate treatment and an untoward outcome. Excellent legibility leads to proper interpretation of the record, especially if introduced as evidence in a court of law.

Documentation is only useful if others can read it. Illegible information may be misinterpreted, resulting in inappropriate treatment and an untoward outcome. Names and dosages of medication may appear similar if the handwriting is unreadable. Excellent legibility leads to proper interpretation of the record, especially if introduced as evidence in a court of law. Legibility is also important when others are reading the documentation for further decision-making or follow-up.

Error Correction

If a documentation error is made, the correction of the error should be made according to nursing standards and the specific organizational policy. The basic nursing standard for correcting an error is to:

❖ Draw one line through the incorrect entry, date (m/d/yr), and sign the error above or next to it.
❖ Initials may be permissible according to organizational policy.
❖ Proceed with documenting the actual entry.
❖ The labeling of the mistake as "error" or "mistaken entry" may or may not be part of your policy.
  o Example:

Correct:	5/31/98 J. Smith, RN
	~~LUQ~~ LLQ abdominal pain

Incorrect:	5/31	(year is missing)
	JS	(who is the nurse)
	~~LUQ~~	(multiple cross-outs)

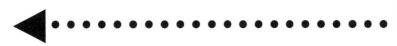

- ❖ If the error is large, such as a sentence or paragraph, the reason for the error should be indicated.
  - o Example:

  Error – wrong patient 5/31/98 J. Smith, RN

Entries should never be removed using erasable ink, correction fluid, or tape. Original entries should remain visible to dispel any presumption of altering or tampering of the medical record.

Signature

The encounter note should be signed at the end of the documentation. Many standardized telehealth documentation forms have a designated line for signatures that correlate with initials. Subsequent entries at a later date or time on the same documentation tool also require an appropriate signature, even if it is by the same nurse.

On some occasions, other health care providers may consult or follow-up with the patient. Their signatures must also be on the documentation form. All health care provider signatures should consist of the following components:

- ❖ Complete first name or initial of first name (according to organizational policy).
- ❖ Full last name (Note: initials can be used in the documentation as long as there is a signature that correlates with the initials).
- ❖ Professional licensure (RN, FNP, LPN).

Late Entries

If the nurse remembers an important aspect of the encounter long after completing the documentation, caution should be taken in documenting a late entry. The proper method for adding a late entry is as follows:

- ❖ State the entry as a "late entry" or "addendum."
- ❖ Date and time the late entry.
- ❖ Document the entry on the next available line.
- ❖ Do not skip lines or squeeze the entry in vacant spaces or the margins of the note.

The intent of a late entry is to add information that is pertinent to the patient's assessment and disposition. Late entries should not be documented in a manner that might provoke suspicion. For example, if major pieces of information are added, a reader may wonder if the nurse handled the encounter appropriately.

The intent of a late entry is to add information that is pertinent to the patient's assessment and disposition. Late entries should not be documented in a manner that might provoke suspicion.

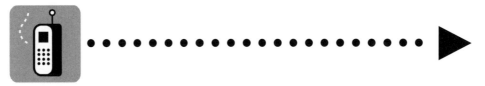

Rewriting Telehealth Notes

If there is a need to rewrite a telehealth note (for example, notes that are unreadable due to spills, tears, or multiple mistakes), the original documentation should not be discarded. The new documentation should be identified by stating, "recopied note from 5/28/08" (Iyer, & Camp, 2005). The original note should be attached to the recopied note.

The intention of these guiding principles for effective documentation is to assist in producing valuable documentation that communicates the telehealth interaction. Thorough documentation and the integrity of the record will enhance defensibility of the nurse and the health care organization in the event of legal action.

DOCUMENTATION FORMATS

The nurse is obligated to become acquainted with the organization's documentation standard(s) and use these consistently, thoroughly, and completely when charting.

Use of the documentation tool and a method for charting must be well-defined by the organization. The nurse is obligated to become acquainted with the organization's documentation standard(s) and use these consistently, thoroughly, and completely when charting.

Universal documentation practice and standards do not exist among nursing professionals and organizations that practice telehealth nursing. A variety of documentation tools are available. Some forms are as short and simple as a telephone log, while others are longer and more complex. The best form is one that is time-efficient, easy to follow, and prompts the nurse to obtain complete information. These forms need to correspond to and complement the symptom-based decision support tools used in that setting. The documentation tool, in conjunction with written decision support tools, can prompt the nurse to obtain applicable information that might otherwise be forgotten while talking to the caller.

Information that should be documented (no matter what type of documentation form is used) includes:

❖ **Encounter Characteristics**
  o Date/time of encounter.
  o Telephone number from where patient is calling (in case of disconnecting).
  o Telephone number of where the patient can be reached.
  o Name and title of nurse (and any assistive personnel) processing the encounter.
❖ **Patient Characteristics**
  o Patient name (full first and last name).
  o Date of birth (month, day, and year).
  o Gender.
  o Past medical history.
  o Allergies.
  o Current medications.

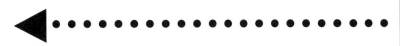

- ❖ **Contact Characteristics**
  - ○ Contact person's name (if not the patient; full first and last name).
  - ○ Relationship to patient.
- ❖ **Reason for Encounter**
  - ○ Reason for the encounter.
  - ○ Chief symptom, complaint, or information desired.
  - ○ Presence or absence of symptoms.
  - ○ Whether the patient has called before with a similar complaint or information request.
- ❖ **Nursing Actions**
  - ○ Assessment of symptoms and situation.
  - ○ Specific decision support tool used.
  - ○ Plan of action.
  - ○ Intervention or information given.
  - ○ Referrals to services, providers.
  - ○ Coordination of care.
- ❖ **Follow-Up Actions**
  - ○ Patient understanding.
  - ○ Refusals to care.
  - ○ Nurse's rebuttal and patient's response to rebuttal.

Additional information that may be required, depending upon the nature of the encounter and/or the patient, includes:

- ❖ Last menstrual period.
- ❖ Pregnancy status.
- ❖ Breastfeeding status.
- ❖ Home care measures tried previous to the encounter.

DOCUMENTATION TOOLS

There are a variety of documentation tools that a telehealth nurse can use. Development of the perfect documentation tool may take some trial and error. Tools should be developed to meet the needs of the specific health care environment and patient population while decreasing the nurse's legal risks (see Table 8-1).

There are a variety of documentation tools that a telehealth nurse can use. Tools should be developed to meet the needs of the specific health care environment and patient population while decreasing the nurse's legal risks.

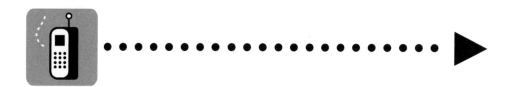

Table 8-1.
Summary of Documentation Methods and Tools

DOCUMENTATION METHOD	DOCUMENTATION TOOLS	FEATURES	ADVANTAGES	DISADVANTAGES
NARRATIVE	❖ Blank Form ❖ Standardized Form ❖ Telephone Log ❖ Progress Note	Can include normal and abnormal subjective data from the patient	❖ Documentation is in fragments or complete sentences ❖ Easier to write	❖ Paragraphs can be long with unnecessary words ❖ Data is not in a structured or logical order ❖ Promotes ambiguity
SOAP	❖ Blank Form ❖ Standardized Form ❖ Progress Note	Problem-specific	❖ Reflects the nursing process ❖ Follows a systematic, organized format	❖ Objective data is limited ❖ Inability of nurse to state assessment as working/ nursing diagnosis ❖ Cumbersome for data organization
FOCUS	❖ Blank Forms ❖ Progress Notes	Problem/behavior/ concern-specific	❖ Flexible ❖ Reflects the nursing process ❖ Systematic and organized ❖ Format easy to follow ❖ Reflects health care issues in addition to problems ❖ Documents normal and abnormal results	❖ Can easily become a narrative note if unable to sort data
DOCUMENTATION BY INCLUSION	❖ Check-Off Form ❖ Blank Form ❖ Progress Note ❖ Standardized Form	Includes normal and abnormal responses from the patient	❖ Gives a more complete picture of the patient's situation	❖ Time consuming ❖ Lengthy notes
DOCUMENTATION BY EXCEPTION	❖ Blank Form ❖ Telephone Log ❖ Progress Note	No record of normal responses by the patient	❖ Succinct documentation ❖ Less time spent documenting	❖ Does not give a complete picture of patient's situation ❖ Assumes standard questions were asked and answers were normal

Telehealth Nursing Practice Essentials © American Academy of Ambulatory Care Nursing, 2009

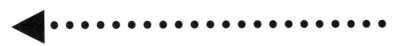

Telephone Logs

The telephone log is usually a short form that may have a carbon copy for duplication. Several forms or entries can occupy a page that may or may not be in a logbook. The log has limited space for minimal information. Therefore, thorough documentation of assessment, consultation, and follow-up is almost impossible. The information gathered must be concise, simple, and clear. The telephone log format is not useful for documenting assessments or consultative and follow-up criteria, but it works when minimal information is elicited, such as when an appointment is given. Telephone logs can be useful for medication refills as well as requests for referrals to other services or providers.

These logs are helpful for gathering data about the number and type of encounters being received because all encounters are together. The carbon copy of the form can remain as a backup to the logbook for easy retrieval. When a logbook is completed, the dates of the first message through the last message are written on the cover of the book and stored. Although telephone logs are convenient because all encounters are listed within one book, the information does not get entered into each individual patient's record. This means that the provider does not have easy access within the patient's chart to his/her prior telephone encounters.

The telephone log is usually a short form that may have a carbon copy for duplication. The information gathered must be concise, simple, and clear.

Chief Complaint Check-Off Forms

The check-off format is specific for the chief complaint. A separate form must be developed for each set of symptoms or guideline typically used. An organization may choose to have specific check-off form for their most frequent 10-20 symptoms. This type of documentation form contains check-off boxes for the primary and associated symptoms. The tool is in a yes/no format with space available to describe abnormal responses. The check-off form includes very few, if any, narrative lines for documentation of consultation and follow-up instructions.

Documentation on check-off forms is less time-consuming and promotes easy data compilation for the most common symptom complaints. However, multiple forms need to be developed, and there is no guarantee that all encounters will match the appropriate symptom forms. This form type produces a large amount of paper for print and storage.

Standardized Forms

Standardized forms have prompts or triggers that sequentially cue the nurse to gather specific information. They allow the nurse to interview and document the telehealth encounter in a logical and systematic sequence. This type of form can have boxes for data, such as last menstrual period (LMP), allergies, etc. Check boxes can be used to mark whether the patient was triaged as emergent, semi-urgent, or non-acute. Specific areas on the form can be used for writing clear and concise descriptions on the

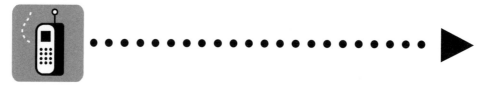

reason for encounter, assessment, symptoms, measures tried for symptom relief, interventions, and plan of care. Many standardized forms have 10-20 defined areas that must be completed for each encounter.

When an area on the standardized form is not relevant or not applicable, "NA" is the appropriate way to document. The use of a slash or strikeout (———) crossed through an element of the tool indicates that the questions were not asked. It also obliterates the use of the lines for documentation purposes. Depending on the organization, the slash may not indicate that the element was not applicable ("NA") to the telehealth encounter.

Electronic Forms

In practice settings where computerized software systems are used for documenting calls, the software will direct the data collection and documentation processes. A record of the decision support tool accessed and the disposition will be maintained automatically when these systems are properly installed and used.

DOCUMENTATION METHODS

Narrative Documentation

The narrative method of documentation is frequently used in telehealth nursing practice. This method includes writing sentences, fragments, or paragraphs. Documentation is free-flowing in story format, according to the caller's responses and the interview style.

The narrative method of documentation is frequently used in telehealth nursing practice. This method includes writing sentences, fragments, or paragraphs. Documentation is free-flowing in story format, according to the caller's responses and the interview style. However, free-flowing documentation may cause ambiguities or repetitive information. A disadvantage to narrative documentation is that the nursing process may appear disorganized. In addition, important elements can be missed without trigger words, check boxes, or defined areas on the form.

SOAP Documentation

The SOAP method of documentation is problem-oriented and problem-specific. This method organizes data and promotes a structure that is systematic, reinforcing the use of the nursing process.

*S**ubjective Data.** This information is obtained from the patient's perspective regarding the chief complaint or concern. It includes his/her experience with primary and associated symptoms or events related to the reason for the encounter.

*O**bjective Data.** This information is collected and measured by the nurse. The patient cannot be visually observed, but by listening not only to the words but also the tone of voice and other cues, the nurse can gather verbal and emotional data. Relevant information about the patient from other sources (e.g., other health care providers,

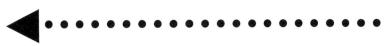

lab/diagnostic findings) can also be considered objective data (past medical history, pregnancy, breast-feeding, and allergies.).

Assessment. This is the impression of the patient's chief complaint or concern based on the subjective and objective data. The assessment can be documented by restating the chief complaint along with the working or nursing diagnosis.

Plan of Care. This is based on the patient's health care information, guideline/protocol, and the judgment and experience of the nurse. The plan may include an emergent or acute visit, home care advice, teaching, and follow-up instructions. The plan also incorporates a recommendation of appropriate actions for the patient to take. This portion of the telehealth documentation should include call-back instructions and the patient's agreement, comfort, or refusal to follow the stated plan.

Decision Support Tools

Clinical decision support tools are frequently used to guide documentation of critical information from both the patient and the nurse. Varieties of methods exist, but most follow the usual sequence of information flow. If the decision support tool is computerized, documentation may occur directly on the computer as information is requested from and given to the patient.

SUFFICIENT DOCUMENTATION

When nurses get together and discuss documentation, the conversation frequently turns to questions on what should and should not be included in documentation. Detailed record-keeping and documentation procedures should be based on the concept that undocumented care is assumed not to have occurred. Whether the documentation tool is a flowsheet, narrative form, or a standardized form, the organization should decide on a style of charting that will be complete and consistently practiced among their nurses. Comprehensive assessment assists the nurse in formulating an appropriate plan of care, and the documentation provides valuable patient information to the health care team. Some institutions believe that *proof of care* can only be shown by including everything in the documentation, while other institutions believe that proof of care can be demonstrated by exclusion.

Documentation by Inclusion

Documentation by inclusion means that all positive and negative responses to questions must be documented. By including all responses, the documentation shows what questions the nurse asked and what questions were not asked. Although this is more time-consuming, it

Detailed record-keeping and documentation procedures should be based on the concept that undocumented care is assumed not to have occurred. Whether the documentation tool is a flowsheet, narrative form, or a standardized form, the organization should decide on a style of charting that will be complete and consistently practiced among their nurses.

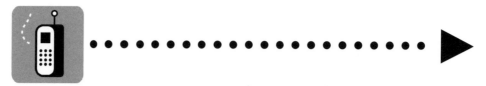

provides a very comprehensive description of the encounter. Additionally, documentation by inclusion helps in justifying why a specific assessment guideline was used and why the triage category chosen.

For example: If the patient has chest pain, the nurse would document all questions asked, even if the patient does not have chest pain symptoms. The nurse would then document, "denies shortness of breath, radiating pain, sweating, and states he is comfortable." This time-consuming documentation helps provide the justification for the care disposition reached by the nurse and patient.

Documentation by Exception

Documentation by exception assumes that standardized questions were asked because they are part of the assessment policy, but the negative responses are not included in the documentation.

For example, if the patient's only symptom were substernal chest pain, the nurse would document "substernal chest pain." It would not be necessary to document "denies shortness of breath, radiating pain, etc."

The risk with documenting by exception is that it does not prove that all assessment questions were asked or the patient's response to these questions. If a facility adopts documentation by exception, it is extremely important to have a detailed policy of what needs to be included and what can be excluded.

The advantage of documenting by exception is time-saving because minimal charting is done. However, the risk with documenting by exception is that it does not prove that all assessment questions were asked or the patient's response to these questions. If a facility adopts documentation by exception, it is extremely important to have a detailed policy of what needs to be included and what can be excluded. At some health care facilities, their policy states that all patients are asked emergent/urgent symptoms until a match of symptoms are found. Then, only the matching symptoms need to be documented. In other words, the nurse does not have to chart, "denies shortness of breath, radiation, chest pain, dizziness." The nurse charts, "Has slight cough only."

Because there are so many documentation methods and tools that can be used, the nurse and the employer will need to decide what best meets their needs. Tools should be developed to support the nurse and the nursing process while being patient-focused.

CRITICAL DOCUMENTATION SITUATIONS

There are also issues of encounter handling that warrant special attention and need to be documented with care.

Variations from Decision Support Tools

If the patient's situation varies from the written clinical decision support tool, or if the patient chooses to deviate from the nurse's recommendation, it is important to always document the reasons for the variation. Some organizations require that a provider be consulted prior to deviating from a decision support tool and require the provider's directions to be documented. If nurses are allowed to deviate from

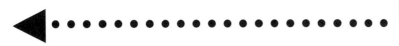

decision support tools using their own clinical decision-making and judgment, the reason for the deviation should be documented. Nurses should keep in mind that they should never downgrade a patient's triage category but may upgrade the triage disposition based on their clinical knowledge and judgment.

Follow-Up Instructions

Some specific decision support tools include *possible complications* of the symptoms or *warning signs and symptoms* for which the patient should watch. The nurse should document the discussion of warning signs, and instructions should be given to patients, including asking them to call back if any of the warning symptoms occur. If specific warning signs are not part of the protocol, the nurse can use the acronym PCWAS (Brown, 2008). PCWAS instructs the patient to call back if there are **P**ersistent, **C**hanging, **W**orsening, **A**nxiety-provoking or **S**pecific symptoms. This opened-ended statement informs the patient to call back if the symptoms do not resolve, if anything new develops, or if they are uncomfortable with the course of the complaint/concern/treatment. The nurse can document, "Instructed PCWAS."

Compliance/Refusal with the Plan of Care

It is important to clarify that the patient understands and will adhere to the recommended appointment, referral, home care advice, or follow-up. If the patient is confused about the plan of care, the nurse documents the patient's response and reiterates the instructions. When a patient refuses to comply with the recommended plan, the nurse states the reasons for non-compliance. For example, the nurse states, "Your child should be seen this morning for his asthma. If you wait until later this afternoon, he runs the risk of developing respiratory difficulty." The caller replies, "I really cannot miss any more work, so I will have to bring him in for either a late afternoon or evening appointment." Document, "Father desires late afternoon/evening appointment due to work constraints. Aware of the risk for developing respiratory difficulty if he waits for appointment later in the day."

Method of Transportation

When the telehealth encounter includes specific instructions to the patient not to drive him/herself, this recommendation should be documented. Also document the recommended mode of transport, such as, "Instructed patient to have wife drive him." If the patient ignores the nurse's instructions, drives himself, and gets in an accident, there will be a record of the nurse's transportation recommendation.

It is important to clarify that the patient understands and will adhere to the recommended appointment, referral, home care advice, or follow-up. If the patient is confused about the plan of care, the nurse documents the patient's response and reiterates the instructions.

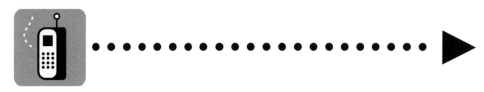

SPECIAL CIRCUMSTANCES TO DOCUMENT

There are numerous special circumstances that require specific documentation. If an administrative policy is in place, the nurse should follow this policy. However, if organizational policies are lacking, the nurse may use the following information for assistance with documentation.

Return or Follow-Up Encounters

If the nurse makes any outbound encounters to the patient, he/she should be aware of the federal regulations contained in the 1996 Telecommunications Act. Additionally, all states have laws regarding telemarketing that apply if a patient is being contacted about upcoming health care events, service offerings, or marketing events. An example is when patients are contacted by the provider's office and the staff shares information about their new office location and that they are offering free blood sugar testing to celebrate the new office. Because this is a "marketing encounter" (a promotional offer), the encounters are subject to the Telecommunications Act. A violation of the Act also occurs when a person asks to be taken off a call list, and the organization fails to abide by this request. The Act includes stipulations, such as calling before 8 A.M. and after 9 P.M. Failure to adhere to the standards contained in the acts leaves the organization or nurse subject to fines.

Prior to implementing outbound encounters, the nurse must be aware of his/her organization's relevant policy. Never *promise* to contact someone, because it is not possible to be *absolutely certain* that you will reach him or her. Instead, inform the patient that you would like to follow up and ask his/her approval to contact him/her or a designated other person by stating, "We may want to contact you in a few days. Is this OK?" Document:

❖   That the patient gave permission.
❖   Who you have permission to speak to.
❖   What times of the day to attempt the encounters.

Lack of permission for the contact should be very clearly documented in the encounter record. Procedures need to be in place to ensure that these patients do not receive a callback.

Lack of permission for the contact should be very clearly documented in the encounter record. Procedures need to be in place to ensure that these patients do not receive a callback. When handling encounters from minors, it is essential to obtain the minor's permission for a follow up. The nurse should also attempt to obtain permission to speak to a parent. Never assume that is appropriate to follow-up with the parent.

For follow-up encounters or callbacks, the nurse must document the following:

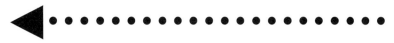

- ❖ Each attempted and completed encounter made with the date and time.
- ❖ The person reached.
- ❖ A summary of the interaction.
- ❖ The plan of care.
- ❖ If a message was left on an answering machine or if there was no answer.

A policy should be developed on the number of follow-up attempts to make, an identified period of time, and what to do if the patient is not reached within the designated timeframe. If the follow-up is for providing important information such as laboratory results, a registered letter may need to be sent if the patient is not reached. When a registered letter is sent, the following should be included in the patient's chart:

- ❖ Document the reason why a registered letter was sent.
- ❖ Place a copy of the letter in the patient's chart.
- ❖ Place the outgoing *registration* form.
- ❖ Place the completed *return receipt* form (shows proof that the letter arrived at the destination).

Patient Complaints

Because the nurse is considered to be a representative of the health care organization, patients may contact the nurse to complain about providers, other members of the health care team, or services they have received.

When handling complaints, the nurse should never make promises to the patient about what is going to be done about the complaint. Additionally, the nurse should not agree with the patient about the complaint but should act as a neutral third party willing to report the complaint information. Upon hearing the complaint, the nurse should ask the patient's permission to document the concern so that it can be forwarded to the appropriate person to handle. Complaint documentation should include:

- ❖ Specifics about the issue.
- ❖ The nurse's response to the patient (such as "informed patient that manager would try to contact him in the next few days").
- ❖ The caller's response to the nurse's action.
- ❖ The nurse's action – who was informed about the complaint.

It is an organizational decision, and should be addressed by policy, as to how or if the complaint is documented in the patient's record. It is important to keep a departmental file of patient complaints in order to

When handling complaints, the nurse should never make promises to the patient about what is going to be done about the complaint. Additionally, the nurse should not agree with the patient about the complaint but should act as a neutral third party willing to report the complaint information.

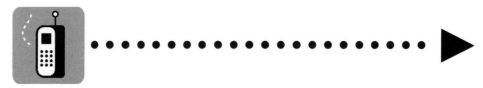

analyze trends and issues. These records need to be stored in a confidential manner similar to *patient incident* reporting.

Reports on Child and Elder Abuse

All states require that health care workers report cases of suspected child and elder abuse and neglect. This includes telehealth nurses. Although the telehealth nurse has not seen the patient, it is a requirement that the nurse report the case because he/she is *aware of or has knowledge of a situation*. The caller should also be instructed to contact the authorities as they have first-hand information of the abuse or neglect. When reporting abuse or neglect, the organization's policy on reporting to authorities must be followed carefully. Documentation should include:

- ❖ Direct quotes from the caller and his/her concerns.
- ❖ Description of symptoms and triage advice.
- ❖ Nurse's plan of action in following through with the patient or caller.
- ❖ Nurse's plan of action in reporting the abuse or neglect, and agency information given to the caller.
- ❖ The state or local reporting agency contacted by the nurse.
- ❖ The name of the person from the agency who took the report, his/her title, and the date and time that the report was made.

Most states have specific forms for abuse and neglect cases that need to be completed along with the encounter documentation. The nurse must know where to mail the report and if copies of the report are kept with the employer. Again, the specifics of this situation should be addressed by organizational policy.

After an abuse/neglect report is filed, a caseworker will be assigned to investigate the issue. After the investigation is completed, many states will send a follow-up letter with information on the state's findings to the party who reported the abuse. The nurse will need to know if these findings should be documented into the encounter record as a late entry. The *findings* letter should be kept, along with a copy of the telehealth note and a copy of the initial report. The nurse will need to know the policy on where these documents are to be stored.

Anonymous Encounters

Occasionally, a patient will want to remain anonymous during the encounter. This is more common in call centers than provider offices. However, the nurse needs to document these encounters regardless of the setting. Anonymous encounters should have a unique identifier for that encounter in order to easily find the encounter information at a latter date. A unique identifier commonly used is the 1) date of the encounter 2) time of the encounter 3) nurse's initials who handled the encounter. For

After an abuse/neglect report is filed, a caseworker will be assigned to investigate the issue. After the investigation is completed, many states will send a follow-up letter with information on the state's findings to the party who reported the abuse. The nurse will need to know if these findings should be documented into the encounter record as a late entry.

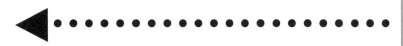

example, in the demographic area for the patient's name, the documentation could be:

Last Name   First Name
10/09/03 3:00 PM   anonymous/mke

Although an encounter may be anonymous, it must include complete documentation. If possible, document why the demographic information was not provided. Policies should provide guidance for managing anonymous encounters.

CONFIDENTIALITY ISSUES

The nurse is responsible for keeping all interactions and documentation confidential in order to protect the patient and the organization. Confidentiality means that all encounter-related information will be regarded as privileged, private, and available to authorized users only.

The patient has a right to confidentiality based on legally enforceable concepts of a trust relationship and invasion of privacy statutes. At no time may the nurse reveal the nature of the encounter to any other party unless the patient gives consent. The patient should be assured of this confidentiality during the course of his/her telehealth interaction, and if confidentiality concerns arise, the nurse should document the patient's concerns. An exception to confidentiality is with child and elder abuse, where state laws mandate that the nurse report information to authorities even if the caller requests confidentiality.

The patient has a right to confidentiality based on legally enforceable concepts of a trust relationship and invasion of privacy statutes. At no time may the nurse reveal the nature of the encounter to any other party unless the patient gives consent.

Release of Encounter Documentation to Patients and Callers

Occasionally, a caller will request a copy of the encounter documentation. For example, documentation may be requested for child custody issues when one parent is trying to prove lack of care by the other, or when the calling parent needs to prove that he/she took appropriate measures for his/her ill child. The nurse must be aware of Health Insurance Portability and Accountability Act (HIPAA) and the organization's specific policies. If no organizational policy has been developed for encounter documentation, the following information may serve as a starting point in developing the policy.

Generally, only a summary and generalities of the telehealth documentation should be released. An example of the released information might be:

"A female called at <time> on <date> identifying herself as <name> and that she was the <relationship> of the patient. She stated that <patient name> had <general (not detailed) symptoms>.

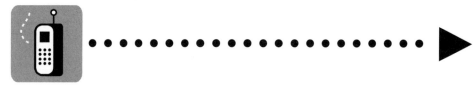

The patient was <assessed>, and the caller was instructed to <disposition of care>. The caller stated that she would follow <the plan of care>."

If a caller wants a summary statement of the encounter, it is very important for this request to be in writing and to follow the organization's *release of medical record* policy. Identification of the requester is important for the organization because there is no guarantee that the person who initiated the original encounter is actually the person requesting the information. Meanwhile, the nurse should add an addendum to the original encounter documentation regarding the caller's request and if the caller will be sending their request in writing.

Full call documentation should be copied and released only according to organizational policy. If the documentation is in a logbook with other patient calls, call documentation must be obscured so only the one specific patient's information is seen.

Release of Encounter Documentation to Provider

When the nurse is part of a service that provides telehealth triaging services for designated providers (such as after-hours services), policies should describe the encounter documentation and mechanism for supplying copies to the providers. Generally, the complete encounter documentation record may be provided. However, policies must include the frequency for sending the documentation (daily, weekly, or monthly) and when the provider should review the documentation. The policy should also define responsibilities for patient follow-up if there are issues that need attention.

If the provider is participating in a quality improvement (QI) project, it is important not to record QI notes on the permanent patient encounter documentation. For example, the after-hours service sends its encounter documentation to the provider, and the provider's QI project is to analyze the appropriateness of the nurse's *triage category and patient disposition*. The provider will review the encounter documentation, write comments agreeing or disagreeing with the triage decision, and place the encounter documentation with his/her QI critique into the patient record. This is problematic when there has been disagreement with the triage decision. The QI result has been written into the record and stays in the patient's permanent file. Instead, a copy of the documentation should be made for the QI project and these records stored separately from the patient's encounter documentation.

Release of Encounter Documentation to Managed Care Organizations

Frequently, callers are members of a managed care organization (MCO). Problems may arise when the managed care organization requests a copy of the encounter documentation. Again, it is very important to

When the nurse is part of a service that provides telehealth triaging services for designated providers (such as after-hours services), policies should describe the encounter documentation and mechanism for supplying copies to the providers.

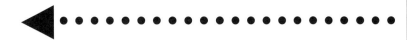

adhere to HIPAA regulations and analyze the appropriateness of sending medical records (encounter documentation) to the MCO. The problem becomes more complicated when the patient tells the MCO that the telehealth nurse sent him/her to the emergency department, but the nurse did not make that recommendation. Meanwhile, the MCO cannot justify the emergency visit and wants the encounter information disclosed. Well-defined policies must be developed on when encounter information may be provided to the MCO. In all cases, the MCO should not receive encounter documentation unless the patient has given written permission for release of information.

Release of Encounter Documentation to Services and Provider Referrals

In the course of the day, the nurse's responsibilities may include referring patients to various providers and services. Again, it is important to safeguard the documentation so that the patient's encounter confidentiality is maintained. Before sending patient information to another office (provider, service, etc.), written permission must be obtained from the patient. For call centers with *physician referral services*, no patient information may be given to the provider unless consent is obtained from the patient.

Release of Encounter Documentation for Mailing Lists

Occasionally, the marketing or communication department of an organization may request lists of callers who have inquired about specific diseases or illnesses. The use of non-identifiable, patient demographic information components (summary of zip codes, ages of callers, sex of callers) to support internal program analysis and program planning is permitted. Identifiable demographic information (name, address, etc.) should never be disclosed without written patient consent.

DOCUMENTATION RETENTION

Telehealth documentation is part of the medical record; therefore, each documented telehealth encounter is treated in the same manner as other documents placed in a patient's chart. Every organization defines its responsibility to maintaining copies of medical records for a specific number of years. Time frames vary from state to state and are determined by:

- ❖ State regulations (from no specific time frame to keeping records permanently).
- ❖ State statutes of limitations for medical malpractice.
- ❖ Organizational policies with input from legal council.

In the course of the day, the nurse's responsibilities may include referring patients to various providers and services. Again, it is important to safeguard the documentation so that the patient's encounter confidentiality is maintained.

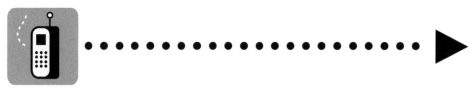

❖ Internal needs for record keeping (medical research, peer review, QI).

Medical record retention for patients who are minors is based on state law for a specified period of time (usually 2 years) after the minor patient reaches majority (usually 21 years old). This means that a telephone call about a newborn would need to be kept for a minimum of 23 years. Many organizations choose to maintain records longer than their state's statute of limitations. Medical records can be retained in their original form by hard copy or electronic storage media. The policy regarding the use of storage media is based on professional practice standards, state regulations, and medical and administrative needs of the organization.

SECURITY

Patients have a right to privacy and this includes maintaining the privacy of the encounter documentation. A violation of the patient's right to privacy can result in a federal and civil liability. The telehealth nurse needs to be very aware of who has access to the telehealth documentation, and to take care there is no unauthorized access to the record. Although the nurse's desk may be in an area shared by other staff members, it is imperative not to allow other employees to peruse the documentation.

TECHNOLOGICAL ISSUES

With the ongoing infusion of technology into the health care arena, new issues have emerged. From use of recording devices to faxes, policies related to documentation must continuously evolve.

With the ongoing infusion of technology into the health care arena, new issues have emerged. From the use of recording devices to faxes, policies related to documentation must continuously evolve.

Recording Encounters

Recording telehealth encounters cannot be used as a substitute for documentation because the record does not show the chain of decision-making used by the nurse. For instance, recording an encounter does not show which decision support tool was used or which symptoms were the key factors that influenced the nurse to make clinical decisions for the patient. With written documentation, the nurse can phrase the charting to show why the clinical decision was made for the patient. With recording, clinical decisions and triage rationale can only be inferred. In most states, recording of encounters is permitted (after informing the caller), but documentation must still include complete details of the encounter.

Computerized Documentation

A fully automated software system allows medical records to be created, modified, signed, and authenticated by computers. However, most regulatory agencies recognize the advantages of computerized medical

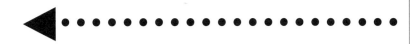

records, such as their storage and retrieval, and approve their use for documentation along with electronic signatures. Objectives for the use of electronic documentation may include (Hannah, Ball, & Edwards, 2006):

❖ To eliminate redundancies and duplication.
❖ To enhance the quality and reporting of clinical care from a multidisciplinary approach through standardization.
❖ To define and standardize common clinical documentation data elements.
❖ To develop an approach for standardizing clinical documentation practices for both automated and manual settings.
❖ To automate an ideal clinical documentation workflow.

Computerized documentation records are organized and legible; therefore, they limit the possibility of misunderstanding a nurse's handwriting. Using computerized records also reduces the risk of lost or misplaced records.

The most significant problem with computerized documentation is the increased risk of improper disclosure and breach of confidentiality. Employees not directly involved in the patient's care (such as other providers and computer personnel) may be able to access the computer records, which results in a breach of confidentiality.

Because of confidentiality, access to computer terminals must be limited only to those authorized. The use of computers for documentation presents a legal risk of mass disclosure of patient information Because of this, security measures for computerized documentation include:

The most significant problem with computerized documentation is the increased risk of improper disclosure and breach of confidentiality.

❖ Using passwords and access codes that are changed regularly.
❖ Limiting access to the specific computer screens based on job classification and responsibilities (for instance, a secretary should not be able to access specific triage encounter documentation).
❖ Having an audit system that detects and tracks unauthorized access to the system.
❖ Having a system that prevents mass copying of records.
❖ Securing the records so that changes to the records can be tracked back to the specific computer user.
❖ Using electronic user codes for signatures that are protected by security.

Faxing and Emailing Encounter Documentation

Facsimile transmissions (faxes) of telehealth documentation are a convenient method of forwarding patient records. However, before faxing, the fax number should be verified and a cover letter with confidentiality notification placed before the encounter documentation. The nurse should ascertain that the receiving fax is in a private area and is not shared by

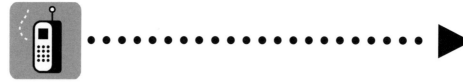

people who do not have rights to the patient's encounter documentation. Only minimal encounter documentation should be faxed. For instance, if the nurse is faxing a prescription order to a pharmacy, the pharmacy should only see the pertinent patient demographics and prescription order. It would be a breach of HIPAA regulations to disclose and fax the assessment and triage notes.

If the nurse works in a setting where provider orders are faxed, it is important to have hard copies of each provider's signature on file. These hard copies should be used to compare to the fax signature.

The nurse should know HIPAA regulations on faxing or emailing encounter documentation (medical record). The nurse must also review The Joint Commission regulations on faxing and emailing under the standards of patient confidentiality.

SUMMARY

When an organization develops documentation policies and procedures, it is important to consider the amount of time allowed for completing the documentation, encounter-handling necessities, the method for acquiring the information, and the need for comprehensiveness of the documentation.

The purpose of documentation is to demonstrate professional nursing and the nursing process. Documentation also informs readers of the nature and acuity of a patient's health care issue. Without complete documentation, fragmentation makes it difficult to convey the linkages of information and events throughout the health care continuum. Registered professional nurses are expected by virtue of state nurse practice acts to use clinical judgment, the nursing process, and verbal and written communication skills when participating in patient care. Nurses have an ethical and legal obligation to develop documentation tools and have skills that demonstrate competency in transforming verbal interactions into written communication.

Telehealth nursing practice addresses a broad range of health care issues and services that must be included in the patient's overall health care picture. The telehealth encounter is a valuable asset in promoting coordination and continuity of patient care, and as such, the nurse must be knowledgeable and professionally responsible for documentation.

With the implementation of HIPAA regulations, patient confidentiality has become a very important part of encounter documentation. Every nurse that handles encounters from patients must be responsible for maintaining confidentiality and an appropriate medical legal record. Based on the unique patient populations, appropriate and specific documentation policies must be developed. Once these policies are in place, it is the professional nurse's responsibility to uphold these standards.

> *If the nurse works in a setting where provider orders are faxed, it is important to have hard copies of each provider's signature on file. These hard copies should be used to compare to the fax signature.*

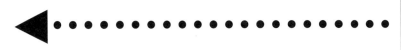

TIPS & PEARLS

☎ If you didn't document it, the presumption is that you didn't ask it, say it, or explain it!

☎ Documentation of the telehealth encounter includes gathering data, utilizing critical thinking skills to analyze the information, defining a plan of care, and then translating the information into a permanent format as a summary of the interaction between the nurse and the patient.

☎ Documentation should reflect that the nurse used the nursing process and followed standards of care.

☎ Documentation should be concise with specific information to qualify and quantify urgency and acuity, as well as to clarify the disposition, consultation, and follow-up.

☎ Use of a documentation tool and a method for charting must be defined by policy of the organization.

References

American Academy of Ambulatory Care Nursing (AAACN). (2007). *Telehealth nursing practice administration and practice standards* (4th ed.). Pitman, NJ: Author.

Brown, J.L. (2008). Telephone care requires use of language that paints clear picture for parent, doctor. *AAP News, 29*(3), 22.

Hannah, K.J., Ball, M.J., & Edwards, M.J.A. (2006). *Introduction to nursing informatics* (3rd ed.). New York: Springer Sciences and Business Media.

Iyer, P., & Camp, N. (2005). *Nursing documentation: A nursing process approach.* St. Louis, MO: C.V. Mosby Co.

Joint Commission on Accreditation of Healthcare Organizations (JCAHO). (2007). *Comprehensive accreditation manual for ambulatory care.* Oakbrook Terrace, IL: Author.

National Committee for Quality Association (NCQA). (2006). *Standards for the accreditation of managed care organizations.* Washington, DC: Author.

Answer/Evaluation Form   AMBP9c06
Continuing Nursing Education Activity
Telehealth Nursing Practice Essentials
Chapter 8: Documentation of Telehealth Encounters

This activity provides 1.4 contact hours of continuing nursing education (CNE) credit in nursing.
(Contact hours calculated using a 60-minute contact hour.)

This test may be copied for use by others.

┌───┐
│   **COMPLETE THE FOLLOWING:**   │
│   │
│ Name: _____   │
│   │
│ Address: _____   │
│   │
│ City: _____ State: _____ Zip: _____│
│   │
│ Telephone number: (Home)_____ (Work)_____│
│   │
│ Email address:_____   │
│   │
│ AAACN Member Number and Expiration Date: _____│
│   │
│ Processing fee: AAACN Member: $12.00   │
│   Nonmember: $20.00   │
└───┘

Answer Form: (Please attach a separate sheet of paper if necessary.)
1. What did you value most about this activity?

_____
_____
_____

2. If you could imagine that you have fully integrated your learning into practice, what would be different about your present practice?

_____
_____
_____

Evaluation	Strongly disagree				Strongly agree
3. The offering met the stated objectives.					
a. Describe five reasons why documentation of telehealth encounters is essential to telehealth nursing practice.	1	2	3	4	5
b. Summarize the essential components of effective telehealth documentation.	1	2	3	4	5
c. Compare and contrast the various types of documentation tools and charting methods available for documenting various types of telehealth encounters.	1	2	3	4	5
d. Summarize procedures to maintain confidentiality of telehealth documentation.	1	2	3	4	5
e. Explain the effect of technology on telehealth documentation.	1	2	3	4	5
4. The content was current and relevant.	1	2	3	4	5
5. The content was presented clearly.	1	2	3	4	5
6. The content was covered adequately.	1	2	3	4	5

7. How would you rate your ability to apply your learning to practice following this activity? (Check one)

☐ Diminished ability ☐ No change ☐ Enhanced ability

8. Time required to complete reading assignment and answer form: ___ minutes
Comments _____

_____

I verify that I have completed this activity:

_____
Signature

Objectives

This educational activity is designed for nurses and other health care professionals who provide telehealth care for patients. This evaluation is designed to test your achievement of the following educational activities.
1. Describe five reasons why documentation of telehealth encounters is essential to telehealth nursing practice.
2. Summarize the essential components of effective telehealth documentation.
3. Compare and contrast the various types of documentation tools and charting methods available for documenting various types of telehealth encounters.
4. Summarize procedures to maintain confidentiality of telehealth documentation.
5. Explain the effect of technology on telehealth documentation.

Evaluation Form Instructions

1. To receive continuing nursing education (CNE) credit for individual study after reading the indicated chapter(s), please complete the evaluation form (photocopies of the answer form are acceptable). Attach separate paper as necessary.
2. Detach (or photocopy) and send the answer form along with a check, money order, or credit card payable to *AAACN* East Holly Avenue/Box 56, Pitman, NJ 08071-0056. You may also send this form as an email attachment to ambp401@ajj.com.
3. Answer forms must be postmarked by December 31, 2011. Upon completion of the answer/evaluation form, a certificate for 1.4 contact hours will be awarded and sent to you.

Payment Options

☐ Check or money order enclosed (payable in U.S. funds to AAACN)

☐ MasterCard ☐ VISA ☐ American Express

Credit Card #:_____

Expiration Date: _____ Security Code:_____

Card Holder (Please print):

_____

Signature:

_____

This educational activity has been co-provided by the American Academy of Ambulatory Care Nursing (AAACN) and Anthony J. Jannetti, Inc. (AJJ).

AAACN is a provider approved by the California Board of Registered Nursing, Provider Number CEP 5336.

AJJ is accredited as a provider of continuing nursing education by the American Nurses Credentialing Center's Commission on Accreditation.

This book was reviewed and formatted for contact hour credit by Sally S. Russell, MN, CMSRN, AAACN Education Director, and Maureen Espensen, MBA, BSN, RN, Editor.

American Academy of Ambulatory Care Nursing
East Holly Avenue/Box 56, Pitman, NJ 08071-0056
Phone: 800-AMB-NURS; Fax: 856-589-7463
Web: www.aaacn.org; Email: aaacn@ajj.com

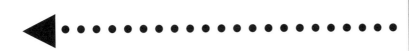

CHAPTER 9
Technology and Other Topics

Objectives

1. Describe future changes in telehealth and the impact on nursing practice.
2. Describe some of the technology used in telehealth nursing.

As our world of health care leaps into the future, nurses will continue to see drastic changes in the delivery of health care. For instance, prior to the 1980s, physicians were considered to be the "captains of the ship." They were in charge of their patients' care, and the patient-physician relationship was not influenced by outside parties. Patients expected their physicians to manage their family's medical needs and care for them. In the 1980s, the emergence of managed care began, along with sophisticated utilization review, concurrent review, pre-approval, and claims auditing. During this time, patients began to notice restrictions from their insurance plans and recognized their lack of power as "consumers" of health care. It was also during this time that patients had very few tools to make educated health care decisions.

In the 1990s, the term *demand management* was developed to describe consumer informed decisions regarding health and medical care. These informed decisions were reached by providing health information and education to patients, along with proactive health management. The key to demand management was and still is managing the *demand* for health care (MacStravic & Montrose, 1998). Demands can include patients who require physician appointments for minor illnesses or patients who wish to use the emergency department for routine care. Management of the demand includes providing health information and education in a way so that patients are satisfied and comfortable enough to care for their symptoms at home while staying alert for worsening symptoms.

The next generation beyond demand management is *medical management*. Medical management is the process of moving from managing the demands of the patient (such as an HMO environment) to a system of patient advocacy and provider support (MacStravic & Montrose, 1998). Medical management consists of concepts such as personal health management, disease management, quality management, and outcome management. With medical management, the delivery system is both patient and provider focused. The patient and provider are no longer in penalty situations where the managed care company scrutinizes the care management decisions. Instead, the patient and providers are given tools that help and enhance care delivery.

Medical management consists of concepts such as personal health management, disease management, quality management, and outcome management. With medical management, the delivery system is both patient and provider focused.

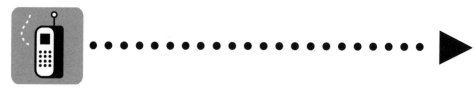

As we move further along in the 21st century, a *paradigm shift* is occurring in health management. Paradigm shifts are described as making or allowing radical changes in the core, basic ways a person thinks about situations. A paradigm shift allows for belief changes after a person has learned more about a situation and has an increased understanding, resulting in changes of perspective and action. *Health care consumerism* is becoming increasingly evident. Patients are consumers who are relatively savvy in terms of health trends. More importantly, they want to make their own choices and value tools that give them the information to do so. Health care providers must be willing to make changes in order to remain successful in this environment. Because of this paradigm shift, health care providers are providing tools that encourage patients or consumers to become more self-directed, self-educated, and participatory in their health care and overall well-being. There is an increased focus on self-care and motivation for making sound health care decisions (Baldwin, 2006). With this paradigm shift in health care, consumers consider their health care providers and telehealth nurses as *consultants* rather than directors or *managers* of their health care needs. Providers (including nurses) are finding satisfaction in partnering with their patients and providing the tools, knowledge, and facilities to improve their health and wellness.

Paradigm shifts are described as making or allowing radical changes in the core, basic ways a person thinks about situations. A paradigm shift allows for belief changes after a person has learned more about a situation and has an increased understanding, resulting in changes of perspective and action.

Because of these paradigm shifts in health care, consumers are very knowledgeable about their own health and medical issues. They actively participate in the management of their health care. Technology systems are used to provide more self-direction with patient education, appointment setting, monitoring, and counseling. Nurses are providing care enhancements for their patient populations via newsletters, e-newsletters, television, radio, video conferencing, online tools, and telephonic tools.

TELHEALTH NURSING CHANGES

Because of increasing competitive pressure, health care organizations continuously seek strategies to remain viable while strengthening relationships with their customers (patients). In order to control costs, one of the most prevalent strategies is controlling the amounts and types of services being utilized (MacStravic & Montrose, 1998). At the same time, health care organizations are focusing on better management of relationships with all customers. These relationships not only include patients, but also physicians, nursing personnel, support staff, pharmacists, physical therapists, providers, and all employees.

Telehealth nursing is a key component in supporting these strategies because of the strongly bonded relationship that develops between the caller and the nurse. Telehealth nursing supports consumer health management through education and expert advice. People desire medical advice from a professional whom they feel they can trust. Because of these

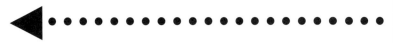

needs, nurses can be key in developing positive relationships and experiences while providing quality, cost-efficient health care for patients. Telehealth nurses enhance the depth, quality, and value of interactions for consumers.

The telehealth nursing practice service is a customer-focused area. This service is defined as any setting where encounters are handled in a formalized method, staffed by one or many hundred nurses and sponsored by a single physician office, multi-physician clinic, managed-care facility, insurance provider, hospital, pharmaceutical provider, or a stand-alone for-profit operation.

Over the past 20 years, there has been an ever-growing number of telehealth nursing encounter services that handle nurse triage, health care information, appointment scheduling (especially for complicated specialist referrals), and care coordination. The nursing contact center has further evolved into a multi-media customer service center that uses a variety of communication devices, such as voice, telephone, Internet, video, computer software, and print media.

As consumers become more self-care driven, new health care technologies and strategies will be offered so that informed decisions can be made. Already, many consumers seek health care information via self-care books, telephone "advice" lines, audio libraries, interactive modules, and the Internet. An explosion of health information and education materials has become available over the last 15-20 years, and future technology has no limits.

Telehealth nursing practice centers utilize technology to link nurses to consumers by many different interactive electronic means. The nurse practice center of today includes the nurse, telephone, and/or Internet, facsimile, email, home monitoring equipment, while the technology of tomorrow will include video and specialty equipment (such as EKG monitors) that integrate and share data. Some of the new cyberspace technology has already arrived, while other technology is still evolving in the minds of engineers for the future. For the delivery of superior patient care, telehealth practice nurses are using various technologies, along with their clinical knowledge, critical thinking, and judgment.

As consumers become more self-care driven, new health care technologies and strategies will be offered so that informed decisions can be made.

TELEPHONE TECHNOLOGY

Part of providing a positive experience for a caller is the delivery tool for the interaction. Traditionally, nurses have used the telephone as their delivery tool. The telephone has become common technology when attempting to gain health care information and advice in a timely and efficient manner.

Most consumers of today's society are quite acclimated to the technological automations in their lives. People regularly use telephones, voice mail, faxes, electronic mail, and other interactive technology to

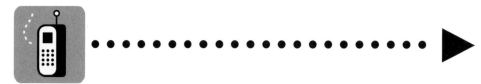

obtain services and products, and to access information. Some consumers use these technologies to a great extent while enjoying the endless capabilities and efficiencies. Other consumers would rather go without these complex technologies but use them reluctantly out of necessity.

To meet the needs of these diverse groups of consumers, the contact center must create and provide quality, efficient services using the best technology available. Some of the telephone technology available includes Internet telephony, call distributors, call routers, and automatic dialing systems.

Voice Over Internet Protocol (VoIP)

Voice over Internet Protocol (VoIP), also called Internet telephony, is the transmission of voice through the Internet. The VoIP system carries voice as a digital audio file (or packet) and can be saved as such. This allows messages left as voicemails to be listened to, emailed to a recipient, forwarded electronically, or saved in a dedicated folder or patient's record.

Because VoIP utilizes the Internet, long distance charges do not exist. Therefore, telehealth nurses on VoIP and with a fast Internet connection no longer need to consider long distance charges when making outbound calls. Likewise, consumers using VoIP no longer need to consider these charges when calling a telehealth nurse out of their immediate telephone service area.

In addition, conference calling, call forwarding, automatic redial, and caller ID, which traditional telecommunication companies charge for, typically come standard with VoIP. Advanced features such as call routing (see *ACDs* on p. 145) and screen pops (see *CTI* on p. 145), integration with video conversation, and message or data file exchange are easier and cheaper to implement since the phone call is on the same data network as the nurse's computer.

As with any technology, there are drawbacks as well as benefits. The contact center or remote nurse who uses VoIP must ensure there is enough available network bandwidth to transmit the voice packets. There may also be issues with reliability because VoIP service is down whenever the Internet is down. Some connections may have dropped packets, which can cause a momentary drop-out of voice. There is an important consideration regarding emergency calls. Due to the difficulty of locating a VoIP caller geographically, a 911 call may not be easily routed to a nearby contact center. The Federal Communications Commission (FCC) has taken steps to require that providers of VoIP services meet Enhanced 911 obligations (E911 systems automatically provide to emergency service personnel a 911 caller's callback number and, in most cases, location information) (FCC, 2008). As this technology matures, it is expected to continue to improve quality and performance (Anderson, 2006).

The contact center or remote nurse who uses VoIP must ensure there is enough available network bandwidth to transmit the voice packets. There may also be issues with reliability because VoIP service is down whenever the Internet is down.

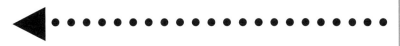

Automated Call Distributors (ACDs)

An Automated Call Distributor (ACD) is a computer-based system that routes calls. ACDs also collect various data regarding the volume and distribution of calls. The ACD works by routing calls based on the availability of agents or nurses. If an appropriate person is not available to take the call, the ACD holds the call in a queue (waiting system). The ACD also distributes the calls evenly among the available staff and collects statistics.

Statistics can include the caller's wait time in the queue before his/her call was answered, how many callers hung up instead of waiting, the length of the call, the number of calls received, and individual agent statistics. This data is used for decisions regarding staffing during peak and low-call times, productivity, and efficiency issues. Physician offices have implemented ACDs as a method of tracking their call volumes and improving processes in their office. Many physician offices have even moved beyond the ACD and are using call routing systems.

Call Routing

Call routing systems are routinely used in many contact centers and physician offices. With this technology, the caller uses voice commands or a touch-tone phone to navigate through the phone system. Call routers move calls quickly to the most appropriate person. For example, when a caller dials the physician's office, the caller hears: "For routine appointments, press 1. If you are having symptoms, press 2. For test results or medications, press 3. For all other calls, please stay on the line." After the caller enters a choice on a touch-tone phone or responds verbally to the prompts, the call is routed to the pre-designated person or phone extension. With successful call routing, a patient with symptoms can speak with the nurse directly instead of first having to explain their reason for the call to the office receptionist, and then waiting for the call to be transferred to the nurse.

Call routing systems are routinely used in many contact centers and physician offices. With this technology, the caller uses voice commands or a touch-tone phone to navigate through the phone system. Call routers move calls quickly to the most appropriate person.

ACDs and call routers are also used for prioritizing calls. In many settings, symptom-based calls receive priority answering over prescription requests and refills. The systems may be designed so callers can leave messages on an answering machine if the appropriate person is not available.

Computer Telephone Integration (CTI)

Another advancement in telephone technology is the use of computer telephone integration (CTI). This is the linking of voice (telephone) and data (computer) systems to allow data to be passed or shared between systems and correctly connecting a telephone call. CTI technology is used in banks when a person uses a touch-tone phone and enters his/her bank account number and personalized identification number (PIN) to check the account balance. Health care organizations use this technology for patients

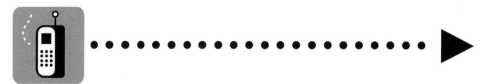

desiring to automatically check their patient account balance. Another example of CTI use is for patients who are members of a wellness program that provides telephone triage and care coordination by membership only. The patient uses the touch-tone phone to enter the membership number, and within milliseconds, the telehealth nurse has the demographic and patient information on the computer screen. The nurse can even greet the patient by name, if desired.

Outbound Dialing Systems

Telephone technology has advanced beyond the outbound telephone appointment and reminder systems. The original systems automatically placed outbound calls to patients via a power dialer. These systems gave scripted reminder messages to patients about their upcoming appointments.

Reminder systems now include technological linkages into other databases. For example, there are systems that read the pharmacy record and analyze if a patient has not refilled prescriptions as frequently as prescribed. If so, the provider is notified and makes treatment plans accordingly. Outbound dialing reminder systems are also being used to remind patients when it is time for immunizations, flu shots, mammograms, prostate examinations, etc. Some systems even track abnormal laboratory results and alert providers if the patient has not called to schedule further treatments or appointments.

There are also outbound systems on the market that query a series of health questions. The patient responds by using a touch-tone phone. For instance, an outbound dialer may be programmed to ask the patient to key in the blood sugar results for the day as well as ask the patient to rank how he/she feels. This data is collected, graphed, and analyzed by nurses and others so that patient care is managed more proactively.

Another outbound dialer example would be one for smoking cessation participants, which gives positive feedback and words of encouragement on a consistent basis. By having proactive contact, these new non-smokers have an increased success rate (Fiore et al., 2000).

Health care organizations throughout the United States are using outbound dialers for assistance in improving the health status of the populations that they serve. Telehealth practice nurses in these settings have expanded their roles to include the monitoring and analysis of the patient results. Nurses utilize these systems as part of their care coordination role in telehealth practice nursing.

Inbound Access Systems

Inbound access systems allow patients to gain access to laboratory or test results by using a personalized access code. This technology is similar to voice mail systems, with patients having their own temporary mailbox.

Health care organizations throughout the United States are using outbound dialers for assistance in improving the health status of the populations that they serve. Telehealth practice nurses in these settings have expanded their roles to include the monitoring and analysis of the patient results.

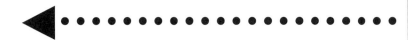

Health care providers have inbound access systems, an efficient tool for providing laboratory results to patients. The benefits include:

* The patient dials in for test results during a time that is most convenient.
* The patient receives a personalized message from his/her provider with health care information and education.
* The provider staff does not have to perform as many outbound calls trying to reach patients.

Telehealth practice nurses may have contact with these patients after they have dialed into the system. This is common when there is an option to speak to a nurse at the end of the message. Nurses may provide further information as well as detailed education and health tips. The nurses also mail out printed materials containing health information so the patient can understand his/her disease process.

Another example of an inbound access system is an automated voice response system for managing diabetes. Automated systems are being implemented when the cost of one-to-one provider-patient phone monitoring is no longer cost effective or efficient. Once patients are identified, the system is coded specifically for that patient to access.

The inbound access system is designed to receive inbound calls from patients, 24 hours a day, 7 days a week. When the patient calls, the system asks a series of questions. The algorithm questions continue based on the patient's answers, which are keyed in with the touch-tone phone. If any of the responses indicate a need for immediate medical attention, the system notifies the health care provider at the end of the call. Encounter data is collected and becomes a part of the patient's medical record. Additionally, the patient has the option of speaking with a health care provider (such as the nurse) if desired. For example, studies have shown that self-reporting programs appear to be effective for HbA1c levels monitoring among youth and adults (Chu-Weininger, Esquivel, Knowles, & Dunn, 2007). Telehealth practice nurses are involved with this type of technology by being available to answer incoming calls from, or proactively conduct outbound calls to patients when blood sugars are abnormal. Telehealth practice nurses may also collaborate with the other health care providers in coordinating the care of these patients.

Telephone Technology Tips
* Automatic Call Distributors, Call Routers, and Computer Telephone Integration help improve call-handling efficiencies. Yet, it is very important that telephone systems are patient-focused and customer-friendly.

Telehealth practice nurses may have contact with patients after they have dialed into the system. Nurses may provide further information as well as detailed education and health tips. The nurses also mail out printed materials containing health information so the patient can understand his/her disease process.

❖ With the implementation of new technology in telehealth practice settings, there must be a commitment to quality and ongoing improvement.

❖ Before implementing any telephone changes, it is important to analyze who will use the system. For example, foreign language options may be helpful in an "English-as-a-second-language" population.

❖ When a patient is affected by telehealth technology changes, the practice should inform the patients beforehand of this change. Office staff can share this information in person with patients when they come in for office visits or by communicating the change via posters, or a mailing.

❖ Changes should be communicated to patients by many different avenues and more than once. The majority of callers are willing to accept new technology if informed and given an explanation on the benefit of the change along with adequate time to adapt.

❖ When utilizing call routing, there should be a very limited number of options for the caller. The general rule of thumb is not to provide more than 3 or 4 "press" options.

❖ If a symptom-based call is not answered immediately and goes into the queue system, a message should instruct the patient to "call 911 if this is an emergency situation."

❖ The phone system should be designed only after understanding why patients are calling and analyzing their needs for information via the telephone.

❖ Data should be collected in order to find high volume and high-risk issues. Once collected, a telephone specialist can assist with designing the most appropriate prioritization and routing of the calls.

❖ Calls must be routed so the patient never ends up orbiting around the telephone world by being "stuck in the queue." In other words, if the nurse is not available to take incoming calls (such as during the lunch hour), the calls should go to another person.

❖ Caution should be taken when allowing callers to leave messages on voicemail for the nurse. If symptom-based messages are left on voicemail, callers must be informed how soon a nurse will be able to respond to their message. In addition, callers should be given an additional message of what to do if they cannot wait for the return phone call.

❖ If calls are recorded, the caller must be informed at the beginning of the call that their call may be recorded for quality assurance or other reasons.

❖ Message systems need to be designed so the nurse is alerted when there are messages in need of a response. The telehealth nurse must have standards in place to assist in prioritizing his/her calls based

Calls must be routed so the patient never ends up orbiting around the telephone world by being "stuck in the queue." In other words, if the nurse is not available to take incoming calls (such as during the lunch hour), the calls should go to another person.

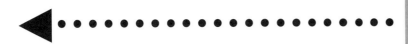

on severity and respond to these messages in a timely manner. It is imperative that messages not build up for extended lengths of time while continuing to take other incoming calls in rapid succession.

❖ As automated systems are installed for the giving and receiving of test results, providers must develop procedures so patients are not at risk when there are abnormal test results.

❖ Ongoing daily, weekly, and monthly analysis of the data received from the phone system needs to be completed. With the implementation of telephone hardware, there should also be a commitment to improve patient care delivery and various telephone reports can provide information for quality improvement changes.

❖ Patients should be surveyed on their satisfaction of call handing changes. Patients feel valued when they can provide input to changes. Additionally, it is important to receive input from callers in order to ensure they will use the service and be satisfied that their needs are met. Many times, the nurse is the first person a customer (patient) has contact with in the health care organization. If the caller has a poor experience, they may form a negative opinion about the entire organization.

❖ Patients need to feel assured that their medical information is kept confidential with any new call handling technology. Additionally, patients need to be acknowledged that they are being treated as an individual person and are valued. Patients will be extremely dissatisfied if they develop the impression that their calls are simply part of a mass production for handling phone calls.

❖ Processes must be developed to ensure that patients are receiving the correct information and are using the inbound or outbound system.

❖ Providers (including nurses) must be willing to evaluate the telephone data and patient satisfaction on a regular basis and make operational changes.

TELECOMMUTING

Many telehealth practice settings now have staff members that telecommute instead of coming into an office on a daily basis. These nurses take calls from their homes or at other sites and should have access to the telehealth database on a desktop computer or laptop with Internet connection, as well as a networked telephone service.

Remote nurses may be used because of high call volumes during peak hours or because it is more cost-effective to redistribute employees versus maintaining a large contact center space. The nurses may be working in the local geographic area or the system may have been designed for calls to overflow to other locations thousands of miles away.

Remote nurses may be used because of high call volumes during peak hours or because it is more cost-effective to redistribute employees versus maintaining a large contact center space.

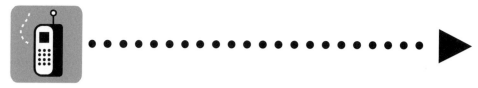

Tips and Issues

❖   Quality assurance and productivity measures must be in place for the remote staff as they are for the staff in the contact center.

❖   All telecommuting procedures must be focused on carefully guarding patient confidentiality.

❖   The nurse working remotely (including after hours) must create a secure and confidential office space allowing for private conversations out of range of other persons, including the nurse's own family members. Additionally, callers should never hear background noise, such as a dog barking, doorbell ringing, or child talking.

❖   The use of cellular phones for handling patient calls may be inappropriate because the conversation is transmitted across public lines.

❖   If modems, virtual private network (VPN), Citrix, terminal server, wireless connections, or other electronic methodologies are used for transmission of computer records, security measures such as firewalls must be used to prevent unauthorized access to records.

ELECTRONIC INTERFACES

As telehealth nursing expands, it will become necessary for patient information to be shared across health care delivery systems. Important patient data will no longer reside in *silos* of independent databases. For example, in many health care delivery systems, the patient's primary care physician may maintain a separate *(silo)* medical record that cannot be accessed by the centralized telehealth triage nurse, the care coordinator at the patient's health plan, or by the case manager of the hospital.

With silo systems, a patient could possibly call each of these nurse providers about a medical problem. The nurse would not know that the other has had contact with the patient. Additionally, each of the nurse providers could be using their silo's own set of clinical guidelines for medical care and decision-making. Sharing databases is essential in improving the care delivered. Telehealth nurses will be hearing more about clinical data repositories and data warehouses, not only for their health care organization, but also the national sharing of patient information throughout the United States.

Fortunately, some health care organizations are building new database technologies to help tear down silos by creating electronic interfaces. This allows users such as telehealth practice nurses to have access beyond their own database. In these settings, contact center nurses can view the medical chart and/or radiology and lab results from provider office visits or hospital admissions. Additionally, the telehealth nurses can view diagnoses, consultations, case management records, and treatment recommendations while communicating with their patients by telephone.

As telehealth nursing expands, it will become necessary for patient information to be shared across health care delivery systems. Important patient data will no longer reside in silos of independent databases.

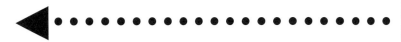

In some contact centers, interfaces are being written so the nurse's computerized documentation can be added to the patient's medical record even though they are in two different databases and computer systems. With these interfaces, there is decreased duplication of services and care because the care providers have access to patient information no matter where or how the interaction took place. Because of these interfaces, the patient has more coordinated and streamlined care. For example, while conversing with the telehealth practice nurse, the patient does not have to repeat detailed information about the office visit because the nurse is able to view this information on the computer. This helps facilitate an easy rapport with the patient, enabling the nurse to support the provider's care plan and increase patient compliance.

In some contact centers, interfaces are being written so the nurse's computerized documentation can be added to the patient's medical record even though they are in two different databases and computer systems.

Tips and Issues

❖ Telehealth practice nurses should proactively seek out new technology and know what technology is available in their facility in order to have the most complete information about their patients.

❖ By interacting with other health care organizations, ideas can be shared and knowledge gained to apply in other practice settings.

❖ There needs to be thoughtful consideration of what information is shared in an interface. Sharing of patient information increases the ability for continuity of care, but at the same time can increase the risk of breach of patient confidentiality.

INTERNET TECHNOLOGY

It is estimated that close to 71% (Internet World Stats, 2008) of United States households have access to the Internet. Within these households, health care information is a high priority for many. Because of this, most health care organizations are turning to the Internet as a method of enhancing their patient-provider relationships.

Health organizations are providing 24-hour, online access to their patients for health care information. By offering another avenue in which to communicate with patients, there may be an improvement in medical management. On an Internet Web site, a variety of medical topics may be offered by the health care facility, such as well-baby care, nutrition, and cancer-related issues. Additionally, online programs have been developed for patients to track their daily health status, medication use, and diet. The health care provider (including the nurse) should carefully monitor this information. Feedback is given to the patient electronically or by phone with the goal of increasing treatment compliance.

Consumers are connecting into their health care organization via the Internet to keep their personal medical records up to date. These authorized consumers access their medical data, including medications,

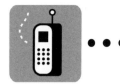

allergies, immunizations, and appointments. Security-tight systems are designed so patients can be more informed consumers. Another Internet offering is a system for the patient and provider to manage wellness and chronic disease together. Studies have shown that when consumers become more involved with the care management, they become more accountable for their health. As Internet capabilities expand for the management and care of patients, the nurse can be intimately involved in developing and utilizing online applications in order to monitor and manage patient outcomes.

Telehealth practice nurses are also connecting into their health care organizations' online electronic medical records remotely. These systems may contain the patient's history, progress notes, prescriptions, treatment ordering (including standing orders), and laboratory and radiological test results. Nurses access the patient's medical record by going into a security-tight password-protected system located inside the organization (Intranet) or outside (Internet). Since the nurse is able to obtain the medical record for the patient remotely, care can be provided in a more efficient and thorough manner both during office hours and after. Medical providers may also use this information in order to provide second-level assessment and advice after office hours.

Health organizations are integrating data to create personalized patient intervention profiles including health risk appraisals, inter-relationship assessments, laboratory results, medical claims, pharmacy usage, triage encounters, disease-state management, and utilization management. These informational tools will allow telehealth nurses the ability to provide personalized patient interventions based not only on the needs of their patients, but also on individual risks and specific patient histories.

The Internet provides a two-way benefit for the patient and the health care organization. Every patient appointment booked online means one less appointment booked manually. Every query handled electronically means one less phone call to field. This is a way for patients to be more involved in their own care (Baldwin, 2006).

The Internet provides a two-way benefit for the patient and the health care organization.

Although the number of Internet users is steadily increasing, there are still a great number of health care consumers who are not computer literate. Senior citizens lag far behind other groups in being able to access the Internet. Telehealth practice nurses may find that their most frequent voice customers are women, and that their most frequent Web customers are men. On the Web, men may be answering questions about their family's health, but may or may not be proactive in their care.

An issue occurring with Internet customers is the lack of verbal interaction with intonations and voice inflections. Telehealth practice nurses must be scrupulous in electronic communications so that their chosen words are not misinterpreted.

Secure portals have been developed for consumers to electronically "chat" with a nurse and receive health information and triage advice.

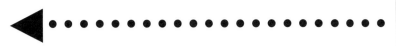

Some of these sites charge for their service while others provide the service as a commitment to their patients and community. Health care organizations have found that telehealth practice nurses have excellent skills for providing this type of Internet service. However, prior to implementing triage over the Internet or even providing medical information and advice, extensive research should be done on the legalities, patient rights, confidentiality, and appropriateness of the service.

Telehealth practice nurses need to be aware of what is being offered in their facility and what their callers want for service. For example, in a setting that is primarily urban with the majority of consumers having Internet access, nurses may find that Internet communications are an efficient way of enhancing patient-provider interactions. Conversely, if very few callers have access to the Internet, it would be inappropriate to provide exclusive types of health care information, education, and triaging via the Internet.

Telehealth practice nurses need to be aware of what is being offered in their facility and what their callers want for service.

Planning for Internet Services

❖ Begin gathering information about callers. How many have computers, modems, and access to email? Talk to your marketing and business planners who most often have a pulse on your community demographics.

❖ Be aware of who callers are, because there will always be two groups of people – the technologically savvy and those who are not.

❖ Begin learning more about callers. Are they interested in an Internet service? Would they feel comfortable using it?

❖ Be visionary in planning telehealth Internet services of the future by requesting hardware and software that has the capacity to grow with your contact center's various communication modalities.

❖ Network on a regular basis to see what other health care organizations are providing their patients. Look at their Web sites.

❖ Attend conferences to glean new ideas.

❖ Be aware of new services that competitors are offering to patients and offer services that are above and beyond.

Tips

❖ Development of an interactive Web site is a strategic initiative. However, stringent safeguards need to be designed to ensure privacy for patients. If the Internet is going to house any personal health information, security measures must be put in place so only the designated patient and his/her caregivers have access to that information.

❖ If health care instructions are given to a patient electronically, a method must be in place to verify receipt of the message and that

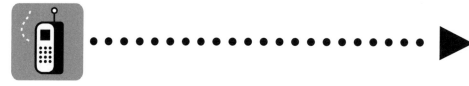

the recipient understands the education. Also, patients and providers must both keep in mind that the Internet is not a substitute for medical care but is used as an adjunct to care.

TELEMEDICINE

The current use of the telephone is already considered to be "low end" telecommunications technology. Telephones were once used to just transmit audio data from one party to another. Now telephones can record and transmit images as well as video. Computers and laptops now routinely come with attached cameras and software that allow consumers to transmit live or recorded video. By integrating technologies and special medical monitoring equipment, a patient can send online data (such as heart rate, blood pressure, temperature, blood sugar, and breathing levels) to providers. A patient simply attaches a heart rate clip to the finger, selects "monitor health" on the television, telephone, or computer screen, and the data is transmitted via the Internet. One location where this technology is being used is in retirement complexes, where older adults need more frequent routine monitoring of health, but not an actual provider visit.

Telemedicine goes beyond computers by integrating computers and telecommunication devices. Telemedicine includes the transmission of medical data via still picture images or actual video movements. One of the earliest telemedicine technologies available was the ability to transmit electrocardiograms across phone lines. For example, hospitals in rural settings utilized telemedicine by having a regional medical setting monitor patients on heart monitors. Other original uses of telemedicine included the ability for physician-to-physician consultations by transmitting x-rays and "still" pictures or images across telephone lines. Today, telemedicine has progressed and moved into the patient's living room, and it includes telehealth nurses. Home-based telemedicine includes not only telemonitoring, but also tele-interacting with patients. A variety of telemedicine devices are now available on the market. These include systems that transmit video images of patients in their homes to the telemedicine nurse located a few blocks or thousands of miles away. Medical peripheral devices (such as stethoscopes, oxygen saturation machines, three lead electrocardiograms [EKG], and blood pressure monitors) are then used for monitoring the patient. For example, the patient at home is given a series of prompts, such as placing the bell of the stethoscope over specific body landmarks (for example, on the apex and base of the lungs). Then, the telemedicine machine records and graphs the results.

Some "in-home" telemedicine systems have moveable video cameras so the telemedicine nurse can assess how a wound is healing or how an intravenous site looks. These images are transmitted back to the

By integrating technologies and special medical monitoring equipment, a patient can send online data (such as heart rate, blood pressure, temperature, blood sugar, and breathing levels) to providers.

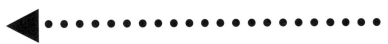

telemedicine office and stored as part of the patient's file. Additionally, these images can be reproduced and sent to a physician's office.

Telemedicine devices may include television-type "touch screens" or buttons that coach patients through procedures, such as central line dressing changes or the correct placement of EKG leads. Some systems even have health status questionnaires as part of their assessment. For example, a congestive heart failure patient could be asked to rank how short of breath he feels that day. He would key in the answer by choosing from a list on the touch-tone screen. The results would be transmitted to the telemedicine nurse for future clinical assessment and decision-making.

Other uses for telemedicine monitoring devices include monitoring of bone marrow transplants, immune deficiencies, neonatal conditions, cardiac disease, diabetes, chronic wounds, and other debilitating conditions with multiple co-morbidities. Patients using telemedicine systems can save time and energy by not needing to leave their homes to have a daily physical assessment. For the health care organization, more resources are available for the actual patient-provider interaction.

There are multiple approaches for health care providers utilizing home-based telemonitoring systems. One approach is through home health agencies where telemonitoring substitutes for home visits. One pilot study showed a 31% reduction in hospital readmission rates in a group of heart failure patients who were monitored remotely, compared to patients receiving usual care (American Heart Association, 2008). These substitute visits include the monitoring of basic vital signs and weight, teaching, and analysis of medication compliance. However, telemedicine cannot substitute for hands-on nursing care, such as occupational health assessment and extensive wound care.

Another use of telemonitoring is for disease management. Because of managed care and capitated fee arrangements, providers are motivated to provide high-quality care for the least amount of the health care dollar. By providing proactive access and monitoring of patients, as well as timely intervention when needed, studies have found that health care utilization costs can decrease by decreasing readmission rates and length of stay for those patients who do need to be admitted (American Heart Association, 2008).

Another use of telemonitoring is for disease management. Because of managed care and capitated fee arrangements, providers are motivated to provide high-quality care for the least amount of the health care dollar.

It is common knowledge that 20% of patients use 80% of the total health care dollars. Of these 20%, about 1% of the patients are considered the most high-risk, high users of health care dollars. Telemedicine is targeted to the top 1% of the patient population.

Additional health care statistics show that:
❖ 95% of the general population consumes 35% of health care dollars for general medical care, such as pap smears and prostate examinations.

- ❖ 4% of the general population consumes 30% of health care dollars because they have chronic diseases, such as hypertension, diabetes, etc.
- ❖ 1% of the general population consumes 35% of health care dollars because of being chronically and critically ill. This 1% can benefit from disease management, intense intervention, education, and family support. Telemedicine is ideal for the 1% of the population because these patients are "frequent flyers" into the emergency departments and high utilizers of health care resources (Institute of Medicine, 2001).

Many health care providers were initially concerned that telemedicine would be a cold and impersonal method of delivering health care. However, some of the positive responses to telemedicine show that the patient has more frequent and consistent access to the health care provider. Usually, a provider contacts the patient on a daily basis via video, and a unique relationship is formed because they see each other and share information face-to-face instead of just by telephone. Additionally, because these telemedicine patients have sophisticated health care tools in their homes and participate in their care, they see the effects of their care more readily.

Even though these are excellent benefits, telemedicine still causes some fundamental changes in the way that health care is delivered. Telemedicine causes a huge paradigm shift because these systems are extensions of the health care provider, yet it allows patients more freedom and decision-making in their care. Basically, telemedicine reverses care. Instead of waiting for the patient to contact the nurse, the nurse becomes proactive and contacts the patient on a regular basis.

Telemedicine is considered a proactive dimension beyond demand management. It offers a more informed and complete assessment rather than a telehealth assessment. It provides proactive education and information, allowing the patients to perform return demonstrations of skills in caring for wounds, catheters, etc.

Telemedicine is re-engineering the health care delivery system in the patient's home. There is improved patient outcome regarding access to care while decreasing hospital utilization rates (American Heart Association, 2008). Telehealth practice nurses have the skills and knowledge to be the providers of telemedicine-based home care. For example, when a patient with congestive heart failure calls with shortness of breath, this new technology can help the nurse assess the patient. The telemedicine nurse can read the home EKG, listen to the patient's heart and lung sounds, and visualize the patient's color on the video monitor. With this information, the nurse then can use decision support tools and critical decision-making skills to arrive at the most appropriate care for the patient.

Telemedicine is considered a proactive dimension beyond demand management. It offers a more informed and complete assessment rather than a telehealth assessment.

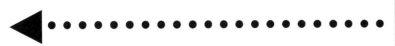

High-risk pregnancies managed at home using mobile ultrasound technology are another example of how telemedicine is easing access, increasing patient safety, and facilitating best practice. This technology is used for women who are well enough to stay home, yet need daily ultrasonography. The nurse assists the expectant mother in monitoring her care, similarly to how nurses provide fetal heart monitoring by phone today.

Remote parts of the country have a need for access to magnetic resonance imaging (MRI) and/or computerized tomography (CT) for head and body scans. Now this technology is made available via mobile CT and MRIs. The nurse can assess the patient further by interacting with him/her so that the provider can arrive at a diagnosis.

TECHNOLOGY OF THE FUTURE

Twenty years ago, it was nearly impossible for a patient to leave the hospital and administer his/her own intravenous antibiotics. Today, it is quite commonplace. In the world of tomorrow, there will be other new technologies available so patients can provide sophisticated care for themselves while staying in their homes. Some technological ideas that are currently being shaped and imagined are outlined below.

Video medicine. A tiny video camera is placed in the patient's home that can peer into ears and throats, and transmit images to a health care provider. This technology might become so commonplace that the camera replaces the need for office visits for minor illnesses (such as for ear pain or inflamed sore throats). The video camera will be an additional assessment tool for the nurse to use in addition to his/her decision support tools. The nurse could then use specific video decision support tools once the verbal and visual assessments are completed.

Soundwave stethoscopes. Advancing the technology of telemedicine stethoscopes, these stethoscopes would be programmed to interpret the sound waves heard when listening to the heart and lungs, and objectively classify wheezing and heart murmurs without human error. The nurses would be able to analyze these objective measurements, and along with verbal assessment and other technologies, arrive at the disposition of care.

Advanced medical image technology. Advanced medical image technology will create high-quality 2-dimensional and 3-dimensional image reformations from CT and MRI scans at a lower cost and at the same time offer tools for manipulation, appearance, measurement, views, history, and help. This technology will provide more information for better assessment and decision-making by providers. As with mobile scanners, nurses would utilize this tool for furthering assessment, answering questions and interacting with the patient so the provider can arrive at a diagnosis and options for treatment.

Twenty years ago, it was nearly impossible for a patient to leave the hospital and administer his/her own intravenous antibiotics. Today, it is quite commonplace. In the world of tomorrow, there will be other new technologies available so patients can provide sophisticated care for themselves while staying in their homes.

These are just a few of the technologies that might be fun to use. With each, there are implications for nurses to consider with encounter management and decision support tools. Telehealth practice opportunities will continue to grow as future technology changes and shapes health care.

OTHER TOPICS IN TELEHEALTH NURSING

Student Nurses

There is a new breed of student nurses who are interested in securing employment in the field of telehealth practice nursing. Many of these applicants have already worked in the customer service field, and have telephone and computer skills, as well as course work in telehealth nursing.

Some curricula now include clinical time in telehealth practice settings. Telehealth nurses may have the opportunity to provide this experience for student nurses.

Some nursing schools are now including telehealth concepts in their curriculum. The nursing students learn how to assess by telephone, use decision support tools for triaging, and how to provide education and information by telephone and electronically. Some curricula now include clinical time in telehealth practice settings. Telehealth nurses may have the opportunity to provide this experience for student nurses. With special headsets or telephone programming, the student nurse can participate in the telephone encounter. However, students are not licensed providers and should not be triaging patients.

Although student nurses and new nursing graduates have an understanding of triaging, they still need to develop critical thinking and judgment skills to accompany their education. Education on the fundamentals of telehealth nursing assessment and advice is not enough. A professional registered nurse who practices telehealth nursing must use critical thinking skills. These skills only come with experience and applied knowledge.

When hiring a new telehealth nurse, course work in telephone triage should never be considered a substitute for clinical experience. In other words, a new graduate nurse who has had telephone triage curriculum experience cannot be expected to function with the same critical thinking skills as a nurse with experience. It is recommended that a nurse have a minimum of 2 years of clinical nursing experience before beginning to work in a telehealth practice setting (Schmitt, 2004).

Alternative Medicine

As the world of health care moves from traditional medical management, nurses will need to transition their practice to keep up with change. There will be increasing practice standards, increasing legal issues, and significant changes in technology and health care.

Some nurses are already practicing in futuristic models, while others are just beginning to see the possibilities of providing telehealth assessment and advice. Some nurses are using technological

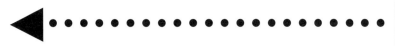

advancements, such as telemedicine and online applications, while others are just starting to consider using decision support tools for assessing patients.

Telehealth practice nursing is changing along with health care in general, with traditional medicine being integrated with holistic and alternative medicine. Part of this integration is due to consumers desiring alternative methods to improve their health outside of traditional medicine. Callers are contacting nurses to discuss therapies involving acupuncture, biofeedback, chelation, detoxification, enzymes, herbal medicine, hyperthermia, and hypnosis. These callers range from those who are just beginning to seek knowledge to those who are well-informed about alternative and naturopathic medicine.

Telehealth practice nurses need to keep up with these changes in medicine and apply them as appropriate to their practice. For instance, decision support tools in some telehealth practice settings now include herbal and alternative remedies for home care measures.

SUMMARY

Telehealth practice nurses must self-direct their scope of practice as health care communication moves beyond the telephone and into the Internet, telemedicine, video conferencing, and virtual medicine. It continues to be the telehealth nurse's responsibility to keep abreast of patient education and care management to integrate clinical information and multimedia technologies into patient care. These new communication methodologies and technologies will ease access to health care, medical information, and the delivery of quality medical care. Challenges remain and need to be addressed, such as reimbursement, health care organizations adapting to new technologies, privacy and security, information overload, and development of new standards.

Enhanced practice standards will need to include these telehealth technologies. Even so, practice standards must continue to be patient-centered. Telehealth nurses must be informed and seek out information on the ever-changing role of telehealth by following today's trends, as well as helping develop the future.

Telehealth practice nurses must self-direct their scope of practice as health care communication moves beyond the telephone and into the Internet, telemedicine, video conferencing, and virtual medicine.

TIPS & PEARLS

☎ A shift in recent years toward health care consumerism has created a need for tools that encourage consumers to become more self-directed, self-educated, and participatory in their health care and overall well-being.

☎ Telehealth nursing supports consumer health management through education and expert advice.

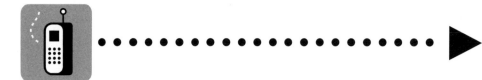

☎ The nursing contact center is evolving into a multi-media consumer service center that uses a variety of communication devices (such as voice, telephone, Internet, video, computer software, and print media) and will have access to shared data across health care delivery systems.

☎ Telemedicine integrates computers and telecommunication devices and includes the transmission of medical data via still picture images or actual video movements.

References

American Heart Association. (2008). *Remote monitoring improves heart failure patients health, may reduce readmissions* [Press release]. Retrieved February 27, 2009, from http://www.connected-health.org/media/1642 10/remote%20monitoring%20improves%20heart%20failure%20patients %20health%205.1.08.pdf

Anderson, N. (2006). *Some VoIP services surpass traditional phones.* Retrieved February 16, 2009, from http://arstechnica.com/business/news/2006/09/ 7806.ars

Baldwin, G. (2006, September 19). The connected patient. *HealthLeaders News.*

Chu-Weininger, M.Y.L., Esquivel, A., Knowles, L., & Dunn, K. (2007). *Telemedicine application in diabetes blood glucose monitoring: A systematic review* [PowerPoint presentation].

Federal Communications Commission (FCC). (2008). *FCC consumer advisory: VoIP and 911 service.* Retrieved February 16, 2009, from http://www. fcc.gov/cgb/consumerfacts/voip911.html

Fiore, M.C., Bailey, W.C., Cohen, S.J., Dorfman, S.F., Goldstein, M.G., Gritz, E.R., et al. (2000). *Quick reference guide for clinicians: Treating tobacco use and dependence.* Rockville, MD: U.S. Department of Health and Human Services.

Institute of Medicine. (2001). *Crossing the quality chasm: A new health system for the 21st century.* Washington, DC: National Academies Press.

Internet World Stats. (2008). *Internet usage statistics for the Americas: Population and telecom reports.* Retrieved February 13, 2009, from http://www.internetworldstats.com/stats2.htm

MacStravic, R.S., & Montrose, G. (1998). *Managing health care demand.* Gaithersburg, MD: Aspen Publishers.

Schmitt, B.D. (2004). *Pediatric telephone advice* (3rd ed.). Philadelphia: Lippincott Williams & Wilkins.

Suggested Reading

Kordoyanni, M. (2006, May 31). Consumerism in healthcare: Changing the healthcare landscape. *Pharmaceutical Business Review.*

Answer/Evaluation Form
Continuing Nursing Education Activity
Telehealth Nursing Practice Essentials
Chapter 9: Technology and Other Topics

AMBP9c07

This activity provides 1.2 contact hours of continuing nursing education (CNE) credit in nursing.
(Contact hours calculated using a 60-minute contact hour.)

This test may be copied for use by others.

COMPLETE THE FOLLOWING:

Name: _____

Address: _____

City: _____ State: _____ Zip: _____

Telephone number: (Home)_____ (Work)_____

Email address:_____

AAACN Member Number and Expiration Date: _____

Processing fee: AAACN Member: $12.00
                 Nonmember: $20.00

Answer Form: (Please attach a separate sheet of paper if necessary.)
1. What did you value most about this activity?

_____
_____
_____
_____

2. If you could imagine that you have fully integrated your learning into practice, what would be different about your present practice?

_____
_____
_____
_____

Evaluation	Strongly disagree				Strongly agree
3. The offering met the stated objectives.					
a. Describe future changes in telehealth and the impact on nursing practice.	1	2	3	4	5
b. Describe some of the technology used in telehealth nursing.	1	2	3	4	5
4. The content was current and relevant.	1	2	3	4	5
5. The content was presented clearly.	1	2	3	4	5
6. The content was covered adequately.	1	2	3	4	5

7. How would you rate your ability to apply your learning to practice following this activity? (Check one)

☐ Diminished ability ☐ No change ☐ Enhanced ability

8. Time required to complete reading assignment and answer form: ___ minutes
Comments _____
_____

I verify that I have completed this activity:

_____
Signature

Objectives

This educational activity is designed for nurses and other health care professionals who provide telehealth care for patients. This evaluation is designed to test your achievement of the following educational activities.
1. Describe future changes in telehealth and the impact on nursing practice.
2. Describe some of the technology used in telehealth nursing.

Evaluation Form Instructions

1. To receive continuing nursing education (CNE) credit for individual study after reading the indicated chapter(s), please complete the evaluation form (photocopies of the answer form are acceptable). Attach separate paper as necessary.
2. Detach (or photocopy) and send the answer form along with a check, money order, or credit card payable to *AAACN* East Holly Avenue/Box 56, Pitman, NJ 08071-0056. You may also send this form as an email attachment to ambp401@ajj.com.
3. Answer forms must be postmarked by December 31, 2011. Upon completion of the answer/evaluation form, a certificate for 1.2 contact hours will be awarded and sent to you.

Payment Options
☐ Check or money order enclosed (payable in U.S. funds to AAACN)

☐ MasterCard ☐ VISA ☐ American Express

Credit Card #:_____

Expiration Date: _____ Security Code:_____

Card Holder (Please print):

_____

Signature:

_____

This educational activity has been co-provided by the American Academy of Ambulatory Care Nursing (AAACN) and Anthony J. Jannetti, Inc. (AJJ).
AAACN is a provider approved by the California Board of Registered Nursing, Provider Number CEP 5336.
AJJ is accredited as a provider of continuing nursing education by the American Nurses Credentialing Center's Commission on Accreditation.
This book was reviewed and formatted for contact hour credit by Sally S. Russell, MN, CMSRN, AAACN Education Director, and Maureen Espensen, MBA, BSN, RN, Editor.

American Academy of Ambulatory Care Nursing
East Holly Avenue/Box 56, Pitman, NJ 08071-0056
Phone: 800-AMB-NURS; Fax: 856-589-7463
Web: www.aaacn.org; Email: aaacn@ajj.com

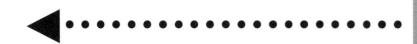

CHAPTER 10
Care of the Telehealth Nurse

Objectives

1. Recognize that self-care is important in order to provide optimal telehealth nursing.
2. Identify sources of telehealth stress and basic methods to more effectively deal with stress.
3. Describe an ergonomic work environment and identify basic steps to transform personal workspace.

There is no doubt that telehealth nursing practice is much more than "talking on the telephone" all day. It is an ongoing process of adapting the traditional nursing process and communication skills to meet the needs of unseen patients. The delivery of health care and nursing care to meet patients' needs is stressful. To be consistently successful in telehealth nursing, the nurse must be able to adapt to diverse expectations and demands. Simply by answering the telephone, the nurse's alarm system is triggered to deal either positively or negatively to the anticipated stress. Typically, nurses fail to acknowledge their own personal needs because of continually focusing their energy on providing care for others. If this behavior continues, the delivery of quality nursing care will be compromised. Additionally, consistently high levels of stress will have negative effects on the nurse's physical and psychological well-being, as well as potentially affecting personal relationships. This chapter is devoted to identifying potential stress specific to telehealth nursing practice with recommendations to minimize the effect. This information is included to encourage all nurses to take care of a very essential component of telehealth nursing practice – the nurse.

Successful nursing relies upon intellectual, clinical, and technical competencies. In addition, the nurse must be proficient in interpersonal skills in order to foster a trusting relationship with the patient. As discussed in other chapters, effective communication is essential in delivering telehealth nursing care. Even a nurse who excels in each of these competencies will be hindered in his/her relationship with the patient if not physically and mentally prepared to meet the challenges of telehealth nursing. Stress will affect the nurse's physical motor skills and critical thinking skills. Competency associated with such skills often influences the nurse's adaptability and coping techniques. The best way for nurses to manage stress is to take control of managing themselves. The first step in this process is identifying the source of stress – physical, emotional, or

Successful nursing relies upon intellectual, clinical, and technical competencies. In addition, the nurse must be proficient in interpersonal skills in order to foster a trusting relationship with the patient.

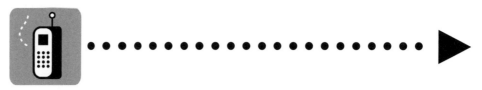

psychological. The nurse can then be prepared to employ one of a variety of strategies to minimize the effect of stress on personal competencies and delivery of quality nursing care.

SOURCES OF STRESS

American workers report that job stress makes them discontent and less productive. A primary reason that people leave their jobs is because of stress. The nurse engaged in telehealth nursing might identify with this because of continuous encounters with various stressors. The requirement to listen attentively to each patient is demanding; when coupled with the repeated expectation of processing information accurately, stress becomes a constant. The nurse's coping skills for stress are further challenged by unknown call volumes, limited sensory perception, ergonomic issues, and inability to follow the patient through the care continuum. The telehealth practice nurse rarely hears about the patient's ultimate outcome unless it is negative feedback.

Physical Stress

With the evolution of technology, nursing skills have become more diverse. Computers have made it possible to process, transfer, and file information efficiently within the work place. However, working with enhanced technology may result in physically stressing work. A significant portion of telehealth nursing in ambulatory care settings (such as a physician's office or call center) requires the nurse to remain stationary. Sitting in one place for extended periods of time places a great deal of physical stress on the neck, back, and legs throughout the day. An awkward posture and repetitive motion will lead to fatigue and discomfort. Over time, these factors will result in Repetitive Motion Injuries (RMIs), also called Cumulative Trauma Disorders (CTDs). To avoid suffering any of these conditions, nurses need to examine their workstations. This includes the desk, chair, and placement of the computer, resource materials, office supplies, and telephone. In addition, nurses must identify proper body positioning and use equipment appropriately to minimize physical stress. The goal is to adjust the workstation to the nurse rather than adjusting the nurse to the workstation.

The nurse should avoid cradling the telephone receiver between the chin and shoulder. This causes musculoskeletal strain on the neck, shoulders and back. Awkward twisting of the body and reaching for items may seem comfortable. Over time, physical symptoms associated with overextension, repetitive force, and muscle tension will result. Carpal tunnel syndrome is a well-documented work-related injury. Any repetitive action can eventually cause pain, resulting in physical and psychological stress. Additional posture problems include slumped shoulders, lack of

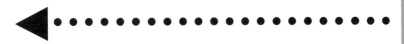

lumbar support, crossed legs, and dangling feet. Again, what may seem like a comfortable position could be causing damage to joints and supporting structures. The nurse's body will feel the stress of telehealth practice from improper positions, limited movement, or tension from a call situation. Muscles with prolonged contraction and stress become fatigued, which affects the circulation to the muscles. In addition, during stressful situations, the nurse's breathing becomes rapid and shallow, thereby lowering the body's level of available oxygen. This can exacerbate muscle tension and fatigue.

Psychological Stress

How the nurse is equipped to adapt and cope with all sources of stress affects the nurse's overall effective delivery of telehealth nursing care. Ineffectual coping may manifest itself with physical symptoms, such as headaches, ulcers, abdominal pain, or other body pains that cannot be linked to attributing physical symptoms. Each nurse needs to be constantly aware of the risk of ineffective coping with job-related stress. The nurse should periodically evaluate his/her psychological stress level, and there are a variety of methods and tools available for this purpose. Tools used to evaluate psychological stress levels typically ask questions such as:

❖ Is eating a planned, relaxed event, rather than wedged between other activities?
❖ Are you frequently feeling run down or ill?
❖ Is exercising part of your daily routine?
❖ Are you able to sleep soundly at night?
❖ Are you able to decline new tasks and maintain sense of control?

Muscles with prolonged contraction and stress become fatigued, which affects the circulation to the muscles. In addition, during stressful situations, the nurse's breathing becomes rapid and shallow, thereby lowering the body's level of available oxygen. This can exacerbate muscle tension and fatigue.

Call Encounter Stress

A primary source of emotional stress for the nurse is the desire to have each encounter result in a perfect outcome. In teleheath nursing practice, the nurse often has considerable influence and responsibility in directing the patient to appropriate care. However, despite the best efforts of the nurse, not all encounters result in the perfect outcome. Regardless of how infrequently this may occur, it can remain one of the most unsettling sources of stress for the nurse. Barriers to the perfect outcome for which the nurse hopes to attain include:

❖ *Noncompliant patient.* The patient will not follow the appropriate recommendation for care, no matter how dire the consequences of noncompliance.
❖ *Negative outcomes.* Not limited to but including the death of the patient, even when it is predictable. The patient may not want to seek additional medical intervention.

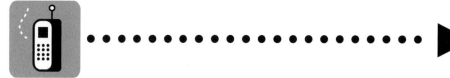

❖ *Lack of patient accommodation or support by the health care system.* When the nurse is unable to secure appropriate resources for the patient; lack of medical supplies or homecare support; or barriers to an appointment in the physician's office.

❖ *Codependency.* When the patient does not want a solution, but only wants to include the nurse in the problem.

Shiftwork Stress

Another common factor affecting the telehealth nurse is the fact that many call centers are open 24 hours a day. This means that many nurses are required to take calls during non-traditional working hours. For many, this could be the first time the nurse has had to work a non-traditional shift. This may create stress for the nurse as well as the nurse's family.

The biggest source of stress is the nurse's ability to sleep effectively. Loss of sleep can lead to a variety of adverse health conditions. The challenge for most is sleeping while one's family is awake and demanding attention. Noelcke (2008) offers the following suggestions to stay well-rested:

❖ Go to sleep as soon as you can after work.
❖ Don't get caught up in chores, errands, and scheduling. Save these for later, when you can devote your full attention to them.
❖ Come home from work and relax in the bath with a book. Then hit the hay.
❖ Avoid caffeine. It may help you make it through your shift, but if you drink caffeine too close to bedtime, you will have a difficult time getting to sleep.

Noelcke also cautions against the use of sleeping aids. They offer a temporary solution, but can cover up larger problems. There is the same caution related to alcohol. She asserts, "It might make you sleep faster, but you won't sleep as soundly."

In each of these examples, the nurse is extremely challenged by aspirations to control and direct the patient in order to have the reassurance of the perfect outcome. This challenge is partially due to the inability of the nurse to direct the outcome to be what is desired, but it is also due to the inability to predict when such events will occur. The nurse is aware of the needed actions to arrive at the appropriate outcome; however, the nurse may not have enough influence over the patient or the health care system for the desired outcome to occur. Even though the nurse has received adequate training and has resources at his/her disposal, the nurse is not prepared for the imperfect outcome and the stress that follows. This results in an overwhelming sense of frustration, guilt, disenchantment, and eventual apathy.

Another common factor affecting the telehealth nurse is the fact that many call centers are open 24 hours a day. This means that many nurses are required to take calls during non-traditional working hours.

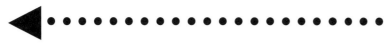

REDUCING STRESS

Role Preparation

Telehealth nursing practice is much more than talking on the telephone all day. Indeed, it is an ongoing process of adapting the traditional nursing process and communication skills to meet the needs of unseen patients. Telehealth nursing practice requires a special blend of communication skills, nursing practice, and the love of helping people who are reaching out through a non-traditional means of medical care. To be consistently successful in telehealth nursing, the nurse must be able to adapt to diverse expectations and demands. Frequently, the telehealth nurse is talking on the telephone, thinking of assessment questions, documenting the call, and planning the care of the patient. For the experienced telehealth nurse, these functions will blend and become almost one seamless action, but new telehealth nurses may find this very stressful. Although actively engaged in a telephone call, the nurse's attention may also be focused on other patient calls taken during the current work shift. The nurse may also be receiving orders from physicians in response to patient calls.

Not all nurses find this form of nursing practice satisfying. Some nurses still feel that it is not "nursing" when face-to-face contact with the patient is not established. Many who have moved from an inpatient setting into telehealth nursing are surprised at the number of nursing decisions that must be made simply by "handling patient telephone calls." Preparation for this type of nursing should include a detailed orientation to telehealth nursing, participating in role playing, reviewing calls, and documenting and researching clinical information on specific patient populations. During orientation, the new telehealth nurse must recognize that the learning curve is steep and learning is ongoing.

Before a nurse accepts a position in telehealth nursing, it is important to consider the various aspects of the job for the "right fit." Lack of fit can be a major source of stress on the job. The nurses should learn about its challenges, educate themselves regarding the transfer of skills, and be able to recognize when it is not the best fit.

PHYSICAL COMFORT

The nurse can decrease physical stress by adjusting his/her work environment. An ergonomic assessment of the work area should be completed along with individualized recommendations on ergonomics for each nurse. Additionally, the nurse may work with administration in developing an appropriate ergonomic environment by making structural and equipment changes. Changes needed may include: replacing worn out or outdated chairs, improving lighting, and updating workstations to accommodate computers. Research by Griffiths, Mackey, and Adamson

Telehealth nursing practice requires a special blend of communication skills, nursing practice, and the love of helping people who are reaching out through a non-traditional means of medical care. To be consistently successful in telehealth nursing, the nurse must be able to adapt to diverse expectations and demands.

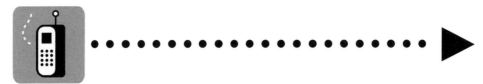

(2007) indicates that work organization is a characteristic of the work environment and deals with the way work is structured and processed, including hours of work, task complexity, skill and effort, job control, and work/break schedules.

Body Position

Poor posture can contribute to physical stress. It is easier to prevent physical stress than to resolve it once it occurs. Good body posture (alignment) is key to minimizing physical stress throughout the workday. Specific adjustments to body position and work equipment will help create a more supportive physical environment. Common recommendations made by ergonomic experts include the following (all of which may be within the nurse's control):

❖ Adjust the chair height so the knee joints form a 90-degree angle with the feet resting on the floor. If it is not possible to lower the chair height, consider placing a step stool or box under the feet.
❖ Adjust the chair backrest so it supports the lumbar curvature of the spine.
❖ Adjust the seat depth so the nurse's knees are at least two to three inches beyond the front of the chair to prevent obstruction of popliteal area.
❖ Adjust the chair armrests to keep the forearms parallel to the floor. The shoulders need to be relaxed with the wrists in a neutral position.
❖ Adjust the keyboard height so the arms and elbows are supported. The wrists and hands should be aligned in a neutral position on top of the keyboard.
❖ Adjust the position and height of the computer monitor so that the neck is kept in a neutral position.
❖ Adjust the chair to the keyboard distance so the shoulders are straight and not rolled forward.
❖ Create an organized workspace in order to have resources (telephone, pens, notepads, books, etc.) within normal reach without overextending, twisting, or bending in an awkward fashion.
❖ Use a headset for conversing with callers rather than the handset. This reduces strain on the neck, shoulders, and back, and it frees both hands for other tasks.

Stretching and Exercise

Even with the best ergonomic workstation and excellent body positioning, the nurse may still need to reduce physical tension throughout his/her shift by implementing a variety of stretching and other exercises. By stretching, the nurse can begin to relieve the muscle tension disseminated throughout the body. Additionally, exercise is probably one

Poor posture can contribute to physical stress. It is easier to prevent physical stress than to resolve it once it occurs. Good body posture (alignment) is key to minimizing physical stress throughout the workday.

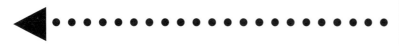

of the most effective ways to reduce muscle tension, in and outside of work. While at work, the nurse should take mini-breaks by simply getting up and standing or walking around the immediate area. By changing positions periodically, muscles are stimulated and will benefit from improved circulation and oxygenation.

The WebMD, Inc. (2007) offers the following stretching exercises that one can perform from their desk:

❖ **Just stand up and sit down—no hands.**
   1. Stand up and sit down while talking on the phone (no one will know).
❖ **Shrug your shoulders to release the neck and shoulders.**
   1. Inhale deeply and shrug your shoulders, lifting them high up to your ears. Hold. Release and drop. Repeat three times.
   2. Shake your head slowly, yes and no.
❖ **Loosen the hands with air circles.**
   1. Clench both fists, stretching both hands out in front of you.
   2. Make circles in the air, first in one direction to the count of ten.
   3. Then reverse the circles.
   4. Shake out the hands.
❖ **Stretch your back with a big hug.**
   1. Hug your body, placing the right hand on your left shoulder and the left hand on your right shoulder.
   2. Breathe in and out, releasing the area between your shoulder blades.
❖ **Do leg extensions.**
   1. Grab the seat of your chair to brace yourself and extend your legs straight out in front of you so they are parallel to the floor.
   2. Flex and point your toes five times. Release.
   3. Repeat.
❖ **Substitute walks for email.**
   1. Instead of emailing a colleague, walk over and talk to him/her whenever possible.

In addition to these stretching exercises at work, any form of exercise outside of work will assist the nurse to feel more relaxed and healthy. To maximize results, ease into an exercise program to gradually build stamina and strength. Some discomfort may occur, especially if stiffness and/or weakness were already present. However, the nurse should remember that if any exercise causes pain or discomfort, he/she should discontinue the exercises and re-evaluate. As with any exercise program, the nurse should consult his/her personal physician prior to starting the program.

In addition to these stretching exercises at work, any form of exercise outside of work will assist the nurse to feel more relaxed and healthy.

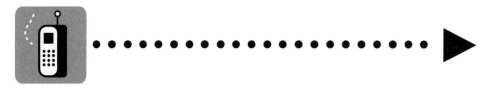

Eye Strain

Besides experiencing tension of the large muscle groups (such as the back), the nurse may also experience eyestrain. This most frequently occurs when the nurse is consistently focusing on a computer monitor throughout a shift. It is key to periodically relax the eyes and reduce eyestrain by redirecting eye focus for a few seconds to an object at least 20 feet away. Additionally, some other techniques to reduce eyestrain include:

- ❖ Rolling the eyes in all directions – up, down, around, and diagonally.
- ❖ Closing the eyes for 10-20 second intervals.
- ❖ Purchasing eyeglasses specifically designed for use with computers.
- ❖ Balancing the lighting in the environment and the computer screen.
- ❖ Adjusting the monitor controls so the contrast between the background and the screen display is adequate.
- ❖ Decreasing light reflection on the computer screen with glare screens, therefore reducing glare from overhead lights and windows.
- ❖ Filtering natural light with window covers or blinds.

Deep Breathing

Another common stress-relieving activity is deep breathing. The intent is to achieve relaxation of the chest and stomach muscles. As noted earlier, when a person is experiencing a stressful situation, breathing patterns become sub-optimal. Stale air is not exhaled effectively, and oxygenation of the tissues becomes incomplete. To avoid this, the nurse should check his/her breathing patterns throughout the day. This means before, during, and after high-pressure situations. If the nurse finds breathing is shallow and is feeling tense, he/she should take several deep, slow breaths:

- ❖ Slowly, deeply inhale through the nose, hold the breath, and then slowly exhale through the mouth.
- ❖ While focusing on breathing, reflect on current thoughts and feelings. Visualize relaxing.

Varying activity is often key to minimizing stress. When pressure begins to mount, take a 5 to 10 minute break to climb some stairs, close your eyes, or simply stretch beside your desk. Telehealth staffing plans should be appropriate not only to meet anticipated call volume, but also to prevent staff burnout. Because telehealth nursing can be fatiguing, shift lengths need to be considered when attempting to avoid burnout.

It is key to periodically relax the eyes and reduce eyestrain by redirecting eye focus for a few seconds to an object at least 20 feet away.

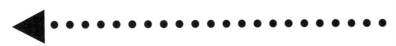

Work Environment – Noise Level

The noise level in the practice setting can increase the level of stress and affect the nurse's ability to work effectively. Besides the obvious concerns with privacy and confidentiality, noise can interfere with being able to focus on the call. Consider the following remedies:

❖ Create a workspace away from high-traffic, high-noise areas.
❖ During conversations with patients, direct your voice away from others in the work area.
❖ Lower the voice if talking to co-workers in the work area.
❖ Use bilateral headsets not only for comfort, but also to help decrease interference from background noise of the office.
❖ Use sound-absorbing partitions, wall coverings, and ceiling tiles to reduce extraneous office noise.
❖ Respect the work area used for telehealth-call handling, and do not use it for social congregating.

Personal Health

The health or wellness of the physical body plays a significant role in the psychological and emotional well-being of the telehealth nurse. The nurse must be as responsible and concerned for personal physical well-being just as much as the well-being of patients. Often, a nurse is so busy caring for patients and handling phone calls that personal physical needs are not considered. Meal breaks should consist of nutritious foods and be enjoyed in an environment conducive to enhancing digestion and providing an opportunity to refocus. There should be opportunity throughout the work shift to have an adequate fluid intake. Ignoring adequate food and fluid intake can result in a variety of physical symptoms, such as constipation or irritable bowel syndrome. By being certain to maintain hydration and eat a balanced diet, the nurse will feel physically better. In addition, the ability to fight off illness is supported by good diet.

The nurse should also consider his/her dietary intake before and after work. At all times, avoid fatty and refined sugar food products. These food types are considered quick energy boosts and will not sustain the body during stress. A commonly used stimulant is caffeine. The nurse should work to gradually eliminate or restrict the amount of caffeine intake. Ideally, water should replace beverages containing caffeine. Each of the above recommendations will offer a healthier defense against the effects of stress.

Not only is nutrition and hydration important in maintaining health and minimizing the effects of stress, but receiving adequate sleep each night is equally important. With reduced sleep, the nurse is ill-prepared to meet the challenges of the workday. This is especially critical to the nurse who

At all times, avoid fatty and refined sugar food products. These food types are considered quick energy boosts and will not sustain the body during stress.

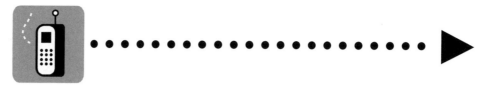

works the late shifts because there is a tendency to try to do more with less sleep. Sleep deprivation has a negative effect on the ability to cope and to use critical thinking skills effectively.

Just as the nurse urges patients to maintain optimal health and receive timely medical attention when indicated, so should the nurse. Often, due to the knowledge the nurse has, personal symptoms may be ignored or minimized until they become more pronounced. More aggressive medical treatments may be needed if the nurse does not seek early interventions. The wise nurse will also practice prophylactic health care by participating in recommended health screenings and immunizations to reduce health risks. Maintaining excellent health is by plan and not by accident, and it allows the nurse to perform at an optimal performance level.

PSYCHOLOGICAL COMFORT

Addressing Stress

Beyond techniques and exercises for physical discomfort, the nurse should be able to identify the core source(s) of psychological and emotional stress. The nurse may be prone to believe it is the fault of others or uncontrolled situations that causes stress. As such, the nurse may feel powerless to address the source of the stress being experienced. To effectively diminish stress, the nurse must first acknowledge responsibility for the emotional response to any given situation. Once this responsibility is recognized, the nurse is positioned to move toward addressing the sources of psychological and emotional stress.

State of Mind

There are constructive methods to cope when the nurse is in a mentally stressful situation. Although these methods may not bring relaxation and comfort to the mind as quickly as stretching allows for a tight muscle, there are ways to overcome the influence of psychological and emotional stress. The way the nurse thinks about a situation can influence whether or not he/she can successfully resolve a crisis. Developing a positive mental attitude and approaching a situation in small increments rather than the whole will often provide the momentum necessary to get through the situation.

One useful method to promote greater peace of mind requires a willingness to view the "big picture" and "not sweat the small stuff." The nurse should begin by setting priorities. The first step is to determine all current demands and develop an action plan to accomplish each task. By breaking a large task into smaller tasks, the nurse can feel more able to accomplish them. This also makes it easier to shift tasks around as priorities change. The nurse should consider delegating tasks to others as appropriate. By doing so, the nurse can further narrow the focus to more

To effectively diminish stress, the nurse must first acknowledge responsibility for the emotional response to any given situation. Once this responsibility is recognized, the nurse is positioned to move toward addressing the sources of psychological and emotional stress.

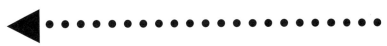

specific issues that demand nursing expertise and full attention. Working together in teams will often ease the stress that a nurse feels when working alone. While it is often difficult for nurses in telehealth practice to share or split work as a floor nurse might, there are opportunities to assist each other. If a nurse overhears a co-worker struggling with a particular call situation and it is his/her area of expertise, assistance may be offered rather than allowing the co-worker to struggle alone.

The nurse can even perform little things to develop and support a positive mental attitude and to reduce the stress level. The nurse needs to determine what can be done to enhance self-image and provide mental relaxation. This can be as simple as meeting a friend for lunch, getting a haircut or massage, or taking a long, relaxing bath or walk. Positive attitude and the ability to cope with stress are not limited to just when the nurse is at work. Typically, events at home and work together create the total climate to which the nurse responds. Balance in the nurse's personal life will help prepare for the work stressors and the ability to cope with the events of the workday.

An individual's choice of a career is often driven by the need to find purpose and position that allows them to experience a personal sense of value and worth. A clearer focus on the benefits that are provided to the patient by telehealth nursing might provide the nurse with a greater sense of respect and value. By reflecting on these benefits, the nurse can also gain positive emotional energy.

To further reduce or control stress, the nurse should take assigned breaks, especially after a particularly stressful call. This helps to clear the mind for a moment and get a fresh start. If it is impossible to physically leave the workstation, the nurse should take a mental break for a few moments.

Self-Affirmation

Self-affirmation relies on the nurse's conscious effort to affect the subconscious. The nurse should frequently repeat positive statements such as, "I can handle this situation," or "I am a good nurse," rather than play negative tapes over and over in his/her mind. By repeating positive statements frequently, it will support the nurse's ability to believe in his/her personal skills and self-worth. To accomplish this, the nurse may consider choosing an affirmation statement each day, memorizing it, and repeating it in spare moments. Alternatively, the nurse might develop a whole written list of affirmations that can be displayed in a visible location, particularly in the workspace. If the nurse finds it difficult to create these affirmation statements, there are a variety of books and articles available to develop personal self-affirmation statements. When belief becomes reality, a more positive attitude with less stress will be the result.

The nurse needs to determine what can be done to enhance self-image and provide mental relaxation. This can be as simple as meeting a friend for lunch, getting a haircut or massage, or taking a long, relaxing bath or walk.

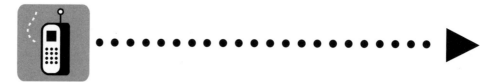

Self-Talk

Typically, self-talk occurs throughout the day, though the nurse may not be cognizant that it is occurring (see Table 10-1).

Table 10-1.
Examples of Destructive and Constructive Self-Talk

Destructive	Constructive
"I'll never get all of these calls done on time."	"If I stay focused and take one call at a time, I'll make steady progress."
"Why did I ever take this job? I'll never get any better at it."	"I am providing a beneficial service to others. I have learned so much already."
"This always happens to me!"	"Everyone must get into this type of challenging situation once in a while."

In each example, the nurse can choose how to react to a situation and what type of mental dialogue or self-talk will occur. This choice will determine how detrimental or supportive the self-talk is, and the nurse chooses to be his/her greatest fan or worst critic.

If the nurse first identifies how the majority of his/her negative self-talk is expressed, he/she can then work to change each negative statement to a more positive one. Scott (2007) offers the following methods to incorporate self-talk into the stress reduction routine:

If the nurse first identifies how the majority of his/her negative self-talk is expressed, he/she can then work to change each negative statement to a more positive one.

❖ **Journal Writing:** Whether you carry a journal around with you and jot down negative comments when you think them, write a general summary of your thoughts at the end of the day, or just start writing about your feelings on a certain topic and later go back to analyze it for content, journaling can be an effective tool for examining your inner process.

❖ **Thought-Stopping:** As you notice yourself saying something negative in your mind, you can stop your thought mid-stream my saying to yourself, "Stop." Saying this aloud will be more powerful, and having to say it aloud will make you more aware of how many times you are stopping negative thoughts, and where.

❖ **Rubber-Band Snap:** Another therapeutic trick is to walk around with a rubber band around your wrist; as you notice negative self-talk, pull the band away from your skin and let it snap back. It'll hurt a little, and serve as a slightly negative consequence that will both make you more aware of your

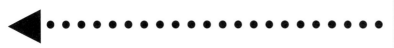

thoughts, and help to stop them. (Or, if you don't want to subject yourself to walking around with a rubber band on your wrist, you'll be even more careful to limit the negative thoughts!)

❖ **Milder Wording:** Have you ever been to a hospital and noticed how the nurses talk about 'discomfort' instead of 'pain?' This is generally done because 'pain' is a much more powerful word, and discussing your 'pain' level can actually make your experience of it more intense than if you're discussing your 'discomfort' level. You can try this strategy in your daily life. In your self-talk, turning more powerful negative words to more neutral ones can actually help neutralize your experience. Instead of using words like 'hate' and 'angry' (as in, "I *hate* traffic! It makes me so *angry*!"), you can use words like 'don't like' and 'annoyed' ("I don't like traffic; it makes me annoyed," sounds much milder, doesn't it?)

❖ **Change Negative to Neutral or Positive:** As you find yourself mentally complaining about something, rethink your assumptions. Are you assuming something is a negative event when it isn't, necessarily? (For example, having your plans cancelled at the last minute can be seen as a negative, but what you do with your newly-freed schedule can be what you make of it.) The next time you find yourself stressing about something or deciding you're not up to a challenge, stop and rethink, and see if you can come up with a neutral or positive replacement.

❖ **Change Self-Limiting Statements to Questions:** Self-limiting statements like "I can't handle this!" or "This is impossible!" are particularly damaging because they increase your stress in a given situation *and* they stop you from searching for solutions. The next time you find yourself thinking something that limits the possibilities of a given situation, turn it into a question. Doesn't "*How* can I handle this?" or "*How* is this possible?" sound more hopeful? Open up your imagination to new possibilities!

In your self-talk, turning more powerful negative words to more neutral ones can actually help neutralize your experience.

Once sensitive to self-talk, the nurse can work toward actively changing subconscious talk. The extent to which the nurse considers him/herself has a lot to do with how well the nurse can relate to patients and co-workers. Consequently, a positive self-image will improve performance and lower the nurse's stress level.

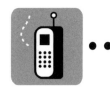

EMOTIONAL RESPONSE

The Crisis Call

At any time, the phone call can be an emergent or urgent situation that causes the nurse to manage a difficult clinical and emotional presentation. The caller may also be anxious, angry, or so ill that he/she loses control. The nurse may be required to exert a great deal of effort to respond in a professional and caring manner.

Of course, there will be times when regardless of the nurse's efforts, things will not go the way intended. In health care, there are negative, unpleasant, or unexpected outcomes. To address the emotions that will result from these types of encounters, nurses should consider:

❖ Acknowledging they are human, and that it is okay to feel emotions in response to a bad outcome.
❖ Engaging in supportive debriefing sessions with co-workers and/or managers.
❖ Preparing for similar situations by reviewing the encounter as part of the ongoing learning process.
❖ Seeking training and skill enhancement to be better equipped the next time similar events occur.

By using a variety of stress-reducing strategies, the nurse can feel in control, even when the situation is out of control. In this way, the nurse can avoid the dangers of personalizing and internalizing negative behaviors or outcomes.

By using a variety of stress-reducing strategies, the nurse can feel in control, even when the situation is out of control. In this way, the nurse can avoid the dangers of personalizing and internalizing negative behaviors or outcomes. However, even with the best coping and stress-busting skills, there may be times when further assistance is needed. This is especially important when the nurse is feeling that he/she can no longer deal with the stress being experienced. At these times, it is vital to seek professional assistance. The earlier the need for intervention is recognized, the sooner the healing can begin. There are many different kinds of professionals experienced in listening and suggesting interventions that can assist the nurse to come to terms with their emotional and psychological needs.

SUMMARY

The ability to perform quality telehealth nursing will often be challenged by a number of stressors. Each nurse's career can be viewed as an ongoing process of adapting to stressful situations. A nurse's degree of happiness and job satisfaction will depend on how successfully he/she can adapt and his/her ability to overcome stress.

Tension and stress are an inevitable part of nursing. For example, almost every ER nurse will acknowledge the "rush" from working in a

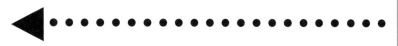

high-paced patient care environment. Most nurses will state that not every nurse is meant to be an ER nurse. The same is true for telehealth nursing. The patient care environment is challenging. Good patient assessment, communication, and interviewing skills are key to successful telehealth encounters, along with meeting and/or exceeding the expectations of the caller, while providing appropriate clinical interventions and remedies.

The intent of this chapter is not to diminish the existence of stress and tension in the role of the telehealth nurse, but to offer remedies and preventative measures that can effectively help the nurse minimize the effects. The end result should increase job satisfaction and the quality of the telehealth nurse's life.

Good patient assessment, communication, and interviewing skills are key to successful telehealth encounters, along with meeting and/or exceeding the expectations of the caller, while providing appropriate clinical interventions and remedies.

TIPS & PEARLS

☎ Nurses, in general, focus their energy on caring for others and fail to acknowledge their own personal needs.

☎ Stress in the work environment will affect the nurse's physical motor skills and critical-thinking skills.

☎ Job stress for telehealth nurses can result from a variety of factors, including call encounters with less than desirable outcomes or from working non-traditional shifts.

☎ Reducing stress through physical comforts (such as good ergonomics, stretching and exercise, deep breathing, and good personal health) and through psychological comforts (such as self-affirmation and constructive self-talk) will result in increased job satisfaction and quality of life.

References

Griffiths, K.L., Mackey, M.G., & Adamson, B.J. (2007). The impact of a computerized work environment on professional occupational groups and behavioural and physiological risk factors for musculoskeletal symptoms: A literature review. *Journal of Occupational Rehabilitation, 17*(4), 743-765.

Noelcke, L. (2008). *How to work the third shift and stay healthy.* Retrieved February 20, 2008, from http://www.sparkpeople.com/resource/wellness _articles.asp?id=217

Scott, E. (2007). *Reduce stress and improve your life with positive self talk.* Retrieved February 28, 2008, from http://stress.about.com/od/optimism spirituality/a/positiveselftak.htm

WebMD, Inc. (2007). Stretching exercises at your desk: 12 simple tips. Retrieved February 28, 2008, from http://www.webmd.com/fitness-exercise/features/stretching-exercises-at-your-desk-12-simple-tips?page= 2

Answer/Evaluation Form
AMBP9c08

Continuing Nursing Education Activity

Telehealth Nursing Practice Essentials

Chapter 10: Care of the Telehealth Nurse

This activity provides 1.2 contact hours of continuing nursing education (CNE) credit in nursing.
(Contact hours calculated using a 60-minute contact hour.)

This test may be copied for use by others.

COMPLETE THE FOLLOWING:

Name: _____

Address: _____

City: _____ State: _____ Zip: _____

Telephone number: (Home)_____ (Work)_____

Email address:_____

AAACN Member Number and Expiration Date: _____

Processing fee: AAACN Member: $12.00
                  Nonmember: $20.00

Answer Form: (Please attach a separate sheet of paper if necessary.)

1.   What did you value most about this activity?

_____
_____
_____
_____

2.   If you could imagine that you have fully integrated your learning into practice, what would be different about your present practice?

_____
_____
_____
_____

Evaluation	Strongly disagree				Strongly agree
3. The offering met the stated objectives.					
a. Recognize that self-care is important in order to provide optimal telehealth nursing.	1	2	3	4	5
b. Identify sources of telehealth stress and basic methods to more effectively deal with stress.	1	2	3	4	5
c. Describe an ergonomic work environment and identify basic steps to transform personal workspace.	1	2	3	4	5
4. The content was current and relevant.	1	2	3	4	5
5. The content was presented clearly.	1	2	3	4	5
6. The content was covered adequately.	1	2	3	4	5

7.   How would you rate your ability to apply your learning to practice following this activity? (Check one)

☐ Diminished ability ☐ No change ☐ Enhanced ability

8.   Time required to complete reading assignment and answer form: ___ minutes

Comments _____
_____

I verify that I have completed this activity:

_____
Signature

Objectives

This educational activity is designed for nurses and other health care professionals who provide telehealth care for patients. This evaluation is designed to test your achievement of the following educational activities.

1.   Recognize that self-care is important in order to provide optimal telehealth nursing.
2.   Identify sources of telehealth stress and basic methods to more effectively deal with stress.
3.   Describe an ergonomic work environment and identify basic steps to transform personal workspace.

Evaluation Form Instructions

1. To receive continuing nursing education (CNE) credit for individual study after reading the indicated chapter(s), please complete the evaluation form (photocopies of the answer form are acceptable). Attach separate paper as necessary.
2. Detach (or photocopy) and send the answer form along with a check, money order, or credit card payable to *AAACN* East Holly Avenue/Box 56, Pitman, NJ 08071-0056. You may also send this form as an email attachment to ambp401@ajj.com.
3. Answer forms must be postmarked by December 31, 2011. Upon completion of the answer/evaluation form, a certificate for 1.2 contact hours will be awarded and sent to you.

Payment Options

☐ Check or money order enclosed (payable in U.S. funds to AAACN)

☐ MasterCard   ☐ VISA   ☐ American Express

Credit Card #:_____

Expiration Date: _____ Security Code:_____

Card Holder (Please print):

_____

Signature:

_____

This educational activity has been co-provided by the American Academy of Ambulatory Care Nursing (AAACN) and Anthony J. Jannetti, Inc. (AJJ).

AAACN is a provider approved by the California Board of Registered Nursing, Provider Number CEP 5336.

AJJ is accredited as a provider of continuing nursing education by the American Nurses Credentialing Center's Commission on Accreditation.

This book was reviewed and formatted for contact hour credit by Sally S. Russell, MN, CMSRN, AAACN Education Director, and Maureen Espensen, MBA, BSN, RN, Editor.

American Academy of Ambulatory Care Nursing
East Holly Avenue/Box 56, Pitman, NJ 08071-0056
Phone: 800-AMB-NURS; Fax: 856-589-7463
Web: www.aaacn.org; Email: aaacn@ajj.com

Section 2

Telehealth Nursing Clinical Aspects

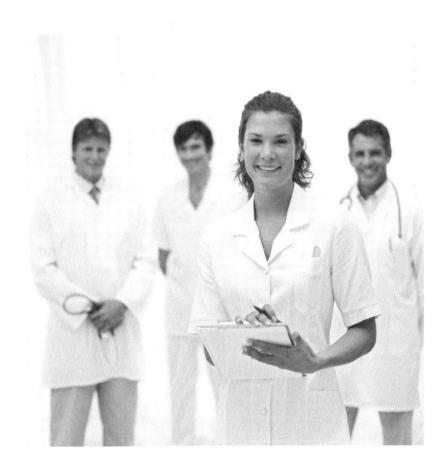

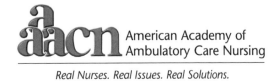
American Academy of
Ambulatory Care Nursing

Real Nurses. Real Issues. Real Solutions.

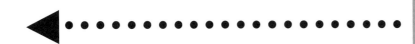

CHAPTER 11
Clinical Knowledge – An Overview

Objectives

1. Summarize clinical competencies needed for telehealth practice.
2. Explain critical clinical questions to consider when interacting with patients in telehealth practice.
3. Describe types of patient situations that should alert the nurse to challenging clinical decision-making events.

When performing telehealth nursing practice either in a formal telehealth call center setting or in an ambulatory care office, the nurse needs to utilize the nursing process, practice effective communication and customer service skills, and apply nursing theory and clinical knowledge appropriate to the presenting situation. The clinical knowledge base must include structured history-taking, disease and age specific care management, risk assessment, counseling and shared decision models, understanding of learning principles, coordination of care through collaboration, and principles of community health nursing. The competencies necessary for telehealth nursing practice should be based on evidence-based practices that identify effective nursing actions, which result in optimal patient outcomes.

In addition to having a firm clinical knowledge base, the nurse must also demonstrate proficiency and technical competency in the use of telephone systems and computer applications – standard tools of the trade – in addition to the traditional health care devices (such as physiologic monitors, stethoscopes, and thermometers). The telehealth nurse must demonstrate interpersonal competency by using effective communication and customer service skills during the patient encounter, which enables the nurse to quickly develop a rapport that encourages the free flow of information.

A telehealth nurse must address patient concerns related to illness (telephone triage, telephone follow-up) and also fulfill a supportive role by helping the patient attain and maintain wellness through patient education (telephone consultation). A telehealth nurse may also promote self-care management (telephone monitoring) using a variety of technology devices based in the patient's home. All organizations with nurses involved in telehealth practice should have organizational policies to support the practice. The organization may consider using the most recent edition of the *Telehealth Nursing Practice Administration and Practice Standards* (American Academy of Ambulatory Care Nursing [AAACN], 2007) as a

> *When performing telehealth nursing practice either in a formal telehealth call center setting or in an ambulatory care office, the nurse needs to utilize the nursing process, practice effective communication and customer service skills, and apply nursing theory and clinical knowledge appropriate to the presenting situation.*

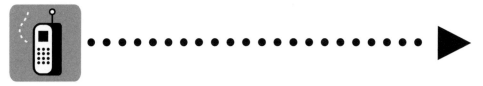

guideline for setting its policies and outlining the core competencies expected of the nurse performing telehealth nursing practice.

CLINICAL COMPETENCY

To function effectively in all nursing arenas, the nurse must possess the ability to utilize critical thinking and knowledge-based judgment in every patient encounter.

The evolution of the role of the clinical nurse continually permits a greater level of autonomy in the decision-making process. Additionally, the nurse is being confronted with increasingly complex health issues and difficult care situations. Therefore, as always, the nurse working in any environment must be clinically competent. Like all specialties in nursing, telehealth nursing has its foundation in basic nursing theory, upon which specific telehealth nursing knowledge is built. The comprehensive knowledge base of a telehealth nurse should include theory related to prevention of illness and health promotion, health risk assessment, disease and age specific care management, as well as self-care management and education strategies. Also required is the ability to use the nursing process and a systematic problem-solving approach to identify and solve health problems in order to meet a patient's health care needs. To function effectively in all nursing arenas, the nurse must possess the ability to utilize critical thinking and knowledge-based judgment in every patient encounter. Many factors (such as changes in health care delivery, advances in technology, increasing diversity, an aging population, and advances in medicine) continually present new challenges and opportunities in the delivery of nursing care. Telehealth nursing practice is only one example of the response within the nursing community to meet these challenges. The ultimate goal of all nursing practice is the delivery of safe, effective care. The methods of delivering the care must respond to the patient's need, whether that care is in person or from a remote location.

As the nurse analyzes the information obtained into a working care plan for the patient, it is important to also employ his/her inherent judgment skills. The six elements of judgment, as defined by Dreyfus (1995), are:

- ❖ *Pattern recognition and the ability to recognize relationships.*
- ❖ *Similarity recognition:* The ability to recognize similarities and dissimilarities.
- ❖ *Common sense understanding:* A deep grasp of the real world and real people's responses to that world.
- ❖ *Skilled know-how:* True expertise – the ability to do something so well that it can be done in a wide variety of different situations.
- ❖ *A sense of salience:* The ability to extract the *truly important* facts from all the information at hand.
- ❖ *Deliberative rationality:* The ability to alter one's perspective and review all the facts from that new perspective.

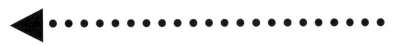

Using Dreyfus' model of skill acquisition, Benner (1984) identified a continuum of nursing abilities ranging from novice to expert. The novice relies on rules to strictly guide the clinical decision-making process, weighs all clinical cues equally, and often over-generalizes from a single cue. The expert works creatively without breaking the rules, uses clinical experience to weigh cues according to potential acuity, and rapidly sorts through multiple cues to focus on the specific problem of the patient. Progression though the stages from novice to expert is a common trait of all nursing specialties. Benner also recognizes these stages when a nurse begins to work in a different specialty of nursing as a novice to that specialty.

TECHNICAL COMPETENCY

Technical skill mastery is essential for efficient, effective nursing practice while demonstrating clinical knowledge. Examples of technical competency can be found in the hospital setting as well as the ambulatory setting. In hospital settings, computers as well as a variety of electronic devices are used to monitor the patient and deliver care. In the ambulatory and telehealth practice settings, some of the very same technology is used to support patient care. Examples include: specially designed software applications, computerized guidelines, email communication, video patient monitoring, and electronic medical records (EMR). Opportunities also exist for other electronic applications (such as the telephone and/or electronic home monitoring devices).

The telehealth nurse must be proficient in the use of the telephone and understand the specific capabilities of the system. This includes mastering how to answer and transfer a call, place a patient on hold, switch to a conference call, and page a physician. All of this must be performed without disconnecting the caller. If applicable to the practice setting, the nurse must also be knowledgeable about the method of call distribution, the call-waiting system (queue), the average wait time, and how wait time is monitored. The nurse should also be aware of his/her own telephone/technology statistics including talk time, wrap time, and how to generate and interpret reports.

Telehealth encounters may require the use of a fax machine. The nurse needs to be knowledgeable on how to send and receive faxes via a stand-alone fax machine or when integrated within the agent's computer.

The use of computers has become the standard rather than an exception in the health care delivery system. A telehealth nurse must demonstrate knowledge and competencies related to the organization's specific computer technology. Minimal computer competency include knowledge of basic computer functions, Windows application, emailing, and the ability to navigate the Internet. Whatever computer, telephone, and

The use of computers has become the standard rather than an exception in the health care delivery system. A telehealth nurse must demonstrate knowledge and competencies related to the organization's specific computer technology.

electronic devices are provided to support telehealth nursing practice, the nurse must be competent and comfortable in the use of each of them.

CLINICAL DECISION-MAKING COMPETENCY

The critically thinking nurse must make certain general inquiries before reaching a clinical decision and decide the best course of action for that patient.

As covered in Chapter 2, "Focus and Roles," critical thinking is a cognitive process involving all thinking modes in purposeful examination and analysis of all available information, and results in sound, accurate clinical decisions. The critically thinking nurse must make certain general inquiries before reaching a clinical decision and decide the best course of action for that patient. With analysis and synthesis of the information gathered, the clinical decision will be influenced by the responses to each of the questions:

1. Who is this patient?
2. Why is the patient seeking assistance?
3. What are the worst possible things that could happen in this situation?
4. What critical information must the nurse obtain?
5. Is there an underlying problem?
6. Is the patient at risk?
7. What are the available resources?

Who is the patient?

The answer to "Who is the patient?" is not simply the patient's name or a medical record number. Local communities are becoming more diverse. As a result, a nurse must begin by thinking more globally when considering this question. A nurse serving patients within a diverse community must be sensitive to the various cultures served in order to best address the specific need of the particular population. Part of the answer to this question may be known even before the nurse's first patient encounter, regardless of the nurse's work setting. The nurse working in a large, regional call center may serve a broader population than a nurse working in a local physician office. Equipped with knowledge about the telehealth clients, the nurse may be able to anticipate the type of symptoms and health care concerns most common for the patient population as shown in Table 11-1.

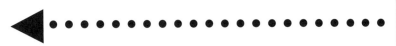

Table 11-1.
Type of Service Area Considerations

Question	Telehealth Application
Is this a rural or urban area?	Suggests types of possible illnesses or injuries.
What are the health care resources?	Suggests patient care treatment and education options.
Where are the medical facilities located?	Suggests time-to-treatment variable.

Detailed responses to each of the population questions in Table 11-2 below will assist the nurse in clarifying the community environment. These responses will vary depending on the medical environment in which the nurse is employed. In larger population areas, the answers may be fairly general. For smaller settings, there may be more detailed knowledge of the patient population. Responses to these questions will help quantify the patient's access to available health care resources and will serve to guide the nurse in determining what other support systems are available in the community to meet the patient's needs. It is necessary to assess the patient in relation to his/her social epidemiological viewpoint so as to enhance compliance with the care directives given.

It is necessary to assess the patient in relation to his/her social epidemiological viewpoint so as to enhance compliance with the care directives given.

Table 11-2.
Populations Served

Question	Telehealth Application
Are there many factories?	Suggests possible workplace exposure or injury risks.
Is there a high unemployment rate?	Suggests restricted resource options.
Is there a significant multi-cultural or ethnic presence?	Suggests strategies for effective patient interview.
What is the geographical location or setting (such as Midwest or coastal area)?	Suggests environment risk: Midwest – frostbite Southeast Coast – marine animal stings or bites

After answering, "Who is the patient?" in relation to the population being served, the nurse can focus specifically on the patient. Each patient is an individual, and possesses both strengths and weaknesses in relationship to his/her health and the ability to maintain health, avoid illness, and when necessary, restore health. For this reason, the nurse

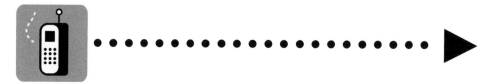

should assess each individual patient's strengths and weaknesses. The individual patient's assets and liabilities will also influence the nurse's management of the patient.

Why is the patient seeking assistance?

What caused this patient to seek assistance? The motivation for the telehealth encounter may often seem obvious, as the patient's opening remarks will indicate what prompted him/her to seek assistance. However, the nurse must be mindful that the reason for the encounter may not be simply what the patient states when asked this question. There may be a need for prompting from the nurse for the patient to give an exact description of what exactly precipitated the encounter. In addition, the patient may be a poor personal historian, leaving out essential relevant details. Occasionally, a patient will give multiple complaints, and the nurse will be required to prioritize the complaints using critical thinking to identify the complaint or symptom(s) that is most likely to result in the most negative outcome in the absence of an intervention. A caller may request help with what appears to be a benign problem and eventually reveal a more critical complaint during the course of the conversation with the nurse. In all situations, the nurse must rely on effective communication techniques, rooted in being an active listener, in order to elicit the perfect balance of quality and quantity of information, to enable the nurse to address the most pressing problem the patient is experiencing.

What are the worst possible things that could happen in this situation?

It is important to remember that the nurse reaches a decision about the appropriate management of the patient, not by evaluating a single symptom, but by thoroughly assessing the patient's current health status and his/her medical history. This is done through the nurse's application of nursing theory, clinical judgment, and critical thinking. In gathering medical history, the nurse must inquire about recent issues that may influence the plan of care, such as recent trauma anywhere on the body, new medications or herbal products, and exposure to anything different in the environment. Vague symptoms may affect the advice that the nurse offers to ensure the safest outcome.

It is very difficult to list the symptoms a nurse would not want to miss, as this would include every emergent or urgent problem that exists. Putting the composite of the patient and the presenting symptoms together (data clustering) is how the nurse assembles the total picture of what is going on with a particular patient at a particular point in time. However, some broad guidance can be provided to recognize priority conditions. If a life-threatening situation is identified, it is essential to immediately respond to presenting symptoms. A directive to activate 911 is warranted if there is severe compromise of any of the following (the "ABCCs"):

It is important to remember that the nurse reaches a decision about the appropriate management of the patient, not by evaluating a single symptom, but by thoroughly assessing the patient's current health status and his/her medical history.

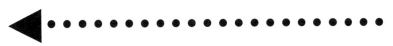

- **A**irway
- **B**reathing
- **C**irculation
- **C**onsciousness

The following symptom sets may or may not indicate an emergency, as the severity of outcome will vary from patient to patient. The association of symptoms and the degree of intensity will ultimately determine the appropriate level of urgency for care. Again, this is not intended to be an all-inclusive list, merely some of the symptoms that might elevate a patient's urgency of care level.

The association of symptoms and the degree of intensity will ultimately determine the appropriate level of urgency for care.

- **ABDOMINAL PAIN**
  With any of the following associated symptoms:
  - Described as constant, localized, severe.
  - Duration greater than 24 hours.
  - Emesis – bright red blood or coffee ground-like material.
  - Bloody diarrhea/black or bloody stools.
  - Fever.
  - History of previous abdominal problems, such as ovarian cysts, thrombosis, spleenectomy, or abdominal aortic aneurysm.
- **SHORTNESS OF BREATH**
  With any of the following associated symptoms:
  - Cough producing bloody sputum.
  - Sudden or recent onset.
  - Wheezing.
  - Unexplained weight gain or new swelling of extremities.
  - Secondary to environmental/inhalant exposure.
  - Associated with possible allergic response.
- **HEADACHE**
  With any of the following associated symptoms:
  - Nausea or vomiting.
  - Visual symptoms (flashing lights, blurry or double vision).
  - Sudden onset of severe headache.
  - Fever.
  - Described as severe pain and change from usual headache symptoms.

What critical information must the nurse obtain?

What information is most essential for the nurse to obtain first? The nurse must first determine that there are not symptoms requiring 911. Is the patient audibly short of breath? Does the patient think they will pass out? Any change in mental status? It would not be prudent to focus on

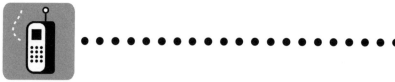

obtaining demographic data at the expense of delaying immediate care. The nurse should obtain the name of the patient and current phone number. This information can be critical if contact with the patient is lost for any reason before the encounter is successfully concluded.

Secondly, the nurse needs to use nursing knowledge and decision support tools to determine what information is most critical in relation to the current symptoms. Again, it is essential to complete a brief initial assessment to address the most critical issues of airway, breathing, circulation, and consciousness. Once the ABCCs are established, the nurse should progress to the organization's guidelines for more detailed assessment of the presenting symptoms. Decision support tools must be organized to assess high priority symptoms to rule out any emergent situation before asking questions that point to less urgent situations.

Is there an underlying problem?

Actively listening when assessing the patient allows the nurse to both hear the words being communicated and pick up other auditory cues. Using this auditory information, a critically thinking nurse may be able to recognize symptoms that the patient has not verbalized or identify the presence of a hidden agenda. To successfully practice active listening, the nurse must be fully focused on the interaction with the patient and avoid all potential distractions. A proficient nurse needs to continually think "big picture" and not focus on only the patient's words. It is essential that the nurse look collectively at what the patient has voiced, how it was voiced, and what other background sounds are audible when communicating by telephone.

❖ Does the patient speak in short, choppy sentences?
❖ Is the emotion verbalized consistent with the presenting symptoms?
❖ Do background noises (other people, environmental noises, etc.) support the patient's presenting story?

Because there is always a risk of unidentified underlying problems or that the patient has not provided complete information or the condition has changed or worsened during a telehealth encounter, it is recommended that the interaction should always end with disclosure statements. These statements inform the patient of the need to contact the nurse again if:

❖ Symptoms are other than what has been discussed during the telephone encounter.
❖ Symptoms persist.
❖ Recommendations do not achieve the expected results in the expected timeframe.

Actively listening when assessing the patient allows the nurse to both hear the words being communicated and pick up other auditory cues. Using this auditory information, a critically thinking nurse may be able to recognize symptoms that the patient has not verbalized or identify the presence of a hidden agenda.

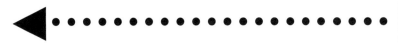

❖ If patient is increasingly concerned about symptoms.
❖ New symptoms develop.

Disclosure statements serve to remind the nurse and the patient that there is a shared responsibility for the desired outcome. Disclosure statements also advise the patient of his/her responsibility to seek further help if symptoms intensify or do not respond to suggested treatments. It is also imperative to verify that the patient clearly understands what the nurse recommended. The most straightforward method is to simply ask, "Do you understand what I have advised you to do?" The disclosure statement, along with verification of understanding, ensures safer patient outcomes and serves as a risk management tool for the nurse as well as the organization.

AT-RISK SITUATIONS

Is the patient at-risk?

Several patient conditions or situations require focused attention by the nurse during the telehealth encounter, because a high level of expertise is needed to sort the various symptoms or cues during the interaction. These patient conditions or situations are considered *at-risk* because there is greater potential for a less than desirable outcome. This overview is not intended to be inclusive of all the at-risk factors, but only to heighten the awareness of particular patient populations. The following at-risk groups are discussed in more detail in other chapters.

Chronic Health Condition

The nurse needs to have an understanding of chronic conditions and affects upon the patient. It is important to remember that chronic disease states affect every aspect of the patient's life as well as the lives of those surrounding the patient. Persons of all ages, cultures, and socioeconomic levels are affected by chronic conditions. More than 90 million Americans live with chronic illnesses (Centers for Disease Control and Prevention, 2008). In addition, chronic conditions often rely on regularly scheduled medication regimens that are necessary to manage the chronic illness. Standard, over-the-counter medications, herbal preparations, or other home remedies have the potential to adversely interact with the daily medications that chronically ill patients take. For that reason alone, patients with chronic illnesses are considered an at-risk population.

The nurse should also remember that the patient with a chronic condition might develop unique coping styles to emotionally handle his/her chronic condition. One patient may be very distressed by a new acute illness, while another patient may shrug off new symptoms and ignore a change in his/her overall medical condition. The nurse should

Several patient conditions or situations require focused attention by the nurse during the telehealth encounter, because a high level of expertise is needed to sort the various symptoms or cues during the interaction.

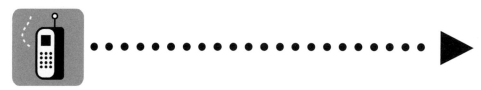

attempt to be aware of each patient's unique coping style and the effect this has on the patient's capacity to share pertinent information. Often a patient talks about his/her chronic health problem(s) in the assessment interview.

History of Recent Surgery

Surgery, whether elective or emergent, places both physical and psychological stress on the patient. A post-surgical patient is at-risk because of possible unexpected outcomes or post-operative complications, such as bleeding, infection, or pulmonary emboli or poor recovery from anesthesia. Changes in post-surgical care have made it increasingly common for the patient to have outpatient surgery or be sent home within a few days of major surgery. "More than 60% of elective surgery procedures in the United States are currently performed as outpatient surgeries. Health experts expect this percentage will increase to nearly 75% over the next decade" (eMedicineHealth, 2006). The percentage of outpatient or short-stay procedures will continue to grow with advancement in procedures, the growth of ambulatory surgery centers, and the influence of insurance providers. Therefore, the ambulatory care and/or telehealth practice nurse must have a thorough understanding of perioperative concepts to support the surgical patient in self-care in the home environment.

Asking the patient for a thorough medical history will be key in determining if the patient has had recent surgery. Knowledge of more distant surgeries can also be of significance if the surgery has a bearing on the current situation. Be aware that the patient may not be comfortable sharing information regarding recent surgical procedures and may consider a past surgery of little or no relevance to the current problem.

Medication History

All medications have side effects, contraindications, and interactions with other medications. It is for this reason that special attention must be paid to the patient who indicates he/she is regularly taking prescribed medications. The nurse also needs to note any over-the-counter, herbal or homeopathic preparations, or recreational drugs used by the patient. The nurse must also be aware of the associated side effects of these preparations. All nurses need to stay informed of new drugs on the market as related to their patient population. Patients should be queried about involvement in clinical studies and the use of experimental drugs (for example, cancer patients). To support their practice, nurses must have immediate access to organization-approved resources, such as written or computer-based drug references, and they should use them appropriately. The resource pool must also include pharmacist resources, because written texts may outdate quickly.

A post-surgical patient is at-risk because of possible unexpected outcomes or post-operative complications, such as bleeding, infection, or pulmonary emboli or poor recovery from anesthesia.

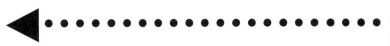

Second-Person or Second-Hand Information

Second-hand information refers to symptom assessment obtained from someone other than the person experiencing the symptom. This may be a necessary situation when an adult is seeking assistance for an ill infant or young child, or an adult who is unable to communicate effectively on his/her own. However, second-hand information increases risk of error in analyzing the presenting problem. Obtaining second-hand information is often more time-consuming and may not be accurate. Whenever possible, the nurse should communicate directly with the patient, if only to verify that the information provided by the other person is accurate. Additional information can be gathered when directly communicating with the patient, including audible wheezing or gasps for air (indicating shortness of breath), or inappropriately answering questions suggesting altered mental status. Under federal guidelines, there has to be consideration for the risk of breaching confidentiality when sharing information regarding an adult or an emancipated minor. If the patient is not present, the nurse needs to know the organization's policy on whether or not a symptom-based assessment can take place in the absence of the person experiencing the symptoms, or if the caller must call back when with the patient, or the if patient themselves should call for triage.

Obtaining second-hand information is often more time-consuming and may not be accurate. Whenever possible, the nurse should communicate directly with the patient, if only to verify that the information provided by the other person is accurate.

Frequent or Repeat Patient

An individual may make repeated contacts with the nurse when experiencing frequent, acute needs or chronic conditions, has an underlying problem or concern that has not been fully addressed, or is feeling lonely or depressed. The nurse must never discount the importance of each interaction with a repeat patient and must be diligent to make a complete assessment with each encounter to determine if the patient needs intervention other than reassurance.

Caution should be used to determine level of compliance and any questions or problems the patient may have regarding prior recommended interventions. The nurse must also determine if there have been any changes in presenting symptoms since the previous telehealth encounter. After this information has been gathered and clarified, the nurse must determine if these are new concerns. The nurse should be wary of the patient who repetitively contacts the nurse with slightly changed symptoms and who has not been compliant with the appropriate, recommended care plan. This patient may be attempting to manipulate the situation toward his/her own agenda. If the encounters with a particular patient develop a repetitive pattern, the telehealth practice nurse should collaborate with other health care professionals to determine what other interventions might be more appropriate to meet the patient's needs, in addition to those available to the telehealth practice nurse.

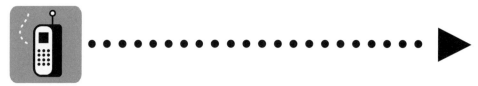

Infant or Young Child

The lack of a fully developed immune system and having little or no verbal communication ability places the infant or young child among those considered at-risk. Due to the immature immune system, a premature infant or an infant under 6 months of age is at greatest risk for frequent illnesses and may also experience a greater risk of a negative outcome from illness. For this reason, most decision support tools require immediate medical attention for fever symptoms when the patient is an infant less than 2 months of age. Lack of fully developed verbal skills makes it impossible for this population to completely convey what is being experienced, requiring that someone else intervene on the child's behalf (see *Second-Person or Second-Hand Information*, previously). The nurse must also consider the emotional status of the second-hand source when involved in a pediatric assessment. There may be higher anxiety or stress related to concerns for the child's health status.

Pregnant or Lactating Woman

A woman in her reproductive years and the unborn child are at-risk due to the potential life-threatening complications associated with known or unknown pregnancies. The nurse must collect specific details from all female patients of childbearing age, determining if the patient is sexually active. Many assessments directly ask, "Are you pregnant?" Birth control information and the date of the patient's last menses should be included. If applicable, it is essential to ask about the possibility of breast-feeding. The patient should understand the implications related to medication use. In each of these scenarios, the risk is increased because the well-being of two patients is in the balance: mother and child.

Geriatric Patient

With aging, the average patient is more likely to have one or more chronic illnesses. Whereas the older adults experience fewer acute illnesses than the younger population, they may suffer more complications with an acute illness due to other pre-existing conditions. Symptoms of the older adult with either a chronic or acute illness tend to be subtle. In addition, chronic illnesses may result in the older patient using more over-the-counter medications than a healthier, young adult patient would. Therefore, the elderly are more at risk for problems related to drug interactions as a result of taking multiple medications. Many chronically ill older adults are on sophisticated drug regimens, and may find it difficult to pay for necessary medications due to a fixed-income status. The geriatric patient may also believe that the side effects of the medication do not offset the potential benefit. These dilemmas may result in noncompliance and thereby place the geriatric patient at greater risk for serious illness or negative outcome.

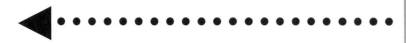

Communication Barriers

A communication barrier exists any time a nurse and a patient are not able to discuss the patient's health concerns easily using a language common to both parties. When either the patient or the nurse is speaking in a second language, there is increased risk that symptoms may not be conveyed accurately and that the nurse's questions or instructions may not be understood. Unless a nurse who fluently speaks the language of the patient and can effectively communicate is present, the patient is placed at risk.

Other communication barriers placing the patient at risk are speech or hearing deficit(s), being intellectually challenged, or under the influence of mind-altering drugs or substances. Additional barriers to effective communication are the quality of the electronic connection, use of cellular telephones, voice volume, line static, and background noises for either the nurse or the patient.

Federal legislation mandates that provisions be made so that language and physical challenges do not impair the patient's access to health care. A qualified language interpreter should be available as needed. Devices to facilitate communication with the hearing and speech impaired should also be available. Each facility should have policies and procedures in place detailing how to handle each of these situations. The nurse should have a plan on how to resolve each type of communication barrier before the patient contacts him/her for assistance. There is no time to resolve this when a patient presents with a life-threatening crisis.

A qualified language interpreter should be available as needed. Devices to facilitate communication with the hearing and speech impaired should also be available.

What are the available resources?

During initial orientation to an organization, the nurse should have a general understanding of the available resources of the community being served. Does the community have enhanced 911? What health care facilities are available and how close are they to the patients being served? Is there a hospital, regional trauma center, or burn center in the community close to the patients? Are there after-hour services and/or walk-in clinics, or are the patients limited to emergency department services only? The nurse must have a broad knowledge base or immediate availability to references regarding community resources, and he/she must possess an ability to work collaboratively with other members of the health care team. A general understanding of how the patient is able to pay for their health care can be useful in determining appropriate resources for the patient and may enhance compliance if certain facilities or goods are covered by the patient's medical insurance plan.

Many different types of agencies provide community services for patients. These can be official, publicly-funded agencies, non-profit agencies, proprietary chains, or health care facility-based programs. Funding for each of these may be in part from Medicare, Medicaid, private

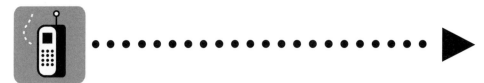

insurance, or direct payment by patients. Patients often must meet specific requirements to be eligible for the services offered by each agency. With the rapid rate of change in the health care system today, the funding of services frequently changes, along with the resources available, eligibility requirements, and associated costs. It is essential to have a directory of facilities and programs available to serve the uninsured and indigent members of the community. The nurse needs to keep abreast of fundamental changes to facilitate the most effective resource utilization for the patient. Utilization of the multidisciplinary approach and collaboration with all health care members promotes shared participation, responsibility, and accountability necessary to meet the complex health care and resource needs of the patient.

Another resource the nurse should be aware of is health information libraries. These often are available to the patient and can be employed by the nurse to assist in providing health education and promote appropriate self-care. In additional to traditional libraries, this resource may be accessible through integrated voice response (IVR) technology or various Internet Web sites. IVR technology requires the patient to have access to a touch-tone telephone, while Internet applications require computer access and skill sets. These health information libraries provide a directory of the available topics accessible to the nurse and the health care consumer. The nurse may assist the patient in choosing the best source for information based on the patient's resources and comprehension level. All resource information should be reviewed regularly to maintain accuracy and currency. As with any resource, the nurse should suggest only those that the organization has approved for recommendation to the patient.

The nurse practicing telehealth nursing should also have professional resources available that reflect the patient population services provided. It is the nurse's responsibility to know personal and professional limitations and to know where to go for acceptable resources to aid in the support and management of the patient. Resources to supplement organization-approved guidelines may include:

❖ Texts or other medical printed materials that have been approved for use.
❖ Regional poison control call centers and suicide hotline numbers.
❖ Other local and state agencies that have an interest in the patient's well-being (such as various crisis lines, children and family services, and public health districts).
❖ Knowledge and expertise of other health care professionals, including fellow nurses, pharmacists and physicians.
❖ Case managers, social workers, or home care nurses as appropriate.

All resource information should be reviewed regularly to maintain accuracy and currency. As with any resource, the nurse should suggest only those that the organization has approved for recommendation to the patient.

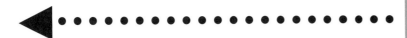

SUMMARY

Telehealth nursing practice requires a complex application of nursing practice with emphasis on unique competencies. This practice requires a blend of a vast clinical knowledge base, effective communication skills, and customer-centered service skills. This all is enabled by technical competencies. The mix of these ingredients will vary depending on the practice setting and the resources available – from a regional call center to the physician office setting. The clinical knowledge base of the telehealth practice nurse must prepare the nurse to assess each patient remotely via technology, regardless of the setting. The assessment must be a systematic review of who the patient is, and all the symptoms and circumstances that are currently affecting the health status of the patient. During the interview process, the nurse must continually evaluate the information provided by the patient to judge if this is an at-risk situation. Based on the information gathered, the nurse must then determine the best intervention for the patient using the most appropriate resource at the most appropriate time. Organization-approved guidelines and standards must provide support and guidance for this process.

Excellent communications skills are essential, not only to determine the complete picture of the patient's needs, but also to enable the patient to understand the directives provided for care and the significance of compliance, including the potential risks associated with noncompliance. In summary, through clinical experience, the nurse demonstrates expertise in using the nursing process, thinking critically, and applying clinical judgment. The nurse must also exhibit competency levels with technology supporting the autonomous practice environment experienced in many telehealth nursing practice settings.

The assessment must be a systematic review of who the patient is, and all the symptoms and circumstances that are currently affecting the health status of the patient.

TIPS & PEARLS

☎ Telehealth nurses must demonstrate technical, clinical, and intellectual competencies and set expectations for others to be competent.

☎ Never underestimate the patient or his/her presenting needs.

☎ Perform a complete assessment with each encounter.

☎ Listen, Listen, and Listen – The nurse will be amazed at what is learned when actively listening to the patient.

☎ Think "big picture" with every encounter. Has the total patient been addressed?

☎ Use only organization-approved guidelines and resources to advise patients.

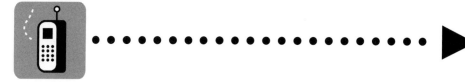

References

American Academy of Ambulatory Care Nursing (AAACN). (2007). *Telehealth nursing practice administration and practice standards* (4th ed.). Pitman, NJ: Author.

Benner, P. (1984). *From novice to expert: Excellence and power in clinical nursing practice.* Menlo Park, CA: Addison-Wesley.

Centers for Disease Control and Prevention. (2008). *Chronic disease overview.* Retrieved February 23, 2008, from http://www.cdc.gov/nccdphp/overview.htm

Dreyfus, H.S. (1995). *Mind over machine: The power of human intuition and expertise in the era of the computer.* New York City: Free Press.

eMedicineHealth. (2006). *Outpatient surgery.* Retrieved February 23, 2008, from http://www.emedicinehealth.com/outpatient_surgery/article_em.htm

Answer/Evaluation Form AMBP9c09
Continuing Nursing Education Activity
Telehealth Nursing Practice Essentials
Chapter 11: Clinical Knowledge – An Overview

This activity provides 1.3 contact hours of continuing nursing education (CNE) credit in nursing.
(Contact hours calculated using a 60-minute contact hour.)

This test may be copied for use by others.

COMPLETE THE FOLLOWING:

Name: _____

Address: _____

City: _____ State: _____ Zip: _____

Telephone number: (Home)_____ (Work)_____

Email address:_____

AAACN Member Number and Expiration Date: _____

Processing fee: AAACN Member: $12.00
                  Nonmember: $20.00

Answer Form: (Please attach a separate sheet of paper if necessary.)
1. What did you value most about this activity?

_____
_____
_____
_____

2. If you could imagine that you have fully integrated your learning into practice, what would be different about your present practice?

_____
_____
_____
_____

Evaluation	Strongly disagree				Strongly agree
3. The offering met the stated objectives.					
a. Summarize clinical competencies needed for telehealth practice.	1	2	3	4	5
b. Explain critical clinical questions to consider when interacting with patients in telehealth practice.	1	2	3	4	5
c. Describe types of patient situations that should alert the nurse to challenging clinical decision-making events.	1	2	3	4	5
4. The content was current and relevant.	1	2	3	4	5
5. The content was presented clearly.	1	2	3	4	5
6. The content was covered adequately.	1	2	3	4	5

7. How would you rate your ability to apply your learning to practice following this activity? (Check one)
    ☐ Diminished ability ☐ No change ☐ Enhanced ability

8. Time required to complete reading assignment and answer form: ___ minutes
Comments _____

_____

I verify that I have completed this activity:

_____
                Signature

Objectives

This educational activity is designed for nurses and other health care professionals who provide telehealth care for patients. This evaluation is designed to test your achievement of the following educational activities.
1. Summarize clinical competencies needed for telehealth practice.
2. Explain critical clinical questions to consider when interacting with patients in telehealth practice.
3. Describe types of patient situations that should alert the nurse to challenging clinical decision-making events.

Evaluation Form Instructions

1. To receive continuing nursing education (CNE) credit for individual study after reading the indicated chapter(s), please complete the evaluation form (photocopies of the answer form are acceptable). Attach separate paper as necessary.
2. Detach (or photocopy) and send the answer form along with a check, money order, or credit card payable to *AAACN* East Holly Avenue/Box 56, Pitman, NJ 08071-0056. You may also send this form as an email attachment to ambp401@ajj.com.
3. Answer forms must be postmarked by December 31, 2011. Upon completion of the answer/evaluation form, a certificate for 1.3 contact hours will be awarded and sent to you.

Payment Options
☐ Check or money order enclosed (payable in U.S. funds to AAACN)

☐ MasterCard   ☐ VISA   ☐ American Express

Credit Card #:_____

Expiration Date: _____ Security Code:_____

Card Holder (Please print):

_____

Signature:

_____

This educational activity has been co-provided by the American Academy of Ambulatory Care Nursing (AAACN) and Anthony J. Jannetti, Inc. (AJJ).
AAACN is a provider approved by the California Board of Registered Nursing, Provider Number CEP 5336.
AJJ is accredited as a provider of continuing nursing education by the American Nurses Credentialing Center's Commission on Accreditation.
This book was reviewed and formatted for contact hour credit by Sally S. Russell, MN, CMSRN, AAACN Education Director, and Maureen Espensen, MBA, BSN, RN, Editor.

American Academy of Ambulatory Care Nursing
East Holly Avenue/Box 56, Pitman, NJ 08071-0056
Phone: 800-AMB-NURS; Fax: 856-589-7463
Web: www.aaacn.org; Email: aaacn@ajj.com

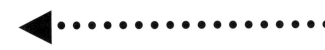

CHAPTER 12
Clinical Knowledge – Special Situations

Objectives

1. Describe critical information to collect when receiving a crisis call.
2. Compare and contrast two major ways to activate Emergency Medical Services in a crisis situation.
3. Propose specific telehealth nursing actions for calls related to cardiopulmonary resuscitation, poisoning/overdose, abuse, sexual assault, and suicide.

It is a normal reaction for a telehealth nurse, as first responder to abuse, rape, or suicide calls, to experience anxiety because of the possible serious outcome of the situation and lack of familiarity with handling these situations. Abuse and suicide calls are frequently very lengthy calls that create stress for nurses, who more often than not have other patients waiting for them to respond to their needs. Crisis calls cannot be short-changed and require tremendous emotional and intellectual energy to manage.

Unfortunately, even when managed by the most skilled telehealth nurse, not all crisis intervention calls have positive outcomes. The goal of this chapter is to help telehealth practice nurses prepare for and understand some basic telephone communication techniques and skills to utilize when challenged with a crisis call.

Abuse and suicide calls are frequently very lengthy calls that create stress for nurses, who more often than not have other patients waiting for them to respond to their needs. Crisis calls cannot be short-changed and require tremendous emotional and intellectual energy to manage.

IMPORTANCE OF POLICIES/GUIDELINES FOR SPECIAL SITUATIONS

It is important for an organization to have policies/guidelines governing special situation calls and for nurses to be familiar with those policies/guidelines. For example, laws for reporting abuse situations and sexual assault vary from state to state. Nurses are more likely to respond appropriately and with confidence if an organization policy/protocol has been written and implemented. Frequent review of the policy/guideline is essential.

A well-written policy/guideline should include:

- ❖ Definitions.
- ❖ Intervention procedures and referrals.
- ❖ Medical record documentation.
- ❖ Plan for staff education.

Most policies/protocols will also guide the telehealth practice nurse on advising the patient about expectations of the clinic/police/crisis unit visit; this may include screening procedures and collection of evidence and photographs.

RECEIVING THE CRISIS CALL

Most telehealth nursing statistics demonstrate that "Call 911" or "Go to the Emergency Room" call dispositions are a small percent of the total call dispositions given by the nurse. The largest disposition of telephone calls is usually evenly divided between home care advice and referral for provider appointment.

As the telehealth nurse begins assessing a crisis call pertaining to poisoning or respiratory or cardiac arrest, obtaining the address where the patient is presently located and the telephone number is important.

As the telehealth nurse begins assessing a crisis call pertaining to poisoning or respiratory or cardiac arrest, obtaining the address where the patient is presently located and the telephone number is important. Obtaining the patient's name is secondary. Patients with issues of abuse, sexual assault, or suicide may be more reluctant to give demographic information. The nurse may need to talk for a period of time until the patient feels more comfortable giving the information. At no time should the nurse risk the possibility of the patient hanging up due to perceived pressure from the nurse to divulge identifying information. The most critical reasons for requesting such information are to maintain connection in case the telephone line should become disconnected or the patient becomes incapacitated (for example, respiratory arrest, cardiac arrest, or the abuser returns), and the nurse must notify the EMS system of the crisis situation. The nurse should be honest with the patient about the reasons for wanting the requested information. However, if the patient is still unwilling to divulge an address and telephone number, the nurse must continue helping the patient.

Telehealth nurses who have access to patient medical records (such as in a primary care practice) or use computerized telehealth advice programs are frequently directed to obtain demographic information at the start of the telephone transaction. Their patients expect to give demographic information and will usually provide it without questioning. This also allows the nurse to access medical records or visit the history of the patient at the beginning of the case, which can be quite helpful.

NOTIFYING EMERGENCY MEDICAL SERVICES (EMS)

The organization should have a policy on whether the nurse or the patient should notify EMS services when indicated. There are advantages and disadvantages to both alternatives.

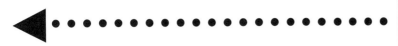

The Telehealth Nurse Notifies EMS

Staying on the line with a patient in crisis to ensure safe, appropriate, and effective disposition of the problem is a standard of crisis intervention. The crisis intervention nurse stays on the line with the patient until the appropriate referral has occurred, the emergency service is dispatched, or the crisis situation is stable.

Nurses may be hesitant to ask the patient to hang up and dial 911 because they fear that the patient may be incapacitated and unable to complete the call requesting emergency services. For example, the patient who complains of chest pain may suffer an arrest before completing the call to 911.

Another risk that nurses take by not placing the 911 call is that patients may be unwilling to contact emergency services. Patients may be trying to protect their privacy. Perhaps patients are afraid of the financial implications of utilizing the ambulance service. Patients frequently express concern that they will be embarrassed if the EMS arrives, and there is really nothing wrong with them. No patient experiencing an acute crisis should be encouraged to drive him/herself to emergency care. It is potentially hazardous to the patient and others if the patient in crisis experiences a debilitating symptom or utilizes poor judgment while driving to seek emergency services. Hysterical parents, caretakers, friends, and spouse of the patient also should not be driving.

A telehealth service providing assessment and advice for a large area or for multiple states needs to ask for the area code as part of the demographics. Because rural areas may have volunteer emergency medical services that employ numbers other than 911, it is important to ask patients in rural areas what number should be accessed for their emergency medical services. If the call is interrupted or the telehealth nurse must notify the EMS for a patient, emergency medical services may be found by dialing the patient's area code, 555-1212, and then asking the operator for assistance in locating and notifying the appropriate emergency services.

Once the patient's address and telephone number are obtained, the best methods for activating the EMS system are to utilize either a direct dial line, conference/linked line, or transfer line. If these telephone modalities are not available, the nurse may need to ask another person to notify the EMS system while the nurse continues to converse with the patient. Even if the nurse is only able to obtain the telephone number from where the patient is calling, the EMS dispatcher will usually be able to use the telephone number to locate the address of the patient. The nurse should never transfer the patient to the EMS without first insuring that:

❖ The call did not get disconnected and that communication between the patient and EMS has been established.
❖ The EMS does not need any additional information from the telehealth nurse.

> *No patient experiencing an acute crisis should be encouraged to drive him/herself to emergency care. It is potentially hazardous to the patient and others if the patient in crisis experiences a debilitating symptom or utilizes poor judgment while driving to seek emergency services.*

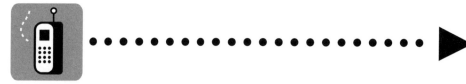

Information that the emergency dispatcher may ask the telehealth nurse or the patient includes:

1. Chief complaint of patient.
2. Age of patient.
3. Is the patient conscious?
4. Is the patient breathing?

The Patient Notifies EMS

The emergency medical system is able to trace the precise location of a call if the community/city is utilizing Enhanced 911 (E911). The patient must place the call to 911 for E911 to be effective. When a call comes in to EMS that utilizes E911, the call is linked via a computer system to the patient's address. This is a valuable service if the patient is unable to give the precise address. This may occur with a small child, mentally handicapped individual, or panicked caller. It is a disadvantage when the telehealth nurse calls EMS for a patient, because the E911 system displays the address of the nurse placing the call. If this is the case, the nurse should immediately alert EMS to the situation and give the medical dispatcher the address and telephone number where the patient is located.

When a call comes in to EMS that utilizes E911, the call is linked via a computer system to the patient's address. This is a valuable service if the patient is unable to give the precise address.

PROVIDING TELEHEALTH ADVICE TO PATIENTS IN CRISIS

It is common for people in crisis situations to be hampered in their ability to think rationally and logically. The telehealth nurse needs to implement simple communication guidelines to help the patient.

Reassure the Patient

"You have called the right place." "I can help you find the care you need." "I really want to help you, and I need the following information." The patient in crisis may need to be reassured multiple times throughout the interaction.

Provide Calm and Specific Guidance

A variety of techniques can be used to help the patient manage the crisis. These techniques include the following:

1. Instruct the patient to take a deep breath and listen carefully.
2. Assure the patient that you are able to help him/her.
3. Give the patient instructions in a logical, step-by-step manner that allows him/her to feel productive and more in control. Action is the anecdote for fear. Some additional examples of action items are:
   ❖ Have the patient lie down or place them in a semi-reclining position if the patient is more comfortable.

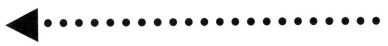

- ❖ Loosen the patient's tight clothing.
- ❖ Turn on the outside light so that the EMS vehicle can locate the address easily.
- ❖ Unlock the front door.
- ❖ Put all pets away so that they do not hinder EMS personnel.

Resource Numbers

It is essential that all telehealth nurses have a list of local crisis intervention telephone numbers and resources. These numbers and resources change over time; therefore, these lists must be updated frequently. Telehealth nurses need to be comfortable with the process utilized to access these numbers and resources. The process should be described in the organization's policies and protocols. Important resource telephone numbers and addresses to have are:

- ❖ Emergency Medical Services.
- ❖ Poison Control Center.
- ❖ Rape Crisis Center.
- ❖ Suicide Crisis Line/Mental Health Triage Line.
- ❖ Child Protective Services.
- ❖ Health and Social Services Department.
- ❖ Adult Protective Services for the Elderly.
- ❖ Nearest Emergency Centers.
- ❖ National Domestic Hotline Number.
- ❖ Intimate Partner (Domestic Violence) Shelters and Programs.

It is essential that all telehealth nurses have a list of local crisis intervention telephone numbers and resources. These numbers and resources change over time; therefore, these lists must be updated frequently.

The following sections review some of the more common special situations that telehealth practice nurses may encounter. Although these types of calls are infrequent, it is imperative for the nurse to have had at least some recent role-playing experience and frequent review of the organization's applicable policies/protocols prior to the occurrence of any of these calls.

CARDIOPULMONARY RESUSCITATION

Each organization should have a policy stating whether or not the telehealth nurse should provide cardio-pulmonary resuscitation instructions. This includes choking or drowning. The American Heart Association (AHA) (2008) states that the most important criteria for improving the outcome of a patient in circulatory arrest is to immediately dispatch emergency medical services. The AHA directs the rescuer to assess the responsiveness of the victim, and if the victim is non-responsive immediately, the rescuer must activate emergency medical services. In accordance with these guidelines, the telehealth nurse or another individual should immediately activate the emergency medical services whenever someone is found to be non-responsive. Once the emergency medical services are activated and trained personnel are on their way, the emergency medical dispatcher or telehealth nurse can then provide *post-dispatch* instructions for cardio-pulmonary resuscitation or implementation of an automated external defibrillator (AED) to the caller according to a written protocol.

OVERDOSE/POISONING

There is a high probability that the telehealth practice nurse will encounter numerous poisoning calls. Poisonings can be grouped into two distinct categories – those that are unintentional and those that are intentional (American Association of Poison Control Centers, 2006; National Center for Injury Prevention and Control, 2008).

There is a high probability that the telehealth practice nurse will encounter numerous poisoning calls.

Unintentional Poisoning Facts
- ❖ In 2005, 23,618 (72%) of the 32,691 poisoning deaths in the United States were unintentional, and 3,240 (10%) were of undetermined intent. Unintentional poisoning death rates have been rising steadily since 1992.
- ❖ Unintentional poisoning was second only to motor vehicle crashes as a cause of unintentional injury death in 2005. Among people 35-54 years old, unintentional poisoning caused more deaths than motor vehicle crashes.
- ❖ In 2006, unintentional poisoning caused about 703,702 emergency department (ED) visits.
- ❖ Almost 25% of these unintentional ED visits resulted in hospitalization or transfer to another facility.
- ❖ In 2006, poison control centers reported about 2 million unintentional poisoning or poison exposure cases.
- ❖ Poison control centers in the United States handle approximately one poison exposure every 15 seconds.
- ❖ In 2004, 95% of unintentional and undetermined poisoning deaths were caused by drugs. Opioid pain medications were most commonly involved, followed by cocaine and heroin.
- ❖ Among those treated in EDs for non-fatal poisonings involving intentional, non-medical use (such as misuse or abuse) of prescription or over-the-counter drugs in 2004, opioid pain medications and benzodiazepines were used most frequently.
- ❖ Men were 2.1 times more likely than women to have an unintentional poisoning. Native Americans had the highest death rate, but Whites and Blacks had comparable rates.
- ❖ The peak age was 45-49 years of age, and the lowest mortality rates were among children less than 15 years old.

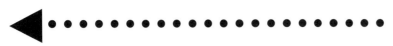

Intentional Poisoning Facts

❖ In the United States in 2005, 5,833 (18%) of the 32,691 poisoning deaths were intentional; 5,744 were suicides and 89 were homicides.

❖ In 2006, intentional poisoning led to about 220,924 ED visits; 216,358 involved self-harm and 3,982 were assaults.

❖ Among the self-harm poisoning ED visits, 75% resulted in hospitalization or transfer to another facility.

❖ Self-harm poisoning was the second-leading cause of ED visits for intentional injury in 2006.

❖ In 2006, poison control centers reported 198,578 cases where the reason for poison exposure was a suspected suicide attempt.

❖ Men were 1.3 times more likely than women to have an intentional poisoning. Whites were 3.6 times more likely than Blacks. The peak age was 45-49 years old.

Poison Control Centers

Poison control centers focus on determining whether a poisoning or toxic substance exposure can be appropriately managed at home. They manage more than 2 million cases of poison exposure annually. A majority of calls to poison control centers can be managed without referral to a health care facility, saving health care resources and improving the quality of service to the community.

Poison control numbers are usually listed on the inside cover of the white pages of telephone books or may be obtained by calling local telephone information services such as 1411 or (area code) 555-1212. Each state's poison control telephone number is also listed on the Internet.

Although poison control centers request a name, telephone number, and address, the information is confidential. Some callers, such as a parent who feels guilty about his/her child's poison exposure, are hesitant to give information because they are embarrassed. A patient who has intentionally overdosed or is contemplating suicide may also be unwilling to provide demographic information. If a patient does not want to disclose demographic information, the center will still help. All documentation is confidential and treated like a medical record.

A majority of calls to poison control centers can be managed without referral to a health care facility, saving health care resources and improving the quality of service to the community.

Carbon Monoxide Poisoning

Common symptoms of carbon monoxide (CO) poisoning are nausea, headache, fatigue, dizziness, and shortness of breath. Incomplete burning of fuels such as natural gas, oil, kerosene, coal, and wood causes CO poisoning. Causes of fatal concentrations of CO are running a car engine in the garage, burning charcoal indoors, and fuel-burning appliances that need repair.

Of particular concern is the high risk of carbon monoxide poisoning in disaster or emergency situations. The public may use alternative sources of power, such as gasoline-powered generators to produce electricity, ovens to heat homes, or charcoal grills while inside a home. These potentially unsafe practices result in several fatalities each year (Centers for Disease Control and Prevention [CDC], 2008).

The Telehealth Nurse's Role

The nurse should immediately assess the overdose/poisoning victim's symptoms. If there is any evidence of circulatory compromise, respiratory failure, or change in mentation, EMS must be notified immediately (see *Notifying Emergency Medical Services*, above).

If the nurse expects carbon monoxide poisoning, the patient should be instructed to get fresh air immediately. Doors and windows should be opened. Based on the acuity of the patient's symptoms, medical help from a same-day provider appointment to emergency 911 care should be recommended.

If there is no immediate need to transport the patient to the emergency room, the nurse or caller should contact the nearest poison control center. Poison control centers are the experts in providing information on treatment of poisonous or toxic material exposures. The best methods of accessing poison control are either by direct dial or conference/link call telephone system.

Sometimes a poison control center suggests using Ipecac with these constraints:

❖ Ipecac is not to be given to children less than 1 year.
❖ It is rarely given to adults, because adults who have ingested poisons are generally poor historians and therefore, the nurse cannot be sure of how much or what they really ingested. The lack of accurate information from adults who have ingested poisons increases the risk of seizures or respiratory arrest, which precludes giving them Ipecac.
❖ Ipecac is rarely given to an individual if the lapsed time between the ingestion of the poison and the call has been greater than 1-1.5 hours.

As with most telehealth advice calls, poison exposure calls frequently present an opportunity for the nurse to educate the patient either at the time of the call or with a follow-up call. Every home should have the poison control center number, along with other emergency numbers posted in an easily accessible place. Safety precautions for storing poisonous substances can also be discussed with the caller.

If the nurse expects carbon monoxide poisoning, the patient should be instructed to get fresh air immediately. Doors and windows should be opened. Based on the acuity of the patient's symptoms, medical help from a same-day provider appointment to emergency 911 care should be recommended.

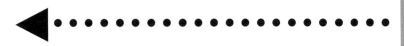

ABUSE

Definition

Abuse can be defined from several different perspectives, all of which have detrimental consequences for the person being abused.

- ❖ *Physical Abuse:* An injury or injuries inflicted through intentional physical force.
- ❖ *Neglect:* The failure to supply children or dependent adults with one or more of their basic needs.
- ❖ *Sexual Abuse:* Any form of sexual contact, either genital or non-genital, which is inflicted upon children (or dependent adults) or upon adults without their consent.
- ❖ *Emotional or Psychological Abuse:* The deliberate use of threats, intimidation, or humiliation in order to inflict mental or emotional anguish.
- ❖ *Exploitation:* Any use of a child that could be damaging physically, emotionally, or socially, such as pornography, financial expectations for income, etc. Exploitation of an adult would be the unjust or improper use of an adult's resources for another's profit or advantage.

Situations That Are High-Risk for Abuse

- ❖ Drug or alcohol abuse in the family or home.
- ❖ Recent stressful situation.
- ❖ Abused person's dependence upon the abuser for basic needs (such as children and the elderly).
- ❖ History of abuse.

Patient Behaviors that May Suggest Abuse

- ❖ Inconsistencies in the history of the injury.
- ❖ Hesitancy to provide information.
- ❖ Lack of appropriate concern for the situation.
- ❖ Delay in obtaining medical advice regarding a serious injury.
- ❖ Making frequent medical appointments for relatively minor complaints or canceling appointments on a regular basis with decreased compliance to the suggested medical regimen.
- ❖ Repeat traumatic injuries. If the nurse has access to the victim's medical record, it would be important to review the record for repeated injuries that may be indicative of abuse. Sometimes health professionals contribute to the abuse process by treating the medical problem and not recognizing the cause of the injury. Since abuse tends to be repetitive, the telehealth practice nurse could analyze prior telephone calls and medical record documentation for previous situations/conditions that may alert the nurse of an abusive situation.

Since abuse tends to be repetitive, the telehealth practice nurse could analyze prior telephone calls and medical record documentation for previous situations/conditions that may alert the nurse of an abusive situation.

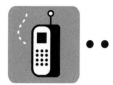

For example, a 5-year-old patient's mother consistently calls every month for some sort of contusion, burn, or accidental poisoning happening to her child. While talking to the mother, the nurse learns that the child is frequently left for long periods of time while the mother goes out with her boyfriend. It is abusive to leave a 5-year-old child alone for extended periods of time without the supervision of a responsible adult. Additionally, multiple calls regarding frequent injuries raise the suspicion of abuse.

Commonly Observed Injuries in Victims of Abuse

Since the telehealth nurse cannot see the injuries, injury information must be obtained by questioning the patient. The patient may be concerned about injuries resulting from the child or dependent adult's visit with a relative, babysitter, or friend. As the nurse collects data regarding a problem, the following information may surface and should alert the nurse to the possibility of abuse:

Since the telehealth nurse cannot see the injuries, injury information must be obtained by questioning the patient.

❖ Burns, especially on the back and buttocks. Be suspicious of burns that are circular or have a pattern.
❖ Unexplained bruises or abrasions, especially to the genitals, inner thighs, lower back, buttocks.
❖ Bruises or cuts on the inner aspect of arms or thighs (unintentional injuries are usually on the outer aspect).
❖ Black or swollen eye(s) or cheeks.
❖ Rope marks or other signs of physical restraint.

Telehealth Nurse Responsibilities

1. **Assess the Symptoms to Determine the Urgency**
   After obtaining the name, address, and telephone number of the patient, the first priority of the nurse is to assess the patient's symptoms to determine the appropriate disposition. If the patient or other household members are in imminent danger, report the situation to 911.

2. **Assess the Lethality of the Situation**
   Exploring the victim's safety is at the center of the lethality assessment for abuse. Violence in abuse situations tends to escalate from verbal to pushing to punching or slapping to physical assaults with bodily injuries to potentially death. To assess the safety of the victim, the following questions may be used:
   ❖ "Are you currently safe?"
   ❖ "Who causes you to feel unsafe?"
   ❖ "Is the abuser there with you now?"
   ❖ "Have there been shouting matches or verbal insults?"
   ❖ "Has [the abuser] threatened homicide or suicide?"
   ❖ "Has there been any time where hitting or punching occurred?"

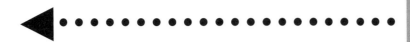

❖ "Have guns or weapons been used, or has their use been threatened in past assaults?"

❖ "Have there been injuries sustained as a result of one of these situations?"

❖ "Has medical care been sought to treat injuries as a result of one of these situations?"

❖ "Does [the patient] feel homicidal or suicidal?"

Since the perpetrator of the abuse is frequently in the same home as the victim, the victim may be calling while in the same vicinity as the abuser. By utilizing the above questions but changing the questions to allow "yes" or "no" responses, a nurse is able to successfully and safely receive information without endangering the patient further. The first few questions could be:

❖ "Are you able to speak freely?"

❖ "Will you answer questions that require only 'yes' or 'no' answers?"

❖ "Are you currently safe?"

❖ "Who causes you to feel unsafe? Is it your husband? Your wife? Your mother?"

Even if the abuser were in the same room as the victim, all that would be heard is "yes" or "no;" at the same time, the nurse would be receiving valuable information about the situation.

3. **Establish a Trusting and Caring Relationship with the Patient**

It is extremely important to establish a trusting and caring relationship with the patient (see Chapter 4, "Communication Principles"). Nurses need to analyze their own feelings and attitudes about abuse so that they can make objective assessments and provide appropriate advice in a non-judgmental, professional manner. Important messages to reinforce with abuse and sexual assault victims are:

❖ "This is not your fault. You did not deserve to be abused (sexually assaulted/raped)."

❖ "There is help available for you."

❖ "I can help you find the care you need."

4. **Direct the Appropriate Action or Follow-Up**

In order to direct the appropriate action/follow-up for an individual who has been abused, the nurse must know the definition of abuse, signs and symptoms of abuse, and situations that are high-risk for abuse. It is important that the nurse recognize patient behaviors that may be suggestive for abuse.

❖ The role of the telehealth nurse in assessing and managing abuse situations is often not clearly delineated; however, the nurse is part of the medical community that has the responsibility to recognize, respond, and educate. Nurses need to know the process for reporting abuse as well as the telephone numbers for Health and Social Services and Child Protective Services, both of which are usually

Since the perpetrator of the abuse is frequently in the same home as the victim, the victim may be calling while in the same vicinity as the abuser. By utilizing questions with only "yes" or "no" responses, a nurse is able to successfully and safely receive information without endangering the patient further.

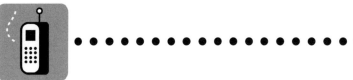

included in the organization's abuse policy/procedure. Most organizations delineate in their *abuse policy* what is reported, to whom it is reported, and who is accountable to report the abuse. If a telehealth nurse is not sure what to do with a suspected case of abuse, the problem should be discussed with a supervisor or attending physician. Legal implications for nurses will be discussed later in this chapter.

❖ Self-help group numbers can be useful resources to offer further assistance to patients, either at the time of the call or later during a follow-up call. Several telehealth resource books are now available that include lists of toll-free numbers for self-help groups. (See page 228 at the end of this chapter for a list of help lines.)

CHILD ABUSE

Incidence

The Children's Bureau of U.S. Department of Human Services developed the National Child Abuse and Neglect Data System (NCANDS).

In partnership with the U.S., NCANDS reported an estimated 1,530 child fatalities in 2006 (Child Welfare Information Gateway, 2006). These fatalities are defined as the death of a child resulting from abuse or neglect or where abuse or neglect was a contributing factor (see Table 12-1).

This translates to a rate of 2.04 children per 100,000 children in the general population. This is a 4.8% increase from the 1,460 fatalities that occurred the previous year. Children younger than 1-year-old accounted for 44.2% of fatalities and 78% of fatalities were children younger than 4-years-old (Prevent Child Abuse New York, 2006).

Long-Term Effects

Sexual and physical abuse either experienced or witnessed places that individual at greater risk for continuing the abusive patterns within their own lives. In a domestic violence study, approximately 33% of the alleged abusers were abused by their parents and about 50% of their parents were themselves involved in battering relationships (Prevent Child Abuse New York, 2003).

Legal

All 50 states require that health professionals report suspected cases of child abuse to a local child protection agency. State laws protect health professionals from liability that may result from reporting "in good faith" a suspected case of child abuse.

In partnership with the U.S., the National Child Abuse and Neglect Data System reported an estimated 1,530 child fatalities in 2006. These fatalities are defined as the death of a child resulting from abuse or neglect or where abuse or neglect was a contributing factor.

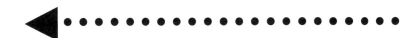

Table 12-1.
Symptoms or Behaviors Specific to Child Abuse

Symptoms or Behaviors
• "Glove" or "stocking" burns on extremities, which may be indicative of dipping an extremity into a hot liquid.
• Urinary discomfort in a young child.
• Sudden aggressive or withdrawn behavior or hyper-sexualized behaviors.
• Injuries inconsistent with the developmental abilities of the child.
• Bruising, fractures, or injuries on the skin that do not match the description of how they occurred, especially if this is a frequent occurrence or the injuries are visible after days away from school.
• Failure to thrive.
• Sexually transmitted disease symptoms.
• Fear or cringing when parents or adults are present.
• Poor physical hygiene or clothing inappropriate for their size or the season of the weather.

Taking the Call

❖ **Be suspicious** if a child calls to discuss his/her own symptoms, especially injuries. Because they are afraid to disclose what is happening to them, teenagers will sometimes call under the guise of "a friend" who has the described problem.

❖ **Ask open-ended questions** like, "How did you burn yourself?" or "How did your child happen to burn himself?" Be careful not to insinuate that the caller caused the injury with statements like, "How did *you* burn your child?"

❖ **Refer the patient for a primary care provider visit.** Even if the symptoms are not otherwise indicative of a health care visit, a nurse who suspects possible child abuse should instruct the parent to have the child seen by a physician or midlevel provider. The child's own primary care provider would be the preferable provider to evaluate the child's condition/situation. If possible, discuss the situation with the provider prior to having the child examined. If the caller refuses to seek professional care for a potentially maltreated child, the telehealth nurse will need to follow the organization's policy/protocol for reporting to Child Protective Services.

❖ **Consult an experienced co-worker or professional** if unsure or inexperienced in assessing child abuse. It can be extremely detrimental to a child and his/her family if a false report is turned in. On the other hand, it is essential to stop child abuse when it is occurring.

Even if the symptoms are not otherwise indicative of a health care visit, a nurse who suspects possible child abuse should instruct the parent to have the child seen by a physician or midlevel provider.

DEPENDENT ADULT OR ELDER ABUSE

Definition

The U.S. National Academy of Science defines elder abuse and mistreatment as intentional actions that cause harm or create a serious risk of harm to a vulnerable elderly person. This harm may be accidental or intentional and usually occurs from another person in a trusting relationship and includes neglect, confinement, cruelty, physical pain, emotional or mental anguish, withholding critical care elements, and misuse of finances. (Bonnie & Wallace, 2003). Simply stated, it is physical, psychological or financial/material abuse or neglect of an elderly individual (see Table 12-2).

Incidence

In 2004, a survey of state Adult Protective Services (APS) sponsored by The National Center on Elder Abuse found that there were 565,747 reports of elder and vulnerable adult abuse for persons of all 50 states and territories.

The National Center on Elder Abuse found that there were 565,747 reports of elder and vulnerable adult abuse for persons of all 50 states and territories.

❖ APS reported that there was a 16.3 % increase in the number of reports of elder and vulnerable adult abuse for victims of all ages when 2004 data was compared to 2000 data.
❖ Self-neglect was the most common category of investigated reports, followed by caregiver neglect and financial exploitation.
❖ A majority of the reported victims of abuse were female (65.7%). Of the victims aged 60 years or more, 42.8% were 80 years of age and older and their abusers tended to be female and under the age of 60 years.

It is believed that elder abuse is under-reported. The under-reporting is partially due to the victim's feelings of embarrassment and intimidation. These feelings increase if the abuser is a family member. Elderly victims may also be concerned that if they report abuse by the family member who is caring for them, they may have to move to a nursing home or worse living arrangements.

Legal

All 50 states have some form of elder abuse prevention laws. Although the laws and definitions of terms vary considerably from one state to another, all states have set up reporting systems.

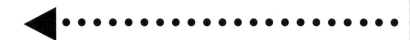

Table 12-2.
Symptoms or Behaviors Specific to Dependent Adult/Elder Abuse

Symptoms or Behaviors
• Bruises, pressure marks, broken bones, abrasions, and burns, which may be an indication of physical abuse, neglect, or mistreatment.
• Unexplained withdrawal from normal activities, a sudden change in alertness, and unusual depression, which may be indicators of emotional abuse.
• Bruises around the breasts or genital area, which can occur from sexual abuse.
• Sudden changes in financial situations, which may be the result of exploitation.
• Bedsores, unattended medical needs, poor hygiene, and unusual weight loss, which are indicators of possible neglect.
• Behavior such as belittling, threatening, and other uses of power and control by spouses, which are indicators of verbal or emotional abuse.
• Strained or tense relationships and frequent arguments between the caregiver and elderly person are also signs.

Taking the Call

It will be infrequent that elderly persons will call and discuss the abuse that is occurring to them because of the above stated reasons. More often, a relative, friend, neighbor, or another family member will call to talk to the nurse about the situation. The nurse can share with the caller how to report the situation, but if the nurse feels like the situation will not be taken care of by the caller, the nurse should follow the organization's policy/protocol for reporting the suspected elder abuse. Elder abuse is generally reported to the state's Adult Protective Services.

INTIMATE PARTNER VIOLENCE (IPV)

Definition

In the past, the term *domestic violence* has been used to describe the physical and/or emotional violence used by an individual to control or intimidate an intimate partner. Domestic violence has come to include other forms of violence, such as child abuse and dependent adult/elder abuse. The CDC also believes that the term *domestic violence* leaves out the controlling violence that may occur among same-sex partners and male victims. *Intimate partner violence* (IPV) is the term that the CDC is currently using to describe physical and/or emotional abuse by a spouse, ex-spouse, boyfriend/girlfriend, ex-boyfriend/ex-girlfriend, or date (see Table 12-3).

Intimate partner violence (IPV) is the term that the CDC is currently using to describe physical and/or emotional abuse by a spouse, ex-spouse, boyfriend/girlfriend, ex-boyfriend/ ex-girlfriend, or date.

Incidence

Facts gathered by National Coalition Against Domestic Violence (2005) suggest that there is a huge personal and national price paid each year regarding domestic partner abuse.

❖ The majority (73%) of family violence victims are female. Females were 84% of spousal abuse victims and 86% of abuse victims at the hands of a boyfriend.

❖ Females who are 20-24 years of age are at the greatest risk for intimate partner violence.

❖ Less than one-fifth of victims reporting an injury from intimate partner violence sought medical treatment following the injury.

❖ 76% of femicide (female homicide) victims had been stalked by the person who killed them.

❖ Intimate partner violence results in more than 18.5 million mental health care visits each year.

❖ 1 in 6 women and 1 in 33 men have experienced an attempted or completed rape.

Other Facts:

❖ 1 in 12 women and 1 in 45 men will be stalked in their lifetime.

❖ 81% of women stalked by a current or former intimate partner are also physically assaulted by that partner.

❖ Boys who witness domestic violence are twice as likely to abuse their own partners and children when they become adults.

❖ 30-60% of perpetrators of intimate partner violence also abuse children in the household.

❖ The cost of intimate partner violence exceeds $5.8 billion each year, $4.1 billion of which is for direct medical and mental health services.

❖ All races are equally vulnerable to attacks by intimates; however, a study completed in Oklahoma in 2002 showed that black women had a rate of injury 4.7 times higher than that of white women (CDC, 2005).

❖ The prevalence of intimate partner violence among gay and lesbian couples is approximately 25-33% (Rainbow Response, 2008).

Legal

Intimate partner violence is a crime in all 50 states; however, each state's laws are slightly different.

❖ Intimate partner violence is a crime in all 50 states; however, each state's laws are slightly different (American Bar Association, 2003).

❖ Federal laws require that states provide restitution for the victim's losses and strengthen federal penalties for sexual abuse.

❖ There are several circumstances in which health care providers may be open to liability if they act or fail to act in domestic violence situations (Orloff & Siu Chung, 1996):

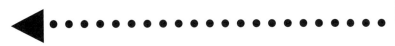

- o Reporting abuse to the police without permission of an adult victim of abuse.
- o Negligence in identifying victims of domestic violence (diagnosis), documenting their injuries, properly treating victims, providing them with information about their options to counter domestic violence (including safety planning), and making referrals to specialists (domestic violence experts).
- o Failure to warn potential victims about the threat of assault from an abuser when the health professional learns that there is a danger of harm to an identifiable victim or victims by a patient who is perpetrator of domestic abuse.

Table 12-3.
Symptoms or Behaviors Specific to Intimate Partner Violence

Symptoms or Behaviors
• High users of health care services for multiple problems that could be related to stress or tension, such as headaches/migraines and gastrointestinal problems.
• Frequent injuries.
• Suicide attempt.
• Depression or withdrawal.
• Drug or alcohol abuse.

The Telehealth Nurse's Role

Some patients may initiate a conversation with a concern about an abusive relationship. However, there are many situations in which patients are not able to admit, even to themselves, that they are in an abusive relationship. If the telehealth nurse suspects abuse, it is appropriate to approach the situation directly. By addressing the problem openly, it gives the patient permission to discuss with the nurse their abuse issues. Because there is no face-to-face interaction, telehealth nurses are frequently viewed as a non-threatening medical person to whom a patient can divulge his/her concerns. Listed below are some examples of how to ask a patient about his/her situation:

- ❖ "I have received a number of calls lately from patients who are being abused. Is this happening to you?"
- ❖ "We have recently had training about intimate partner violence/ domestic violence. We learned that there are a lot of people in this country that have been abused by their partners. Is this happening to you?"

If the telehealth nurse suspects abuse, it is appropriate to approach the situation directly. By addressing the problem openly, it gives the patient permission to discuss with the nurse their abuse issues.

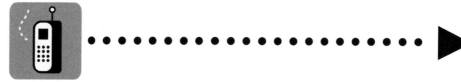

Intervention

Since recent data show that victims of IPV are frequently high users of health care services, health care providers and nurses need to be involved in developing a treatment plan to attack the "real" problem of IPV. In the past, many health care providers and nurses have treated the inflicted symptoms without even recognizing that the patient is in an abusive situation.

The Joint Commission now requires that organizations seeking accreditation demonstrate that they have and utilize protocols to identify and treat victims of IPV. Research has shown that health care professionals *can* make a difference in the lives of IPV victims by identifying domestic violence, reinforcing the victim's own strengths, helping the victim develop a safety plan, and referring the victim to a program.

It may take several telephone or provider visits before the victim is able to break away from the abuser, if ever. The success of the telephone interaction should not be based on whether or not the victim was able to discontinue their situation of abuse. It is a well-known fact that most abused persons need to hear that there is "help" available many times before they can act to change their lives.

The goal of the telehealth nurse should be to provide an emotionally safe encounter along with information and guidance for medical treatment. "Just by inquiring and expressing concern, we begin to build bridges, decrease isolation, and create hope. First and foremost, the abused patient must be able to rely on nonjudgmental and supportive interpersonal communications to enable her/him to participate in the complex but necessary medical and legal evaluations" (Bouquin & Johnson, 1998).

In addition to other interventions for abuse victims, it may be necessary for the telehealth nurse to help the victim develop a safety plan. Domestic violence shelters, safe shelters, physician offices, emergency rooms, and a variety of Internet sources will have written safety plans that a nurse could use to help educate a victim of IPV. A safety plan may include the following advice:

❖ Tell your neighbors or close friends about your concerns. Ask them to call the police if they notice anything suspicious at your house.

❖ Find a safe place where you can go, even if it's 2:00 a.m.

❖ Pack a suitcase containing an extra change of clothes for you and your children, small familiar toys or cherished items for the children, money, a supply of prescription medicines, and an extra set of house and car keys. Leave the suitcase at the home of a trusted family member or friend.

❖ Collect important documents, like birth certificates, social security cards, restraining orders, work permits/Green cards, visa, or passport. Don't forget ATM or debit cards that can be used for immediate cash.

> *Since recent data show that victims of IPV are frequently high users of health care services, health care providers and nurses need to be involved in developing a treatment plan to attack the "real" problem of IPV. In the past, many health care providers and nurses have treated the inflicted symptoms without even recognizing that the patient is in an abusive situation.*

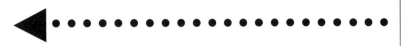

❖ Teach your children how to call 911 for help. Tell them that their job is to protect themselves, not you.

❖ Have your own banking account. The statements should be sent to a relative's or friend's address.

Anyone who has known or suspected abuse occurring in their life should be provided with a list of local shelters or crisis intervention phone numbers. The national hotline for victims of domestic abuse is 1-800-799-SAFE (7233). This line provides 24-hour information, referrals, escape planning, and general information for residents of all 50 states and Puerto Rico.

SEXUAL ASSAULT

Definitions

The Rape, Abuse & Incest National Network (RAINN) defines rape as forced sexual intercourse, including vaginal, anal, or oral penetration. Penetration may be by a body part or an object. Survivors of rape and sexual assault may be forced through threats or physical means. In about 8 out of 10 rapes, no weapon is used other than physical force. Anyone may be a victim of rape: women or men, adults or children, straight or gay (RAINN, 2008).

The phrase *sexual assault* is sometimes used interchangeably with *rape*, but can also convey an attack that stops short of rape and may include fondling, mouth to genital contact, or other unwanted sexual advances. Many experts who currently are working with survivors of sexual assault no longer utilize the term *victim*.

Many experts who currently are working with survivors of sexual assault no longer utilize the term "victim."

Common Misconceptions about Sexual Assault

It is very important that telehealth nurses understand the facts about sexual assault. They need to analyze and evaluate their own feelings so that they can provide an objective and caring assessment and advice to sexual assault survivors.

❖ Sexual assault is not about passion or sexual gratification. It is an act of violence. It is about anger, power, and control.

❖ It is not the survivor's fault that he/she was sexually assaulted. It is not about how a woman or man dresses. It is the offender's responsibility for the assault.

❖ Approximately 75% of all sexual assaults are planned (Albuquerque Rape Crisis Center, 1997).

❖ Sexual assault occurs equally across all age groups, genders, ethnic, social, and economic backgrounds.

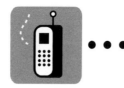

Incidence

RAINN is a comprehensive clearinghouse for information and the nation's largest anti-sexual assault organization. In 2008, RAINN reported that:

❖ Somewhere in America, someone is sexually assaulted every 2 minutes.

❖ While 1 out of every 6 American women are survivors of an attempted or completed rape in her lifetime, about 3% of American men have experienced an attempted or completed rape in their lifetime.

❖ It is estimated that 93% of juvenile sexual assault victims know their attacker and approximately one-third of those attackers were family members.

❖ 50% of all rapes occur either at the victim's home or within one mile of his/her home.

❖ Looking at longer-term data, victims of sexual assault are **3 times** more likely to suffer from depression, **6 times** more likely to suffer from post-traumatic stress disorder, and **4 times** more likely to contemplate suicide.

❖ Many people think of rapists as crazed strangers, yet most rapists (73%) know their victims. The majority of rapists are male, approximately 31 years of age, Caucasian, and have committed a crime before. 1 in 3 is also intoxicated with either alcohol or drugs at the time of the assault.

❖ 60% of rapes/sexual assaults are not reported to the police. Those rapists, of course, never spend a day in prison, according to a statistical average of the past 5 years. Factoring in unreported rapes, only about 6% of rapists ever serve a day in jail.

The Telehealth Nurse's Role

Emotional reactions of the survivor vary from denial, anger, revenge, panic, and anxiety to feelings of helplessness, humiliation, embarrassment, and even absolute composure. Concerns about their reputation, respectability, and their family's reactions are common. Shock, disbelief, or fear may occur initially, but it is important to know that coping mechanisms will vary and there is no right or wrong way to handle the situation. This was a life-changing experience in which he/she had no control of what was happening, and each person must be allowed to grieve and deal with emotions in his/her own way.

The telehealth nurse's role is to quickly assess if the patient needs 911 and assist the patient in seeking immediate medical care. The nurse should not ask details regarding the assault but focus on the *care* of the patient and getting the patient to the appropriate facility for care.

The survivor may want to know what the medical examination consists of and why it is necessary. In most cities, medical examinations for sexual

Emotional reactions of the survivor of sexual assault vary from denial, anger, revenge, panic, and anxiety to feelings of helplessness, humiliation, embarrassment, and even absolute composure.

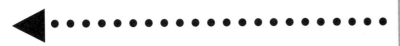

assault are done in emergency rooms or by special sexual assault team units. In rural areas, the examination may be done in the medical provider's office. Trained professionals use the required Sexual Assault Evidence Collection Kit as part of the medical exam. Specimen collection consists of different samples of blood, hair, vaginal mucous, etc. Usually the clothing associated with the assault is collected and sent to a crime lab. An excellent program, Sexual Assault Nurse Examiners (SANE), was developed by a group of nurses in Tulsa, Oklahoma. It has resulted in more humane treatment of sexual assault survivors and has been highly successful in sexual assault prosecution. This federally funded program is staffed by volunteer nurses 24 hours a day and has been implemented in many states. The medical examination includes:

- ❖ General physical examination to make sure no other trauma occurred.
- ❖ Tests to rule out sexually transmitted diseases or blanket treatment for sexually transmitted diseases.
- ❖ "Day-After" birth control pill.
- ❖ Evidence gathering.

The following advice was adapted for telephone advice from a patient education pamphlet developed by the New Mexico Coalition for Sexual Assault Programs, Inc. (Klein & Farr, 1994).

- ❖ **Reassure the survivor that he/she is not alone.** Sexual assault is the most frequently committed of violent crimes. Many other people have gone through what the survivor is going through.
- ❖ **Remind the survivor that he/she is alive** and whatever he/she had to do to stay alive was the right thing. The survivor should not feel guilty that he/she couldn't do more to prevent the sexual assault. He/she used instinct to do what he/she could to stay alive.
- ❖ **Tell the survivor that it is normal** for him/her to have reactions to what happened, and that those feelings may take a long time to resolve.
- ❖ **Advise the survivor that it will be important for him/her to receive counseling** to help deal with the feelings that will occur following the sexual assault.
- ❖ **If the survivor asks about AIDS**, give reassurance that although AIDS can be contracted by sexual assault, this is extremely rare. A baseline HIV test should be obtained. AIDS testing related to the sexual assault will occur 3 months later.
- ❖ **Encourage the survivor to obtain a medical examination as soon as possible.** The survivor does not have to prosecute. Survivors do not have to decide before the medical examination and evidence collection that they want to prosecute. If evidence is to be collected, it

Trained professionals use the required Sexual Assault Evidence Collection Kit as part of the medical exam. Specimen collection consists of different samples of blood, hair, vaginal mucous, etc. Usually the clothing associated with the assault is collected and sent to a crime lab.

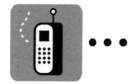

must be done within 72 hours after the assault. If the survivor chooses not to prosecute, the evidence kit will be destroyed. All the information in the kit remains completely confidential. Most states will cover the costs of the evidence collection kit and some costs associated with related medical expenses.

❖ **If the survivor decides to obtain a medical examination**, provide the following *interim* instructions:
  o Do not to eat or drink anything until after the examination, this includes smoking a cigarette.
  o Do not shower or douche before the exam.
  o Bring the clothes associated with the sexual assault to the examination.
  o The state will hire an attorney if the survivor decides to prosecute.

SUICIDE

Overview

Every suicide call needs to be treated like a medical emergency. Although there are patients who have learned to manipulate the system and are just lonely or anxious, most suicide calls result from patients who are extremely distressed. Suicide calls are usually very time-consuming calls to assess and to advise. This can be very frustrating for a nurse who is expected to return a high volume of calls, but it is a *reality* of telehealth nursing and must be dealt with appropriately. Suicide calls are a "code blue" for telehealth nursing. It is important that nurses have time to debrief with peers and evaluate the "good" and the "could use improvement" situations following a suicide call.

All nurses who provide telehealth assessment and advice will eventually have to respond to a suicide call. Suicide calls come from all areas of medical practice. For example, cardiac patients are often severely depressed; postpartum patients struggle with the postpartum blues; adolescent males are known to be high-risk for suicide; and male patients greater than 85-years-old are the most at-risk.

If someone is absolutely determined to kill him/herself, there is nothing that the telehealth nurse can say or do to stop him/her. However, the fact that a call was initiated to the telehealth nurse demonstrates the patient's ambiguity about dying. The patient is not sure about dying, but is feeling very negative about living. The patient is asking for help and reassurance that life is worth living. By demonstrating warm, genuine concern for the patient, the telehealth nurse may be able to tip the scale in favor of life (Gronseth & Marek, 2000).

The Telehealth Nurse's Role

Request the patient's telephone number and address. When the nurse asks for demographic information, the response may be, "I'm afraid that if I

> *Every suicide call needs to be treated like a medical emergency. Although there are patients who have learned to manipulate the system and are just lonely or anxious, most suicide calls result from patients who are extremely distressed.*

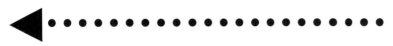

give you my telephone number or address, you will call the police." The nurse may respond, "I will only call the police if I feel like you are not safe, and I will tell you if I am going to call." Most police departments have *crisis teams* that will respond to an impending suicide. (Refer to *Receiving the Crisis Call,* earlier in this chapter, for more information.)

Assess the extent of the injuries. If a suicide attempt has already occurred, assess the patient's injuries and then utilize the appropriate disposition. If an emergency exists, it is preferable to stay on the line with the patient until the EMS arrives. (Refer to *Notifying Emergency Medical Services,* earlier in this chapter, if an emergency exists.)

Engage the patient. The nurse can say to the patient, "You've called the right place. I can find the help you need." As the nurse begins assessing the situation, questions should be framed so that the focus is not on how the patient is feeling. Focus on concrete happenings versus irrational feelings.

> *If a suicide attempt has already occurred, assess the patient's injuries and then utilize the appropriate disposition. If an emergency exists, it is preferable to stay on the line with the patient until the EMS arrives.*

❖ Ask the patient, "What is happening for you now?" versus "How are you feeling?"

❖ "Have you eaten today? What did you eat?"

Establish suicide ideation. Ask, "Are you thinking about killing yourself?" or "Are you thinking about committing suicide?" Many nurses are uncomfortable questioning the patient about his/her suicide intentions; however experts state that directly asking about suicide normalizes the patient's feelings and allows them to talk about their situation (Stoney, 2001).

Assess lethality of the situation. Lethality of the situation means how likely it is that suicide will occur. The decision on whether a suicide call is low, medium, or high lethality is made after the nurse assesses the risk factors and current situational risks. It's also important to try to ascertain if the caller is alone or if they have others in the home or around them at that moment.

Risk Factors for Suicide

❖ Known history of mental illness.

❖ History of substance abuse.

❖ Serious physical illnesses.

❖ Age, with particular attention paid to teens and the elderly.

❖ History of trauma, abuse, or physical assault.

❖ Family history of suicide or a previous attempt at suicide.

❖ Loss of a job, relationship, or financial security.

❖ Local clusters of suicide.

❖ Easy or current access to firearms or other lethal methods for death (Suicide Prevention Resource Center, 2008).

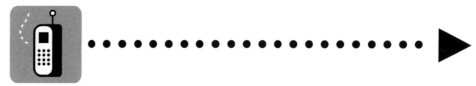

Situational Risk Factors

❖ Is there a detailed plan of how the suicide will happen? The more detailed the plan (as to time, place, and method), the more lethal the situation.

❖ Does the patient have the means available to implement the suicide plan, for example, have a gun, pills, knife, etc? The more available the means of suicide, the more lethal the risk.

❖ How lethal is the planned method of suicide? A loaded gun is more lethal than slashing one's wrists or overdosing on medication.

❖ Refusal or hesitation to make a "no suicide contract" increases the patient's suicide risk (see below).

Make a "no suicide contract" with the patient. An effective tool in delaying and hopefully avoiding a suicide attempt is "contracting." The nurse and the patient together negotiate a contract for delaying the suicide attempt. Most suicidal thoughts are time-limiting. If the nurse can contract with the patient for a specified time, then hopefully, the desire for suicide may diminish. Examples are:

❖ "Will you promise me to put the gun down until we are through talking?"

❖ "Will you promise me that you will not harm yourself until your appointment with your doctor in 2 hours?"

❖ "Will you call me back in 2 hours and let me know how you are doing?"

❖ "Will you promise me that you will call me if you ever feel like committing suicide again?"

Most suicidal thoughts are time-limiting. If the nurse can contract with the patient for a specified time, then hopefully, the desire for suicide may diminish.

Encourage social connection. Help suicide-ideation patients focus on upcoming events, people that matter, or religion as a way to dissuade them from the anguish of the current moment. Allowing patients to generate their own alternatives and suggestions gives them a feeling of self-esteem and control.

❖ "Is there anyone else in there with you? Do they know how you are feeling?"

❖ "Have you thought about how your children would feel if you killed yourself?"

❖ If a person is religious, "Have you thought about how your religion would view you killing yourself?"

Refer the patient to expert resources. Suicide help lines, mental health triage experts, and the patient's own mental health provider are all excellent resources for referral. An excellent example of this service is *The Samaritans,*

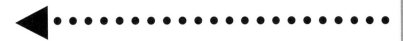

an Internet and phone advice service that provides emotional help to people who are depressed and/or suicidal, and provides education to the public about these two conditions. It is staffed by trained volunteers 24 hours a day.

Additionally, many city and state organizations have local organizations that provide much of the same services and these telephone numbers should also be available to the telehealth nurse. The Suicide Prevention Resource Center has a helpful Web site (http://www.sprc.org/) that provides up-to-date information, as well as a list of important phone numbers for each state. If the patient is struggling with a particular problem (cancer, heart disease, obesity, etc.), there are many self-help groups that are excellent sources of friendship and support. Many of the newer nursing telehealth guideline manuals list dozens of national self-help resources. If the patient lives in a large metropolitan city, there are self-help groups for almost any problem.

You may call the police and ask for a "well-person check." The police will check within the next two hours to make sure that the person is safe. Tell the patient that you are going to request the check so that trust between the nurse and the patient will not be destroyed.

Many of the newer nursing telehealth guideline manuals list dozens of national self-help resources. If the patient lives in a large metropolitan city, there are self-help groups for almost any problem.

Suicide in the United States

❖ In 2003, there were 31,484 suicides in the U.S. (86 suicides per day; 1 suicide every 17 minutes). This translates to an annual suicide rate of 10.8 per 100,000.

❖ Suicide is the eleventh leading cause of death.

❖ Suicide rates in the U.S. can best be characterized as mostly stable over time. Since 1990, rates have ranged between 12.4 and 10.7 per 100,000.

❖ Rates of suicide are highest in the intermountain states. 8 of the top 10 suicide rates are from those states.

❖ Males complete suicide at a rate 4 times that of females. However, females attempt suicide 3 times more often than males.

❖ Elderly adults have rates of suicide close to 50% higher than that of the nation as a whole (all ages).

❖ Youth (ages 15-24) suicide rates increased more than 200% from the 1950s to the late 1970s. From the late 1970s to the mid 1990s, suicide rates for youth rank third as a cause of death among those ages 15-24.

❖ Firearms remain the most commonly utilized method of completing suicide by essentially all groups. More than half (54%) of the individuals who took their own lives in 2003 used this method. Males used it more often than females.

❖ The most common method of suicide for all females was poisoning. In fact, poisoning has surpassed firearms for female suicides since 2001.

❖ Caucasians (12 per 100,000) have higher rates of completed suicides than African Americans (5.1 per 100,000).

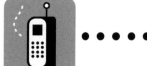

❖ Suicide rates have traditionally decreased in times of war and increased in times of economic crises, and rates are higher among the divorced, separated, and widowed (South Dakota Suicide Prevention, 2008).

FACTS

Data suggest a possible inter-relatedness between poisoning/overdose, abuse of all kinds, sexual assault, suicide, and mental illnesses. The telehealth nurse should be cognizant of this inter-relatedness when assisting patients with these issues/problems.

Data suggest a possible inter-relatedness between poisoning/overdose, abuse of all kinds, sexual assault, suicide, and mental illnesses. The telehealth nurse should be cognizant of this inter-relatedness when assisting patients with these issues/problems.

❖ Los Angeles County Department of Health Services (2001) reported 617 poisoning deaths and 7,153 people who experienced a non-fatal poisoning incident serious enough to require hospitalization. "Among the 617 poisoning deaths in 1997, 76% were unintentional, 20% were due to suicide, 3% undetermined intent, and 1% from homicide. However, when non-fatal poisonings are considered, 53% were suicide attempts, 44% were unintentional, 3% undetermined intentionally, and less then 1% assaultive in nature."

❖ In the United States, about 50% of all poisonings in teenagers are suicide attempts (Litovitz et al., 2001).

❖ Exposure to domestic violence as a child can be associated with problems experienced as an adult. These issues have been suggested to be varying degrees of depression, low self-esteem and posttraumatic stress syndrome in both men and women (Edleson, 2006, p. 175).

❖ Those who have suffered abuse are more likely to develop drug addictions, have alcohol addictions, suffer psychiatric illnesses, and be arrested and incarcerated.

❖ According to a 2-year research effort by the U.S. Department of Justice, personal crime is estimated to cost Americans $105 billion annually in medical costs, lost earnings, and public program costs related to victim assistance (Prevent Child Abuse New York, 2003).

❖ Adults who were abused as children are likely to grow up to become abusers themselves, perpetuating a cycle of inter-generational abuse or neglect (Prevent Child Abuse New York, 2003).

❖ Sexual assault survivors are 3 times more likely to be depressed than non-victims, 4 times more likely to attempt suicide, and have a higher rate of both alcohol and drug addictions (RAINN, 2008).

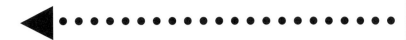

TIPS & PEARLS

☎ Patients experiencing acute crisis should not drive themselves to the place of medical care.

☎ Role-playing is an excellent way to practice dealing with special situations before they happen.

☎ Participate in frequent reviews of the policies/protocols that instruct telehealth nurses on how to manage special situation calls.

☎ Know how to proficiently place a conference (link) call.

☎ Review CPR pre-arrival instructions regularly if the organization has decided to provide pre-arrival CPR instructions.

☎ Attend inservices given by experts who frequently field calls dealing with these special circumstances.

☎ Perform literature review on a regular basis to keep references and emergency phone numbers updated.

HELP LINES

Abuse, Assault, Sexual Assault
o   Childhelp National Child Abuse Hotline
      1-800-4-A-CHILD or 1-800-422-4453
o   National Sexual Assault Hotline (operated by RAINN)
      1-800-656-HOPE or 1-800-656-4673
o   National Domestic Violence/Child Abuse/Sexual Abuse Hotline
      1-800-799-SAFE or 1-800-799-7233

Alcohol and Substance Abuse
o   Alcohol Abuse Treatment Referral Hotline
      1-800-234-0246

Eating Disorders
o   National Association of Anorexia Nervosa and Associated Disorders
    (ANAD)
      1-847-837-3438 (long distance)

Runaways
o   National Runaway Switchboard
      1-800-RUNAWAY or 1-800-786-2929

Suicide Prevention
o   National Suicide Prevention Lifeline
      1-800-273-TALK or 1-800-273-8255
o   The Samaritans Suicide Hotline
      1-800-893-9900 or http://www.capesamaritans.org/

Youth Hotlines
o   National Youth Crisis Hotline
      1-800-442-HOPE or 1-800-442-4673
o   Girls and Boys Town National Hotline
      1-800-448-3000
o   National Call Center for At-Risk Youth
      1-818-710-1181 (long distance)
o   National Children's Alliance (for help in finding a local Children's
    Advocacy Center)
      1-800-239-9950

*Phone references have been provided by The Second Mile, courtesy of their
Web site (http://www.thesecondmile.org).*

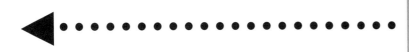

References

Albuquerque Rape Crisis Center. (1997). *Rape: Myth vs. fact.* Albuquerque, NM: Author.

American Association of Poison Control Centers. (2006). *Annual poisoning data reports: 2006 report.* Retrieved October 1, 2008, from http://www.aapcc.org

American Bar Association. (2003). *Know your rights: Domestic violence.* Retrieved October 1, 2008, from http://www.abanet.org/publiced/ domviol.pdf

American Heart Association (AHA). (2008). *Home page.* Retrieved October 1, 2008, from http://www.americanheart.org

Bonnie, R.J., & Wallace, R.B. (2003). *Elder mistreatment: Abuse, neglect, and exploitation in an aging America.* Washington, DC: National Academies Press.

Bouquin, E., & Johnson, W. (1998). *New Mexico health care provider's guide to domestic violence.* New Mexico: Frost Foundation.

Centers for Disease Control and Prevention (CDC). (2005). *Intimate partner violence injuries – Oklahoma, 2002.* Retrieved October 1, 2008, from http://www.cdc.gov/mmwr/preview/mmwrhtml/mm5441a2.htm

Centers for Disease Control and Prevention (CDC). (2008). *Environmental hazards & health effects: Carbon monoxide poisoning.* Retrieved October 1, 2008, from http://www.cdc.gov/co/basics.htm

Child Welfare Information Gateway. (2006). *Child abuse and neglect fatalities: Statistics and interventions.* Retrieved October 1, 2008, from http://www.childwelfare.gov/pubs/factsheets/fatality.cfm

Edleson, J. (2006). *Emerging responses to children exposed to domestic violence.* Retrieved October 1, 2008, from http://www.tricountyfamilyviolence prevention.org/

Gronseth, D., & Marek, A. (Eds.). (2000). *Guidelines for nursing telephone assessment and advice.* Albuquerque, NM: Lovelace Health Systems.

Klein, M., & Farr, J. (1994). *From victim to survivor: An information brochure for victims of rape.* Albuquerque, NM: New Mexico Coalition of Sexual Assault Programs, Inc.

Litovitz, T.L., Klein-Schwartz, W., White, S., Cobaugh, D., Youniss, J., Omslaer, J., et al. (2001). 2000 annual report of the American Association of Poison Control Centers' toxic exposures surveillance system. *American Journal of Emergency Medicine, 19*(5), 337-396.

Los Angeles County Department of Health Services. (2001). *Poisoning statistics.* Retrieved October 1, 2008, from http://www.lapublic health.org

National Center for Injury Prevention and Control. (2008). *Poisoning in the United States: Fact sheet.* Retrieved October 1, 2008, from http://www.cdc.gov/ ncipc/factsheets/poisoning.htm

National Center on Elder Abuse. (2004). *The 2004 survey of state Adult Protective Services: Abuse of adults 60 years of age and older.* Retrieved October 1, 2008, from http://www.ncea.aoa.gov/NCEA root/Main_Site/pdf/2-14-06% 20FINAL%2060+REPORT.pdf

National Coalition Against Domestic Violence. (2005). *Domestic violence fact sheets.* Retrieved October 1, 2008, from http://www.ncadv.org/resources/ FactSheets_294.html

Orloff, L., & Siu Chung, M. (1996). *Physician's tort liability: Potential legal liability for health professionals for actions or inactions in domestic violence cases.* Washington, DC: Ayuda, Inc.

Prevent Child Abuse New York. (2003). *The costs of child abuse and the urgent need for prevention.* Retrieved October 1, 2008, from http://www.prevent childabuseny.org/pdf/cancost.pdf

Prevent Child Abuse New York. (2006). *2006 child abuse and neglect fact sheet.* Retrieved October 1, 2008, from http://www.preventchildabuseny.org/pdf/ 2006CANFactSheet.pdf

Rainbow Response. (2008). *What is intimate partner violence?* Retrieved October 1, 2008, from http://www.rainbowresponse.org/myths.html

Rape, Abuse & Incest National Network (RAINN). (2008). *Statistics.* Retrieved October 1, 2008, from http://www.rainn.org/statistics

South Dakota Suicide Prevention. (2008). *Home page.* Retrieved October 1, 2008, from http://sdsuicideprevention.org/

Stoney, G. (2001). *Information: FAQ.* Retrieved October 1, 2008, from http://www.rochford.org/suicide/inform/faq/answers/3.shtml

Suicide Prevention Resource Center. (2008). *Home page.* Retrieved October 1, 2008, from http://www.sprc.org/

Answer/Evaluation Form
AMBP9c10

Continuing Nursing Education Activity
Telehealth Nursing Practice Essentials

Chapter 12: Clinical Knowledge – Special Situations

This activity provides 1.3 contact hours of continuing nursing education (CNE) credit in nursing.
(Contact hours calculated using a 60-minute contact hour.)

This test may be copied for use by others.

COMPLETE THE FOLLOWING:

Name: _____

Address: _____

City: _____ State: _____ Zip: _____

Telephone number: (Home) _____ (Work) _____

Email address: _____

AAACN Member Number and Expiration Date: _____

Processing fee: AAACN Member: $12.00
                  Nonmember: $20.00

Answer Form: (Please attach a separate sheet of paper if necessary.)

1. What did you value most about this activity?

_____
_____
_____
_____

2. If you could imagine that you have fully integrated your learning into practice, what would be different about your present practice?

_____
_____
_____
_____

Evaluation	Strongly disagree				Strongly agree
3. The offering met the stated objectives.					
a. Describe critical information to collect when receiving a crisis call.	1	2	3	4	5
b. Compare and contrast two major ways to activate Emergency Medical Services in a crisis situation.	1	2	3	4	5
c. Propose specific telehealth nursing actions for calls related to cardiopulmonary resuscitation, poisoning/overdose, abuse, sexual assault, and suicide.	1	2	3	4	5
4. The content was current and relevant.	1	2	3	4	5
5. The content was presented clearly.	1	2	3	4	5
6. The content was covered adequately.	1	2	3	4	5

7. How would you rate your ability to apply your learning to practice following this activity? (Check one)
☐ Diminished ability ☐ No change ☐ Enhanced ability

8. Time required to complete reading assignment and answer form: ___ minutes

Comments _____

I verify that I have completed this activity:

_____
Signature

Objectives

This educational activity is designed for nurses and other health care professionals who provide telehealth care for patients. This evaluation is designed to test your achievement of the following educational activities.

1. Describe critical information to collect when receiving a crisis call.
2. Compare and contrast two major ways to activate Emergency Medical Services in a crisis situation.
3. Propose specific telehealth nursing actions for calls related to cardiopulmonary resuscitation, poisoning/overdose, abuse, sexual assault, and suicide.

Evaluation Form Instructions

1. To receive continuing nursing education (CNE) credit for individual study after reading the indicated chapter(s), please complete the evaluation form (photocopies of the answer form are acceptable). Attach separate paper as necessary.
2. Detach (or photocopy) and send the answer form along with a check, money order, or credit card payable to *AAACN* East Holly Avenue/Box 56, Pitman, NJ 08071-0056. You may also send this form as an email attachment to ambp401@ajj.com.
3. Answer forms must be postmarked by December 31, 2011. Upon completion of the answer/evaluation form, a certificate for 1.3 contact hours will be awarded and sent to you.

Payment Options

☐ Check or money order enclosed (payable in U.S. funds to AAACN)

☐ MasterCard ☐ VISA ☐ American Express

Credit Card #: _____

Expiration Date: _____ Security Code: _____

Card Holder (Please print): _____

Signature: _____

This educational activity has been co-provided by the American Academy of Ambulatory Care Nursing (AAACN) and Anthony J. Jannetti, Inc. (AJJ).

AAACN is a provider approved by the California Board of Registered Nursing, Provider Number CEP 5336.

AJJ is accredited as a provider of continuing nursing education by the American Nurses Credentialing Center's Commission on Accreditation.

This book was reviewed and formatted for contact hour credit by Sally S. Russell, MN, CMSRN, AAACN Education Director, and Maureen Espensen, MBA, BSN, RN, Editor.

American Academy of Ambulatory Care Nursing
East Holly Avenue/Box 56, Pitman, NJ 08071-0056
Phone: 800-AMB-NURS; Fax: 856-589-7463
Web: www.aaacn.org; Email: aaacn@ajj.com

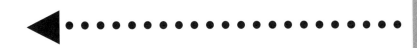

CHAPTER 13
Clinical Knowledge – At-Risk Populations

Objectives

1. Describe nursing actions related to interacting with patients who have at-risk conditions.
2. Explain challenges when interacting with at-risk patients within the telehealth environment.
3. Summarize strategies for implementing effective nursing actions when dealing with at-risk patients.

Many of the telecommunications the nurse receives from patients are symptom-based. Patients contact the telehealth center with symptoms they are experiencing and request help from the nurse to decide what they should do or where they should go. These symptom-based contacts require additional concern for the nurse if these symptomatic patients also have certain diseases or conditions. Areas of concern for the nurse could include the following:

❖ **Medical conditions that have an increased risk of serious outcome or present with atypical signs and symptoms.** For example, atypical signs and symptoms of myocardial infarction (MI) may occur in the postmenopausal woman or the young adult using cocaine.

❖ **Disease states that decrease, eliminate, or mask symptoms of another unrelated condition.** For example, the patient with diabetes neuropathy will frequently be unable to feel pain associated with foot injury or infection.

❖ **Seemingly minor symptoms that may be more serious when associated with high-risk conditions.** Examples include the patient with diabetes who is insulin-dependent and experiences vomiting and diarrhea, and the ambulatory oncology patient with a low-grade fever. Both may be experiencing major side effects associated with their underlying diseases or perhaps developing an opportunistic acute infection.

❖ **Medical conditions that manifest physiological internal environments that may foster rapid progression of other diseases.** For example, an upper respiratory infection may rapidly progress to pneumonia in a patient with an underlying lung disease such as COPD.

❖ **Medical conditions that have a bearing on the disposition and/or treatment.** Take, for example, the 30-year-old woman with abdominal pain. Through the assessment process, the nurse determines that the woman has missed her last menstrual period and is sexually active. The

Patients contact the telehealth center with symptoms they are experiencing and request help from the nurse to decide what they should do or where they should go. These symptom-based contacts require additional concern for the nurse if these symptomatic patients also have certain diseases or conditions.

nurse suspects possible ectopic pregnancy. With many illnesses, the nurse instructs patients to increase their fluid intake. This advice should be not given to patients who contact the nurse with a change in menstruation status and abdominal pain because immediate surgery for ectopic pregnancy may occur.

❖ **Conditions or diseases that preclude certain medication usage.** For example, pregnant or potentially pregnant women should not be given medications that may be damaging to the fetus. Another example would be mothers who are breastfeeding; they should not be given medications that can be transferred via breast milk to the nursing infant. During the assessment of women with menses, ask the date of the last menstrual period (LMP) to determine the possibility of pregnancy, and if appropriate, determine the breastfeeding status.

The concerns discussed above should reinforce for every nurse the importance of inquiring about past and chronic conditions, current medications, allergies, information about LMP, status of pregnancy, and breastfeeding.

CHRONIC DISEASES AND DISORDERS

A patient with a chronic illness or disease requires continuing medical care and education to prevent acute complications and to reduce the risk of long-term complications. Therefore, it is essential for the telehealth nurse to understand the complications of chronic illnesses.

A patient with a chronic illness or disease requires continuing medical care and education to prevent acute complications and reduce the risk of long-term complications. Therefore, it is essential for the telehealth nurse to understand the complications of chronic illnesses in order to incorporate self-management teaching and appropriate intervention of medical care into the nursing assessment and advice.

The remainder of this chapter will detail the following potpourri of at-risk concerns:

❖ Patients with diabetes.
❖ Patients that are immunosuppressed.
❖ Patients with bleeding disorders.
❖ Atypical presentations for MI.

DIABETES

The Center for Disease Control (CDC) stated that in 2005, 20.8 million people reported that they had been diagnosed with diabetes. Both Type 1 and Type 2 diabetes will be discussed in this chapter.

Type 1 diabetics most frequently require insulin delivered by injection or an infusion pump. This accounts for 5% to 10% of all diagnosed cases. Type 1 diabetes usually strikes children and young adults, but can occur at any age (CDC, 2005). Because pump patients may need assistance with pump

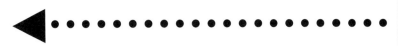

settings, telehealth nurses should be familiar with the following insulin pump terms: basal rates, boluses, insulin to carbohydrate ratio, and blood sugar to insulin sensitivity. The nurse will then have a better understanding when a patient reports their readings.

Type 2 diabetics account for 90% to 95% of all diagnosed cases of diabetes. Many people can control their blood glucose by following a healthy meal plan and exercise program, losing excess weight, and taking oral medication. Diabetes self-management education is an integral component of medical care (CDC, 2005).

Recent statistics show 575,000 *new cases* of diabetes among people ages 60 and older. 10.3 million (20.9%) of *all people* in this age group have diabetes (National Institute of Diabetes and Digestive and Kidney Diseases, 2005). This means that the nurse will have frequent opportunities to interact with patients who have diabetes. Diabetes is discussed in this chapter not only because of the number of patients who have the disease, but also because it affects almost every system of the body – renal, circulatory, neurological, respiratory, endocrine, and sensory. Patients with diabetes require careful monitoring and frequent education to prevent acute complications and reduce the risk of long-term complications. Patients with diabetes are at higher risk for infections, neuropathy conditions, eye disease, renal disease, and cardiovascular disease.

Patients with diabetes require careful monitoring and frequent education to prevent acute complications and reduce the risk of long-term complications. Patients with diabetes are at higher risk for infections, neuropathy conditions, eye disease, renal disease, and cardiovascular disease.

Infection

Poorly controlled diabetes decreases the ability of white blood cells to fight infections. As a result, diabetic patients are more susceptible to infections and are at risk for developing the following types of infections (National Diabetes Education Program [NDEP], 2007):

❖ Bladder and kidney infections.
❖ Mouth infections and thrush.
❖ Fungal infections.
❖ Vaginal infections.
❖ Wound and feet infections (neuropathy may also lead to infections).

The symptoms of infection could be white, painful patches on the tongue, vaginal discharge, burning or painful urination, fever, a minor injury that is not healing, or just that the patient is "not feeling well." The nursing intervention would be to schedule an appointment with a provider or member of the diabetic team and to provide interim advice until the patient is seen. The time frame along with disposition of the encounter would depend upon the acuity of the assessment.

For example, the husband of 30-year-old Mrs. Jones calls the contact center and informs the nurse that his wife has had flu-like symptoms for 2 days. She has been vomiting, has a fever of 100-101° F, and is complaining

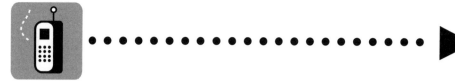

of abdominal pain and shortness of breath. As the nurse continues to gather data, the assessment reveals that Mrs. Jones is a diabetic and takes insulin; however, she has not taken any in the past 24 hours, nor has she monitored her blood sugar. Mrs. Jones feels too ill to talk with the nurse and is described as weak. From the nurse's assessment and knowledge, the nurse advises that Mrs. Jones needs to be seen immediately in the ER for medical evaluation and care. She recognizes that diabetic ketoacidosis (DKA) is a medical emergency associated with Type 1 diabetes, and it can be precipitated by any major physiologic stress, such as infection. Omission of insulin is mismanagement of an ill insulin-dependent diabetic.

Neuropathy

Diabetic neuropathy is a complication that affects the nerves. The most common type of diabetic neuropathy affects the peripheral nerves. The symptoms of peripheral neuropathy include (American Diabetes Association [ADA], 2004):

- ❖ Numbness and loss of feeling (usually first in feet or hands).
- ❖ Weak muscles.
- ❖ Slower reflexes.
- ❖ Pain, which varies from discomfort or tingling sensations in fingers and toes to severe pain.

Often, the patient contacts the telehealth nurse in the middle of the night complaining of lack of sleep due to sharp pain or deep aches in the legs and feet.

Often, the patient contacts the telehealth nurse in the middle of the night complaining of lack of sleep due to sharp pain or deep aches in the legs and feet. The diabetic patient complains that the skin is so sensitive to touch that the sheets on the bed cause discomfort to the feet. Or, in contrast, the diabetic with neuropathy may not notice injuries because of not feeling pain in the affected area (NDEP, 2007). Coupled with poor circulation to the legs and feet due to peripheral vascular disease, an unnoticed foot injury can quickly become infected and cause very serious foot problems. If the patient has a foot injury or a red area under a corn or callus, a same-day appointment is needed for medical evaluation. Comprehensive foot care can reduce amputation rates by 45-85% (NIH, 2005).

Autonomic Neuropathy Changes with Diabetes Mellitus

Autonomic neuropathy is a common change in the diabetic patient. It affects nerves that regulate autonomic function, such as digestion, heart rate and blood pressure. This neuropathy can create problems with bowel or bladder control, and even with the ability to recognize low blood sugar reactions. Autonomic neuropathy can also cause erectile dysfunction in men and the inability to climax in women (ADA, 2004). The nurse needs to have clinical knowledge about the neuropathy changes that alter the body systems in

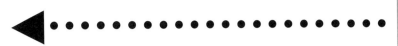

order to adequately assess the diabetic patient and make the appropriate interventions.

Eye Problems

Diabetes is the leading cause of blindness among adults ages 20-74 (CDC, 2005). The longer someone has diabetes, the higher the likelihood of diabetic retinopathy. Between 40-45% of Americans diagnosed with diabetes have some stage of diabetic retinopathy (National Eye Institute [NEI], 2007). Prolonged elevated blood sugars contribute to eye problems. The bleeding of blood vessels that supply the retina causes retinopathy and if not treated, serious retinal changes may occur. Often there are no symptoms with retinopathy until the eyes are damaged. Cataracts occur in persons with diabetes and at an earlier age (NEI, 2008). A cataract is a thickening of the lens of the eye that keeps light rays from passing through to the retina, causing cloudy vision. Visual complaints such as blurry, spotted, or flashing vision require immediate medical evaluation for both the diabetic or non-diabetic patient. The teaching role of the nurse is crucial in preventing eye complications, and annual eye exams for the patient with diabetes should be encouraged.

Diabetes is the leading cause of blindness among adults ages 20-74.

Cardiovascular Disease among Diabetics

Cardiovascular disease directly causes 65% of deaths among people with diabetes (National Heart, Lung, and Blood Institute [NHLBI], 2008). Cardiovascular disease is caused by changes in the blood vessels due to arteriosclerosis and/or atherosclerosis. Three types of this disease are:

1. *Peripheral vascular disease* refers to diseased blood vessels in the legs and feet that cause a decrease in the blood flow to the extremities. Symptoms for a partial obstruction of the blood vessels include leg cramps, weakness, "charley horse," or pain in the legs when walking. Severe pain with coldness and paleness of the leg could signal a complete obstruction of an artery.
2. *Coronary artery disease* refers to diseased heart arteries. For partial obstruction of the coronary artery, the patient will experience angina. Complete blockage of an artery results in MI.
3. *Cerebral vascular disease* refers to diseased arteries in the brain. Partial blockage may result in a transient ischemic attack, and complete blockage of a blood vessel would result in a cerebral vascular accident.

The nurse's role includes teaching the patient how to reduce the risk of cardiovascular disease by encouraging the patient to do the following:

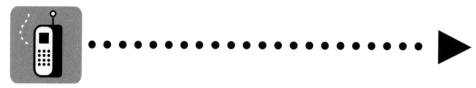

- ❖ Maintain control of blood sugar.
- ❖ Maintain normal blood pressure and emphasize the importance of taking medication for hypertension.
- ❖ Lose extra pounds if overweight.
- ❖ Reduce fats and cholesterol in diet.
- ❖ Exercise regularly (after consulting with your provider).
- ❖ Do not smoke.
- ❖ Continue to see your provider regularly.

When assessing a patient with chest pain, diabetes is a risk factor. However, if a patient has elevated cholesterol, hypertension, and diabetes, the risk of having a heart attack is over 7 times greater than if the patient only had diabetes. Neuropathy from diabetes can mask the severe chest pain that is the classic symptom of a heart attack (ADA, 2004). Assess for other warning signs of heart attack, such as nausea, perspiring, indigestion, or shortness of breath. If the patient with diabetes experiences a combination of these symptoms, or if any one symptom is severe or persistent, consider a MI.

If a patient has elevated cholesterol, hypertension, and diabetes, the risk of having a heart attack is over 7 times greater than if the patient only had diabetes. Neuropathy from diabetes can mask the severe chest pain that is the classic symptom of a heart attack.

Patient Teaching for Sick Day Management

The telehealth nurse who assists the patient with diabetes to manage sick days at home is a vital link in preventing serious complications or outcomes. Diabetic sick day management guidelines are required for safe and consistent home management. An overview of a sick day management of diabetes stresses the following points (University of Arkansas For Medical Sciences, 2006):

- ❖ Never omit the insulin, even if unable to eat.
- ❖ Test blood sugar every 4 hours or more often if symptoms indicate.
- ❖ Type I diabetics must test urine for ketones every 4 hours.
- ❖ How to substitute liquids for solid foods if patient is experiencing vomiting or diarrhea.
- ❖ Rest – do not exercise.
- ❖ Know when to contact his/her provider, diabetic nurse, or telehealth advice nurse.
- ❖ Know when to go to the medical office.

DISORDERS OF THE IMMUNE SYSTEM

When the body's self-defense against foreign invasion fails to function normally, a state of immune deficiency occurs. The body is unable to launch an adequate immune response and is at a greater risk for infection. The primary clinical clue to immunodeficiency, whatever the cause, is the tendency to develop recurrent infections. Some causes of acquired immunodeficient diseases are acute viral infections, malignancies, and

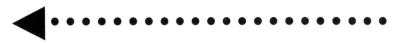

autoimmune disease (such as lupus, erythematosus, and rheumatoid arthritis), chronic diseases, aging, and malnutrition. Many treatments and interventions aimed at helping patients cause immunodeficiency. Patients who may be immunosuppressed tend to become sicker more quickly with poorer outcomes than other patients with the same symptoms. In an immunodeficient patient, signs and symptoms of infection are often atypical, masked, or absent. The telehealth nurse should be aware that a slight increase in body temperature could be significant. Another warning sign of infection is a decrease in nutritional intake or decrease in activity level. The telehealth nurse should report these symptoms to the provider in order to determine if the patient should be brought in for an appointment. Therefore, patients with the following disease states or on the following medications should be watched closely with frequent follow-up contacts, consultation with the patient's provider, and/or by having the patient come in for an appointment (WebMD, 2008a):

- ❖ Patients with HIV.
- ❖ Patients who have received or are receiving radiation therapy or chemotherapy.
- ❖ Patients on steroids.
- ❖ Elderly patients.
- ❖ Transplant recipients.

ATYPICAL SIGNS AND SYMPTOMS FOR CARDIOVASCULAR DISEASE

Some diseases or conditions may contribute to atypical presentation of cardiovascular problems, such as postmenopausal women, patients with diabetes, or young cocaine abusers. Most people picture an older, overweight or overstressed man when they think of a likely candidate for cardiovascular disease. But men are only half the story. Heart disease is the number-one killer of American women and is responsible for half of all the deaths of women over the age of 50 (WebMD, 2008b). The symptoms for a MI in a postmenopausal woman may not be the classic symptoms. The following warning symptoms may occur in both women and men:

Heart disease is the number-one killer of American women and is responsible for half of all the deaths of women over the age of 50.

- ❖ Uncomfortable pressure, fullness, squeezing, or pain in the center of the chest that lasts more than a few minutes or goes away and comes back.
- ❖ Pain that spreads to the shoulders, neck, or arms.
- ❖ Chest discomfort with lightheadedness, fainting, nausea, or shortness of breath.

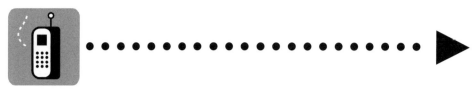

Postmenopausal women sometimes experience different warning signs, which are often more subtle. These symptoms include (Office on Women's Health, 2007):

❖ Atypical chest pain, or stomach or abdominal pain.
❖ Nausea or dizziness.
❖ Shortness of breath and difficulty breathing.
❖ Unexplained anxiety, weakness, or fatigue.
❖ Palpitations, cold sweat or paleness.

Since these symptoms can be vague, they can easily be mistaken for other ailments; therefore, the nurse could easily overlook them when assessing the patient. Men also may present with atypical signs and symptoms for MI; however, it is more common for postmenopausal women to present with atypical symptoms (Office on Women's Health, 2007).

Other cardiovascular diseases that increase in the postmenopausal woman are atherosclerois, hypertension, angina, and cardiovascular accidents. It is necessary for the telehealth nurse to be aware of the health issues of postmenopausal women and be able to correlate this information into the assessment and intervention.

Men also may present with atypical signs and symptoms for MI; however, it is more common for postmenopausal women to present with atypical symptoms.

COCAINE ABUSE

Young adults who are using cocaine are another high-risk population. Cocaine is a cause of MI that should be considered in young adults experiencing chest pain without risk factors. Cocaine can induce MI by causing coronary artery vasoconstriction or by increasing energy requirements (WebMD, 2006). When the nurse assesses the young adult with symptoms of chest pain, the nurse should ask if the person has used cocaine. When cocaine use is associated with chest pain, this becomes an emergent encounter.

OTHER HIGH-RISK ASSESSMENT ISSUES

Hematologic Disorders

Patients with hematologic disorders are potentially high-risk for emergencies, as these are usually chronic conditions with periodic crisis. Hematologic disorders include disseminated intravascular coagulation (DIC), thrombocytopenia, and hemophilia. A brief review of these blood disorders follows.

❖ *Disseminated Intravascular Coagulation (DIC)* is a grave disruption of blood clotting. This disorder is a complication of some other underlying problem, such as infection (gram-negative or gram-positive septicemia), obstetric complications (abruptio placentae or retained dead fetus),

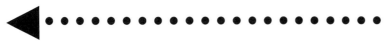

neoplastic disease (acute leukemia or metastatic carcinoma), cardiac arrest, or poisonous snakebite. The most frequent signs and symptoms are bleeding and hemorrhaging from any or several body parts. Bleeding from the GI tract, vaginal bleeding, red or cloudy urine, unexplained bruising, or severe abdominal or back pain due to bleeding into the body organs are the common signs of bleeding from DIC. Patients with this condition are often desperately ill and require emergency intervention (WebMD, 2007).

❖ *Thrombocytopenia* is a deficiency of platelet cells in the blood. It may be congenital or acquired and is the most common hemorrhagic disorder. Platelet count may be reduced in several ways, such as acute infection, ingestion of aspirin or other nonsteroidal anti-inflammatory drugs, blood transfusion, excess alcohol consumption, or preeclampsia. The nurse should assess for the following signs and symptoms: abnormal bleeding that may have a sudden onset, petechiae or bruising, bleeding in the mouth, nosebleeds, heavy or prolonged menstrual periods, or blood in the urine. The patient will also experience malaise, fatigue, general weakness, and lethargy. Severe blood loss would indicate an emergency situation. Medical treatment will vary depending on the underlying cause; however, the patient will need to be seen by a health care provider to begin a treatment plan (NHLBI, 2006).

❖ *Hemophilia* is a hereditary bleeding disorder that results from a lack of a specific clotting factor (Factor VIII) and causes the patient to have episodes of dangerous bleeding. It affects 1 out of every 5,000 males born in the United States. The most frequent signs and symptoms include painful and swollen joints, swelling in the leg or arm when bleeding occurs, frequent bruises, excessive bleeding from minor cuts, spontaneous nosebleeds, and blood in urine. The nursing intervention would be emergency treatment for severe or unusual bleeding episodes. Bleeding episodes can be controlled by infusions of concentrates of Factor VIII. It must be given as soon as possible after bleeding starts. Factor VIII can also be taken as a preventive measure and patients can be trained to administer the treatment themselves. The patient would need to be seen for injury with swelling, bleeding that isn't quickly controlled, or tender, painful, swollen joints (National Hemophilia Foundation, 2006).

Patients Taking Anticoagulants

Nurses must give special consideration to the patient on anticoagulants (such as coumadin or heparin). Anticoagulants are given to patients who are at risk of developing thromboembolic disease. When the therapeutic dosage is exceeded, hemorrhaging may result. The nursing assessment will be emergent. Signs and symptoms of hemorrhaging include:

Nurses must give special consideration to the patient on anticoagulants (such as coumadin or heparin). When the therapeutic dosage is exceeded, hemorrhaging may result.

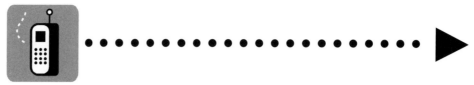

- ❖ Persistent mucosal bleeding.
- ❖ Persistent epistaxis.
- ❖ Frank or occult bleeding in stool, urine, vomitus, or sputum.
- ❖ Bruising and petechiae.
- ❖ Deteriorating mental status.

During the medication history, the patient may report taking other medication (such as antibiotics) or over-the-counter medications (such as aspirin or other salicylates), which can inhibit clotting mechanisms and may cause an anticoagulant overdose. The nursing role with patients with bleeding disorders would be (Briggs, 2007):

- ❖ Assess patient for acuity level of bleeding.
- ❖ Recognize the signs and symptoms of drug overdose for patients on anticoagulant therapy.
- ❖ Collaborate with the health care provider for appropriate disposition.
- ❖ Educate the patient to initiate treatment as soon as signs and symptoms of bleeding occur.

Frequent Encounters

Careful assessment is required for the patient who contacts the telehealth nurse frequently with numerous concerns. It is easy to discount the importance of an encounter when the patient does so frequently with minor concerns. The nurse must always take the time to complete an adequate and thorough assessment to determine if there is a real medical problem.

There are many reasons why patients may contact the telehealth center so frequently. Some may have chronic illnesses that require frequent medical interventions or they may be unsure about managing their care. Many patients want to receive reassurance from the nurse. Persons who frequently contact the telehealth nurse can be lonely and need someone to listen and talk with about their problems. Some patients may contact the telehealth nurse because of not accepting the directive given by their health care provider. In this situation, it is important to collaborate and reinforce the provider's directives.

With effective communication skills and pertinent nursing assessment of the health issue(s), the nurse will be able to determine the primary reason for the contact. If the nurse determines that the patient is lonely and/or lacks family or friend support of their health issue, the telehealth nurse should be able to offer community resources. These resources may be internal or external to the health organization, such as education classes or support groups for chronic illnesses, "warm lines," or referral to case manager or home health agency for medical or nursing problems.

There are several other interventions that the nurse may utilize when dealing with these patients. For example, the patient may be having difficulty focusing on the main reason for the encounter. They may wander and talk

Careful assessment is required for the patient who contacts the telehealth nurse frequently with numerous concerns. The nurse must always take the time to complete an adequate and thorough assessment to determine if there is a real medical problem.

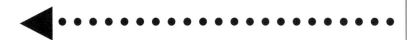

about issues that are not related to the medical problem. The nurse should use communication techniques to obtain the main reason for the encounter. The nurse may courteously interrupt the patient's rambling and then ask what is most concerning for the patient at this time. Example, "Mrs. Jones, I apologize for interrupting. Please tell me what is disturbing you most at this time."

Assess the acuity of the problem by asking the patient to compare. Example, " Mrs. Jones, are you coughing more today than yesterday?"

The nurse should never assume the reason for the encounter, but should always collect the data for assessing the problem. If the telehealth nurse is unable to obtain a clear assessment or is unsure about the patient's condition, consult with the patient's health care provider or make an appointment for the patient. Always err on the side of safety.

The nurse should never assume the reason for the encounter, but should always collect the data for assessing the problem.

SUMMARY

Certain high-risk areas have been identified because some diseases or conditions have increased risk of serious outcomes associated with them. The telehealth nurse should carefully and thoroughly analyze the assessment data to provide the appropriate advice and intervention for disease states/conditions, and thus deter a more serious outcome.

TIPS & PEARLS

☎ Assess to determine that the patient understands and can follow explanations and instructions.

☎ Remember that communication impairments can be due to hearing loss, confusion, misunderstanding the questions, and the patient's ability to articulate the signs and symptoms of the illness or the reason for the encounter.

☎ Be patient and understanding; the geriatric patient takes longer to answer questions and to respond. It takes longer to gather data for a baseline assessment and medical history.

☎ Remember to listen for the subtle changes in physical condition or behavior. Ask what is different today than yesterday or last week. Assess the ADLs and listen for evidence that the patient is beginning to have difficulty with self-care.

☎ Listen for signs of depression and identify risk factors of suicide.

☎ Assess the patient's medications to determine patient compliance and to rule out adverse drug reactions. The geriatric patient needs to be monitored for polypharmacy.

☎ Remember that if the decision support tools are written for the adult patient, they may not address the needs of the older adult who may have atypical presentations of illness.

References

American Diabetes Association (ADA).(2004). National diabetes statistics, diabetic somatic neuropathies. *Diabetes Care, 27*, 1458-1486.

Briggs, J.K. (2007). *Telephone triage protocols for nurses* (3rd ed.). Philadelphia: Lippincott, Williams & Wilkins.

Centers for Disease Control and Prevention (CDC). (2005). *National diabetes fact sheet: United States 2005.* Retrieved February 19, 2009, from http://www.cdc.gov/diabetes/pubs/pdf/ndfs_2005.pdf

National Diabetes Education Program (NDEP). (2007). *What to discuss with patients with diabetes.* Retrieved February 19, 2009, from http://www.ndep.nih.gov/ diabetes/WTMD/discuss.htm

National Eye Institute (NEI). (2007). *Resource guide: Diabetic retinopathy.* Bethesda, MD: Author.

National Eye Institute (NEI). (2008). *Facts about diabetic retinopathy.* Bethesda, MD: Author.

National Heart, Lung, and Blood Institute (NHLBI). (2006). *Thrombocytopenia.* Bethesda, MD: Harvard Pilgrim Health Care.

National Heart, Lung, and Blood Institute (NHLBI). (2008). For safety, NHLBI changes intensive blood sugar treatment strategy in clinical trial of diabetes and cardiovascular disease. Bethesda, MD: Author.

National Hemophilia Foundation. (2006). *Hemophilia A (Factor VIII deficiency).* New York: Author.

National Institute of Diabetes and Digestive and Kidney Diseases. (2005). *National diabetes statistics fact sheet: General information and national estimates on diabetes in the United States.* Bethesda, MD: U.S. Department of Health and Human Services, National Institute of Health.

National Institute of Health (NIH). (2005). *Diabetes, heart disease, and stroke* [Publication No. 06-5094]. Bethesda, MD: National Diabetes Information Clearinghouse.

Office on Women's Health. (2007). *Heart disease: What are the signs of a heart attack?* Retrieved February 19, 2009, from http://www.womenshealth.gov/ faq/heart-disease.cfm

University of Arkansas for Medical Sciences. (2006). *Diabetes sick day management.* Little Rock, AR: Author.

WebMD. (2006). *Substance abuse: Cocaine.* Retrieved February 9, 2008, from http://www.webmd.com

WebMD. (2007). *Disseminated intravascular coagulation (DIC).* Retrieved February 9, 2008, from http://www.webmd.com

WebMD. (2008a). *After the transplant.* Retrieved February 9, 2008, from http://www.webmd.com

WebMD. (2008b). *Menopause guide: Menopause and heart disease.* Retrieved February 24, 2008, from http://www.webmd.com

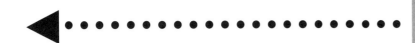

CHAPTER 14
Clinical Knowledge – Pediatric Population

Objectives

1. Describe the special considerations that need to be taken into account when caring for pediatric patients.
2. Explain challenges when interacting with pediatric patients and/or their families within the telehealth environment.
3. Summarize the essential components of an encounter with a pediatric patient.

The setting for telehealth nursing practice in pediatric ambulatory care may vary from a small private practice with one or two pediatricians to a child health clinic within a large university hospital providing multi-specialty pediatric care. It may also be a contact center for a managed care organization or community. However, the role of the nurse does not vary. The role is to respond to the concerns of the parents or caregivers via telecommunication by providing advice that includes (Schmitt, 2006):

❖ *Determining the appropriate disposition.*
  o Call EMS 911 **now**.
  o Go to ED **now**.
  o Go to ED **now** (or to office with PCP approval).
  o Go to provider office **now**.
  o See today in provider office.
  o See within 24 hours in provider office.
  o See within 72 hours in office.
  o See within 2 weeks in office.
  o Home care.
❖ *Directing home care management.* Manage the child's illness or injuries at home.
❖ *Providing anticipatory guidance.* Answer questions about the child's health, behavior, and growth and development.

In family practice offices, many encounters are pediatric in nature. Therefore, the nurse in family practice will also require pediatric expertise and an understanding of guidelines dealing with the pediatric population.

When telehealth nurses who handle pediatric interactions are asked to list the peak encounter times, a pattern emerges. In the early morning, advice nurses receive telecommunications from parents who have been up during the night with a sick infant or child and want an appointment for the child to be

In family practices, many encounters are pediatric in nature. Therefore, the nurse in family practice will also require pediatric expertise and an understanding of guidelines dealing with the pediatric population.

seen. Another peak time is when a school-aged child returns home from school and is ill or feeling worse than earlier that morning. Around 10:00 p.m. or midnight, the advice nurse will receive telecommunications from parents who have been treating a child and are seeking reassurance that they have correctly treated the child.

Monday is usually the peak encounter day of the week. The parent has provided home treatment over the weekend, but the child did not improve or the symptoms worsened; thus, they want the child to be seen by the health care provider. In contact centers, high volumes of pediatric encounters also occur on Sunday evening, as parents start deciding whether to send their child to school the next day.

The telehealth nurse must keep up with current events, such as local outbreaks of communicable diseases like meningitis. Parents may hear this on the news and have questions or be worried that their child has been exposed (Briggs, 2007). The nurse may receive many telecommunications after the newscast. It is important to carefully triage each encounter to determine disposition.

SPECIAL CONSIDERATIONS IN THE NURSING PROCESS WITH ASSESSMENT AND INTERVENTION

Special considerations of assessment and intervention with pediatric telehealth nursing include:

- ❖ Knowing and understanding key factors for assessment that only occur in the pediatric population.
- ❖ Understanding the child's developmental level and the effects of the illness or injury on the child at this stage of growth.
- ❖ Communicating effectively with the child's family and/or the child.
- ❖ Listening to the parent or primary caregivers, because they know the child best.

Assessment of Children

As with all telehealth nursing interactions, it is essential to recognize potentially life-threatening problems that require immediate intervention. Assessing children can be more difficult than assessing adults for several reasons. First, children, especially very young children, may not able to express adequately how they are feeling or their specific symptoms. It is important to develop a trusting relationship with the parent or guardian as they will be the major source for obtaining the assessment and medical history.

A child's response to illness and injury depends on his/her developmental stage. Children may not appear outwardly symptomatic, even when their condition is serious. They may not want others to know, or they can be adept

A child's response to illness and injury depends on his/her developmental stage. Children may not appear outwardly symptomatic, even when their condition is serious.

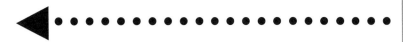

at distracting themselves and may appear pain free. Children also can compensate for impaired functioning for longer periods than adults. Symptoms may be subtle; however, once a child's condition begins to deteriorate, rapid interventions must occur (Springhouse, 2005).

The nursing assessment aids the telehealth advice nurse in determining the immediate problem and necessary intervention. While a complete health assessment may not be possible in an emergency, as much information as possible should be obtained, particularly as it relates to the emergency condition. The history may be completed in the emergency room or primary care facility.

Questions may be direct, open-ended, or leading. Direct questions are quick and useful in yielding specific facts. For example, "Has Susie been vomiting?" Open-ended questions allow more freedom in answering, such as, "Describe or tell me about Susie's vomiting…" Leading questions may be helpful in some situations. For example, "Has Susie ever had a vomiting episode like this before?" However, caution should be exercised when using leading questions because they may bias the child or parents into providing false information to please the telehealth nurse.

Growth and Developmental Level

The telehealth nurse needs to be able to assess the child's growth and developmental level and distinguish normal from abnormal characteristics.

Growth and development are essential parts of the nursing assessment. It is important for the nurse to be familiar with these stages. Many factors can influence growth and development (Springhouse, 2005):

Growth and development are essential parts of the nursing assessment. It is important for the nurse to be familiar with these stages. Many factors can influence growth and development.

❖ **Family.** The way a child has been raised can greatly influence his/her development. If abuse or neglect has occurred, there may be delays in learning trust, disorders of attachment, and problems with feeding and sleeping.

❖ **Health status.** Children with chronic health conditions may be delayed.

❖ **Socioeconomic.** Extra activities may not be possible; parents work long hours to provide basic necessities.

❖ **Cultural background.** A family's cultural beliefs can affect a child's growth and development.

The parent or guardian may contact the nurse with concern because he/she is comparing the baby with a chronic condition to an older, healthy sibling. The nurse needs to provide anticipatory guidance to the mother by explaining that illness and hospitalization can influence the development and achievement of milestones. The nurse then may review the growth and developmental characteristics with the mother. If the baby is within normal limits, the nurse may suggest that the reason the older child met these

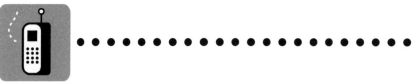

milestones earlier may be because he/she had not had a medical problem like this baby (Springhouse, 2005).

Another reason for understanding growth and development levels is when the nurse is assessing a premature infant. The assessment is different for a 4-month-old infant who was born prematurely versus a 4-month-old infant who was delivered at full-term. For example, the premature infant at 4 months only has the body weight of a 2-month-old infant; therefore, the premature infant is unable to take the same medication dosage as a full-term 4-month-old healthy infant. Nor would the premature infant developmentally be able to tolerate solid foods at the same age as the full-term delivery infant.

Children's perceptions of their illnesses and injuries vary according to their developmental level. Preschoolers are strong magical thinkers. They often believe their illness or injury was caused by them "being bad" or misbehaving. The number one fear of school-age children is injections, so they may minimize their symptoms due to the fear of going to the doctor for a shot. Older school-age children may be sick because of a test at school or may need a day at home with mom. They may also have physical symptoms of illnesses when there are emotional issues. Thus, it is important for the nurse to have a basic understanding of growth and development to meet the needs of the pediatric patient.

Children's perceptions of their illnesses and injuries vary according to their developmental level. Thus, it is important for the nurse to have a basic understanding of growth and development to meet the needs of the pediatric patient.

Communicating Effectively

Depending on the child's age and developmental stage, both the child and the caregiver may be asked to describe the child's current condition. Guidelines for talking with the parent and child are:

- ❖ Ask what the child and caregiver think may have caused any presenting problem and whether either one has any questions or concerns.
- ❖ Listen attentively to the child and caregiver while taking a history.
- ❖ When talking with the child, give special consideration to his/her level of understanding and use vocabulary and questions reflective of that level.

The nurse must remember that the ability to communicate and use language varies with age and that a word may have a different meaning based on a child's background and cognitive level. Direct interaction with the child (particularly the teenager) enhances both the assessment procedure and the success of interventions. Teenagers may initiate an encounter seeking advice for a "friend" when it is actually the teenager who has the symptoms. The wise telehealth nurse will work to build a trusting relationship so that perhaps adolescents will be comfortable sharing what is really happening to them.

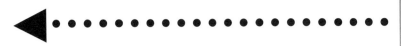

Listening to Caregivers

The nurse should communicate with parents or other caregivers in an understanding, empathetic manner without being judgmental, even if a complaint or question seems trivial. Every encounter is unique, and patience and compassion are required in answering every question.

The nurse should listen to the parents or primary caregivers because they know the child best. A response such as, "I have never seen Tommy this sick," is a major red flag for the nurse. If the child has been injured in an accident, parents or caregivers may blame themselves for the accident and may need emotional support from the telehealth nurse to assist them in coping with the stressful situation.

ESSENTIAL COMPONENTS OF A PEDIATRIC ENCOUNTER

Components of the pediatric encounter include the collection of identifying data, the identification and history of the chief complaint, an update of the past medical history and immunization record, and a description of the patient's daily living activities and developmental history. The next steps are to analyze the information and develop the interventions that are necessary to meet the special needs of the pediatric patient.

Identifying Data

Identifying data include the child's name, date of birth, race, sex, and the name, address, and telephone number of the child's parent(s) or guardian(s). The nurse needs to be aware that the parent initiating the interaction may not have the same last name as the child. The nurse should list the informant (such as mother, father, grandparent, or sitter) and note reliability of the informant to provide accurate information. Non-custodial parents, such as a stepmother who has the child for the weekend, may initiate an interaction seeking advice. When the babysitter or nanny initiates the interaction, the nurse needs to exhibit caution with how much advice or information is given before asking to talk to a parent. Insurance and other information may be obtained, depending on the policy of the health care agency.

The telehealth nurse should also be aware of local legal requirements for consent to provide a minor's medical care. A major difference between pediatrics and adult medicine is that children are minors, and in most jurisdictions, cannot make decisions for themselves. The issues of guardianship, privacy, legal responsibility, and informed consent must always be considered in every pediatric encounter. For example, a nanny initiates an interaction for advice and a same-day appointment for the child is scheduled. The telehealth nurse should check with the nanny to determine if there is written authorization for consent to bring the child in for treatment at the medical facility.

> *The nurse should communicate with parents or other caregivers in an understanding, empathetic manner without being judgmental, even if a complaint or question seems trivial. Every encounter is unique, and patience and compassion are required in answering every question.*

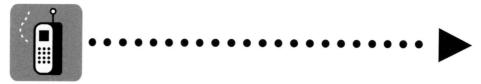

Chief Complaint

The nurse must direct the history-taking toward the chief complaint by asking the parent or child to give a brief account of the problem or reason for seeking care. The chief complaint should be recorded in a brief, concise statement. Does the chief complaint match the symptoms? For example, a parent states that a 1-year-old rolled off the couch onto the carpet; however, the symptoms indicate a fractured leg. This is a red flag for the nurse that warrants further investigation.

Present Illness

A history of the present illness is a chronological account of what has happened to the child since the onset of the illness or injury. The nurse should include influencing factors, duration, symptom chronology, related symptoms, limitations to activity, and location of any pain or discomfort.

It is important to include in the history of the present illness what the parent or child thinks is going on, what the parent already has tried in terms of self-management, and what is most worrisome to the parent. The nurse should work with the parent to identify common disease exposures, including family, friends, school, or daycare, with whom the child has recently come into contact. With infants and children, the child's weight is an important factor in calculating medication doses, assessing for weight loss, and comparing growth and development with the normal growth and development for the child's age. The nurse must ask if the child is receiving medication (prescription or over-the-counter) and if it seems to be effective. The nurse should then decide if the dosage is correct and has been given as prescribed, and ask if there have been any side effects. The nurse needs to be aware that children often react differently to medications. For example, in some children, diphenhydramine hcl causes a "hyper" effect rather than the expected sedating effect. If the encounter is about a breastfed infant who is experiencing symptoms, such as vomiting diarrhea, colic, or lethargy, it is important to consider what foods and medications the mother has recently taken. Be sure to include recreational and herbal drugs or alcohol.

A history of the present illness is a chronological account of what has happened to the child since the onset of the illness or injury. The nurse should include influencing factors, duration, symptom chronology, related symptoms, limitations to activity, and location of any pain or discomfort.

Immunization Status

Immunization history includes whether the child is currently on routine immunizations. This is an excellent opportunity for the nurse to provide information about the importance of immunizations and the diseases that they prevent. If the infant or child has a fever, it is important to assess if the child has received an immunization within the last 24-48 hours because fever is a side effect of some immunizations.

Past Medical History

The nurse obtains an update of the child's medical history, including information about allergies, past illnesses, accidents and injuries, operations

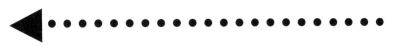

and hospitalizations, and primary source of health care. Allergic history may include questions related to asthma, hay fever, eczema, food allergies, and drug reactions. In the medication history, past significant medications should be recorded. The nurse should get a history of infectious disease, convulsions or any severe illnesses, injuries, or operations for which the child required hospitalization. It is important for the nurse to realize that children can have chronic medical conditions, such as juvenile arthritis, diabetes, and bowel disorders; however, the child may have a completely unrelated illness, such as ear pain or a sprained ankle. Any permanent effects of illnesses, injury, or operations should also be noted, such as an infusion site for intravenous medication regimen or gastrostomy for supplemental feedings.

Developmental History

The nurse must be able to access growth and developmental guidelines, which reflect literature-based normalcy for various age groups. Parents frequently contact the nurse for advice on at what age their child should be walking. They may ask about baby supplies (such as a walker). For liability issues, the nurse should reference approved, printed sources for this information. As discussed earlier, a child's growth and developmental history is vital data for the assessment process. Growth and developmental guidelines also assist the nurse to effectively communicate with the child at his/her level by knowing his/her age-specific competencies (Springhouse, 2005).

Parents frequently contact the nurse for advice on at what age their child should be walking. They may ask about baby supplies (such as a walker). For liability issues, the nurse should reference approved, printed sources for this information.

Activities of Daily Living

When assessing children, information concerning daily living activity is necessary to determine the effects of the illness. This is especially true in the preverbal child. For example, when assessing the activity level of a 2-year-old child, it is important to ask the parent to describe the child's normal daily living activity before determining the nursing diagnosis. If the child is fussy, sleeps at intervals during the night instead of sleeping from 8:00 p.m. until 7:00 a.m. (as usual), will not eat or drink favorite foods or juices, or will not play with favorite toys, these are marked changes in this child's activities of daily living. They are good indicators of behavioral changes. The nurse needs to avoid using vague terms such as "lethargic" or "listless" because these words may mean one thing to the nurse and another to the parent. It is best to have the parent describe the behavior so that the telehealth nurse will have more accurate data. The nurse may ask questions such as, "Is your child acting normal? Is your child eating or drinking? Please describe your child's behavior compared to normal."

HIGH-RISK ENCOUNTERS

With high-risk encounters, the assessment is vital in determining the urgency of the interaction. The parent who is unable to give the nurse the data for assessment due to his/her distress is a high-risk encounter. For example, a mother contacts the nurse crying and sobbing that she does not know what else to do for her baby with colic who has been crying at night for several weeks. She has tried everything that the pediatrician had advised, but the baby continues to cry. The mother complains of lack of sleep. Intervention is required immediately to bring the mother and baby into the clinic for assessment of the mother's mental condition and the baby's physical condition. At this point, the intervention of sending the child to the hospital or medical office right away becomes the priority of the nurse.

> *The parent who is unable to give the nurse the data for assessment due to his/her distress is a high-risk encounter.*

Characteristics That Could Create a High-Risk Encounter

❖ Infants who are under 6 months of age or who are premature are at a greater risk due to their underdeveloped immune systems.

❖ Children with chronic illnesses (such as asthma, HIV, birth defects with multi-problems, and diabetes).

❖ A child who has failed to respond to prescribed treatment should be evaluated. The nurse could also consult with the health care provider for subsequent care.

❖ A parent or caregiver who contacts the nurse more than once within 8-12 hours or within a short time frame is an indicator for a possible high-risk encounter. One of the most important diagnostic indicators for children is the parent's level of concern. If a parent contacts the telehealth nurse repeatedly over a period of hours, this should alert the nurse that the child should be seen; the parent is not reassured or the child is sicker than described (Schmitt, 2006). The nurse needs to assess why this parent is contacting the telehealth center so frequently to be sure the condition has not worsened, or if caregiver is unable to care for the child. This will help nurse to determine appropriate disposition for care.

Examples of Emergencies or Potential Alerts

There are various types of encounters where the nurse assesses that the infant or child requires immediate emergency intervention. Once an emergent disposition is determined, it is important for the nurse to ascertain if it is appropriate for the parent or caregiver to drive. If so, do they have transportation, or should 911 be called for an ambulance? Examples of emergencies or potential emergent conditions are:

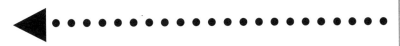

- ❖ Respiratory impairment due to:
  - o Difficulty breathing (cyanosis of fingertips or lips, retractions, persistent rapid breathing, inability to talk due to SOB, wheezing, nasal flaring).
  - o Foreign body blocking the airway (choking episode).
  - o Croup (difficulty breathing and signs of respiratory distress including SOB, color is dusky or blue, nasal flaring, retractions, and strider is present when the child is at rest).
- ❖ Overdose of medication (may be accidental).
- ❖ Dehydration – An infant or child may have signs and symptoms of marked dehydration due to vomiting and/or diarrhea. Signs and symptoms include dry mucous membranes, sunken eyes, sunken fontanel, tenting of the skin, decreased urine output (no urine in 8 hours), and no tears.
- ❖ Accidents/ Injuries (non-penetrating/penetrating injuries).
- ❖ Head injury – An encounter may reveal loss of consciousness, child acting "strange," lethargic or pale, double vision, seizures, clear fluid draining from ears or nose, vomiting, or complaints of severe, persistent headache. If the neck is injured from a fall or blow, the nurse must consider the risk of damage to the spinal cord. Call 911 and instruct the person who initiated the encounter not to move the child.
- ❖ R/O fracture – Protruding bone, shock symptoms, poor circulation to extremity (cold, cyanosis, no color), paralysis, loss of sensation to extremity, deformity, out of alignment, or dislocation are emergent signs and symptoms when assessing for fractures.
- ❖ Burns – Chemical or thermal burns need to be triaged as emergent if there is difficulty breathing, hoarseness, disorientation, lethargy, unresponsiveness, or visual problems. Burns to the face, eyes, neck, genitals, or large burns need to be evaluated emergently. Electrical burns need careful, prompt evaluation.
- ❖ Ingestion of poisons – The following signs and symptoms would require emergency intervention: difficulty swallowing, increased salivation, drooling, gagging, abdominal pain, vomiting, or respiratory distress (Schmitt, 2006).
- ❖ Sexual or physical abuse – The patient needs to be sent to the appropriate facility promptly for evaluation and treatment.
- ❖ Sick infant – Any infant less than 3-months-old who is sick in any way requires medical evaluation to rule out a serious bacterial infection.
- ❖ Severe lethargy – Signs and symptoms that represent lethargy in an infant or child include: stares into space, will not smile, too weak to cry, is floppy, is hard to awaken, poor eye contact, fails to interact with parents, or decreased response to the environment.

Chemical or thermal burns need to be triaged as emergent if there is difficulty breathing, hoarseness, disorientation, lethargy, unresponsiveness, or visual problems.

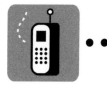

❖ Severe pain – Signs and symptoms that may indicate severe pain in a child include: if a child cries when touched or moved (this could be a symptom of meningitis), constant screaming or inability to sleep, and moaning or high-pitched or unusual cry (may be symptomatic of central nervous system diseases).

❖ Can't walk – Children who lose the ability to stand or walk, walk bent over, or hold their abdomen because of pain need to be seen to rule out a serious abdominal problem.

❖ Tender abdomen – When pressure is applied to the child's abdomen, and the child pushes the hand away or screams in pain, a medical evaluation is required. An emergent medical evaluation is also required if the abdomen is bloated and hard.

❖ Tender testicle or scrotum – A sudden onset of pain and/or swelling in the testicle can be from twisting (torsion) of the testicle and requires immediate disposition to the emergency department. Testicular torsion requires surgical intervention within 6-12 hours (Schmitt, 2006).

❖ Drooling – Sudden onset of drooling or spitting, especially associated with difficulty swallowing, requires immediate medical evaluation.

❖ Fontanel or "soft spot" – If the anterior fontanel is tense and bulging when the infant is not crying, and the infant is quiet and in an upright position, it may be indicative of increased intracranial pressure or congestive heart failure. If the anterior fontanel is depressed, this could be indicative of dehydration. This is an emergent symptom that requires immediate medical evaluation and treatment (Springhouse, 2005).

❖ Stiff neck – To assess for stiffness of the neck, ask the parent to lay the child down, and then lift the head until the chin touches the middle of the chest. If the parent feels resistance or if the child cries or complains of pain, this could indicate nuchal rigidity. Nuchal rigidity is frequently an early sign of meningeal irritation and can be an important clue to the presence of meningitis.

❖ Petechiae – The patient with presence of purple or blood-red spots on the skin, not related to explained bruising, needs intervention and disposition advice to go to the doctor's office **now**. The presence of petechiae associated with fever indicates serious underlying infection and disposition is to call EMS 911 **now** (Schmitt, 2006).

❖ Fever – In a child of any age, a fever of 105° F or greater requires an emergency department visit because there is a 20% risk of bacterial infection (Schmitt, 2006).

❖ Subnormal temperatures in children – A child with a rectal temperature less than 95° F needs medical assessment (Schmitt, 2006). The urgency would largely be based on the infant's behavior and other symptoms.

If the anterior fontanel ("soft spot") is tense and bulging when the infant is not crying, and the infant is quiet and in an upright position, it may be indicative of increased intracranial pressure or congestive heart failure.

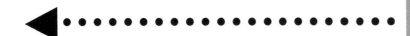

FEBRILE INFANT OR CHILD

One of the most frequent encounters that the pediatric nurse receives is that of the febrile child. Children in the first 2 or 3 years of life have anywhere from 6-10 infectious illnesses each year. Up to one-third of outpatient visits by children to emergency departments and private practitioners are related to fever. 20-30% of after-hours calls to pediatricians concern fever. Although there is no consensus regarding the exact temperature that denotes fever, it is generally accepted that a rectal temperature of at least 100.4° F represents a fever (Schmidt, 2006).

Parents often contact the nurse at the start of a fever and want to know the cause. The nurse needs to provide reassurance that the cause often can't be determined during the first 24 hours of a fever.

It is very important for the telehealth nurse to ask questions to determine the child's activity level. If the parent or caregiver reports that child is limp, weak, not moving, or unresponsive or difficult to awaken, directives are to call EMS 911 **now**. If child has a fever with no signs of infection *and* no localizing symptoms, then the nurse can provide home care advice. The nurse should always provide expectations regarding fever and monitoring instructions so that the parent or caregiver knows if there is need to call back (Schmidt, 2006).

The risk of serious bacterial illness in infants under 3 months of age with fever is generally believed to be higher than in older infants with fever. Serious bacterial illnesses are:

❖ Meningitis.
❖ Bacteremia.
❖ UTI.
❖ Osteomyelitis.
❖ Septic shock.
❖ Pneumonia.
❖ Bacterial gastroenteritis.
❖ Serious skin and soft tissue infections, such as cellulitis.

In some febrile children, fever may be the only complaint, and these children otherwise look fine and behave normally. Other children with fever may appear less interactive, quieter, and less energetic than children of the same age without fever. Their appetite decreases, and they may become fussy. Because young children, especially infants under 3 months of age, have fewer and more subtle behavioral signs when febrile, nurses must be suspicious of a serious bacterial infection, even in the absence of localizing signs (Schmitt, 2006). The nurse needs to question the parents regarding physical findings associated with fever, which could include:

Up to one-third of outpatient visits by children to emergency departments and private practitioners are related to fever.

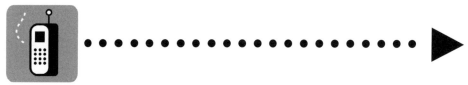

- ❖ Flushed cheeks.
- ❖ Hot, dry skin.
- ❖ Shivering (which is uncommon in the young infants).
- ❖ Cool distal extremities.
- ❖ Tachycardia.
- ❖ Tachypnea.

For example, a mother tells the nurse that she has not taken her infant son's temperature because she has no thermometer. However, she tells the nurse that her baby's skin is hot to the touch, his face is flushed, and she can feel his heart beating faster than usual. These symptoms should be a red flag for the nurse. The nurse recognizes these as symptoms of an elevated temperature and is not surprised about the rapid heart rate because the heart rate increases 10 beats per minute for each degree Fahrenheit of temperature elevation above normal.

Assessment Questions for Fever

Medical history can provide valuable information in the evaluation of children with fever. The history should focus on the onset, duration, pattern, and severity of the fever.

Medical history can provide valuable information in the evaluation of children with fever. The history should focus on the onset, duration, pattern, and severity of the fever. The presence of associated symptoms that may be signs of specific organ system involvement should be noted. The nurse in assessing the child with fever needs to ask the parent the following questions:

1. *How long has the infant/child had the fever, and how high has the temperature been?* The degree of elevation of temperature may correlate with bacteremia, especially if above 105° F (Schmitt, 2006), although a child with a low-grade fever may be septic and one with a high temperature may have a benign course. How the child responds to antipyretics cannot be used as a guide to differentiate septic children from those with viral illnesses. An infant who is septic may respond to antipyretics, whereas those who do not respond may have a mild illness.

2. *Does the infant/child have any other symptoms, such as rash, vomiting, diarrhea, abdominal pain or dysuria, cough, rhinorrhea, or other respiratory symptoms?* All febrile infants (younger than 3 months of age) should receive a medical examination. This is important even when the history may suggest involvement of one organ system. For example, in young children, vomiting and fever may often be the only signs of a UTI, instead of gastroenteritis, as suggested by the history. The presence of petechiae in association with fever indicates serious underlying infection and the child should be sent to the emergency department. Parent or guardian should be directed to call EMS 911 **now** (Schmitt, 2006).

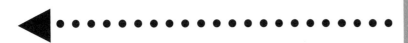

3. *Has the child's activity level changed? Is he/she more sleepy than usual, lethargic, or irritable? Has there been a change in mental status?* As previously discussed, assessment of the well-being of the child is extremely important. The nurse needs to attempt to determine whether the child is behaving and responding in an age-appropriate manner.

4. *Is anyone else sick at home? Any known illness exposures at school or daycare?* It is not unusual for the nurse to hear from the parent about the other children at daycare or school who are having the same symptoms as their child, and they will tell the nurse about this exposure even before the nurse has a chance to ask.

5. *Is the child up-to-date on immunizations? Had the child received an immunization within the last 24 to 72 hours?* If the child is ill, the nurse must triage to determine if child's reaction is to be expected (Schmitt, 2006).

6. *Is the child taking any medications? What treatment has been done at home for the fever?* Febrile children may feel uncomfortable; thus, fever should be reduced to relieve the associated discomfort and malaise. Antipyretics such as acetaminophen or ibuprofen may be used. Aspirin should be avoided in children because of the association with Reye's syndrome and viral illnesses. Unbundling the child aids in fever reduction. Only if the fever is over 104° F (and does not come down with acetaminophen or ibuprofen) *and* it causes discomfort should the parent or caregiver be directed to sponge the child or bathe with tepid water (Schmitt, 2006).

7. *Has there been any recent history of travel, especially outside of the country?* Fever, which is the most important post-travel symptom, should always be carefully and promptly evaluated. Time may be critical. Malaria is the most common cause of fever in the returned traveler.

8. *Has the child ever been hospitalized for an infectious illness?* This will give the nurse insight into the well-being of the child.

9. *Does the child have any medical problems, especially asthma, sickle cell anemia, congenital heart disease, or immunodeficiency?* Febrile children with chronic illnesses require medical evaluation and should be considered high-risk.

Nonspecific signs and symptoms such as irritability, increased fussiness, feeding intolerance, or mild respiratory distress may be the only clues to the presence of serious bacterial infection.

There are two other groups of children with fever that require medical evaluation: infants 3-6 months of age with fever greater than 102° F, and infants and young children 3-24 months with fever over 24 hours without other symptoms (Schmitt, 2006). Nonspecific signs and symptoms such as irritability, increased fussiness, feeding intolerance, or mild respiratory distress may be the only clues to the presence of serious bacterial infection.

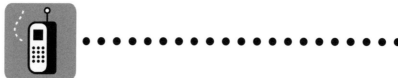

Clinical appearance is the best indicator of the severity of the illness. However, infants less than 3 months of age may not display signs of systemic illness. Thus, any febrile infant less than 3 month of age with fever of 100.4° F or higher needs to be seen immediately by a health care provider.

Fever in most viral illness ranges between 101 and 104° F and may last 2-3 days. About 4% of febrile children will develop a febrile convulsion (Schmitt, 2006).

In summary of the febrile child, the assessment of fever should focus on the onset, duration, pattern, and height of fever. The nurse should determine the associated symptoms, such as vomiting and diarrhea, rash (especially petechiae), breathing difficulty, swallowing ability, or drooling. In addition, it should also be determined if there have been any behavioral changes or decrease in the level of awareness. The nurse should ask about known exposures as well as immunization and travel history. The nurse needs to be more concerned about the 7-month-old with a temperature of 100.8° F who is lethargic and listless, rather than the 3-year-old with a temperature of 101° F who is eating, drinking, and playing with toys.

EVALUATION OF THE ENCOUNTER

The telehealth nurse needs to assess that the parent or caregiver understands the advice given and his/her acceptance and ability to follow the advice.

The telehealth nurse needs to assess that the parent or caregiver understands the advice given and his/her acceptance and ability to follow the advice. A parent may be asked to write down the advice or just to repeat the advice back to the nurse for verification of understanding. Before ending the interaction, the nurse should always ask the parents if they have any other questions. Inform the parent to contact the nurse if the symptoms get worse or the condition changes. The evaluation of the interaction should include the nurse taking a moment after it ends to reflect and analyze if there was anything that might warrant a more severe disposition. If so, it is appropriate for the nurse to contact the parent and reassess the child. It is always better to act on the side of caution. With each encounter, the nurse needs to assess the parent's understanding and willingness to follow the advice given, and then evaluate how well the interaction was managed.

FOLLOW-UP ENCOUNTER

When advice is given for home care, a follow-up encounter may be appropriate to assess if the child is responding to treatment or if a different intervention is needed. When the advice nurse tells a parent or caregiver to call 911, a follow-up encounter within a few minutes to offer assistance until the EMT arrives may provide critical nursing advice and/or emotional support for the parents. A follow-up encounter offers reassurance to the parents regarding the advice given, and provides another opportunity for

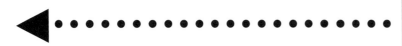

parent teaching and confirming that the situation is being managed appropriately.

SUMMARY

Telehealth nursing practice in pediatric and family practice offices and in contact centers is a vital point of access for parents or caregivers seeking health care advice. The nurse faces many challenges in assessing and intervening to meet the special needs of the pediatric patient. The role of the nurse is to assist parents or caregivers in managing childhood illnesses and/or injuries, and providing anticipatory guidance.

TIPS & PEARLS

☎ Children have great compensatory mechanisms – their symptoms can be very subtle. They may not appear outwardly symptomatic.

☎ Children often have difficulty describing how they are feeling. The nurse must carefully assess the situation based on knowing that the full information may not be disclosed.

☎ A child's response to illness and injury depends on the child's developmental stage.

☎ Parents and/or caregivers may minimize or over-emphasize certain symptoms. However, it is always important to not overlook all symptoms.

The nurse faces many challenges in assessing and intervening to meet the special needs of the pediatric patient. The role of the nurse is to assist parents or caregivers in managing childhood illnesses and/or injuries, and providing anticipatory guidance.

References

Briggs, J.K. (2007). *Telephone triage protocols for nurses* (3rd ed.). Philadelphia: Lippincott, Williams & Wilkins.

Schmidt, B.D. (2006). *Pediatric telephone protocols* (11th ed.). Elk Grove Village, IL: American Academy of Pediatrics.

Springhouse. (2005). *Pediatric nursing made incredibly easy!* Philadelphia: Lippincott, Williams & Wilkins.

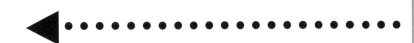

CHAPTER 15
Clinical Knowledge – Geriatric Population

Objectives

1. Describe the importance of change in status of the geriatric patient and other indicators that the telehealth nurse should be aware of.
2. Explain challenges regarding transportation and the care of geriatric patients.
3. Summarize strategies for implementing effective nursing actions when dealing with geriatric patients.

Not only are more people reaching old age, but they are also living longer once they do. The number of people reaching age 70 and 80 has been steadily increasing and will continue to do so. By 2020, there will be 55 million persons ages 65 and older and 7.3 million persons ages 85 and older. (Administration on Aging [AoA], 2007). Telehealth nursing is a vital link between the health care system and the elderly. The nurse offers advice, support, and counseling to the community-based elderly and their families; therefore, older adults increase their self-reliance by providing care for themselves.

While performing a skillful, condensed assessment without being perfunctory, the nurse needs to develop a complete picture of the older adult's situation based on data gathered from the telecommunications interview. The nurse needs to focus on the following specific areas:

> *The number of people reaching age 70 and 80 has been steadily increasing and will continue to do so. Telehealth nursing is a vital link between the health care system and the elderly.*

❖ The immediate concern that triggered the encounter.
❖ The ability of the older adult to exercise safe judgment.
❖ The health history, with emphasis on essential and instrumental self-care abilities.

Telehealth nursing with older adults requires specific nursing knowledge, good listening skills, patience, and good judgment for the nurse to meet the needs of the geriatric patient.

SPECIAL CONSIDERATIONS WITH ASSESSMENT AND INTERVENTION FOR OLDER ADULTS

During the telehealth encounter with the geriatric patient, there are many special considerations for nursing assessment and intervention to consider that are different from the young and middle-aged population. Considerations for the nurse to think about are:

❖ Does the decision support tool address the needs of the older adult?

❖ What are the subtle changes in physical condition or behavior?

❖ Are there atypical presentations of illness?

❖ Can the nurse obtain an accurate assessment of the patient's medical history and medications?

❖ Are there mental health problems that interfere with the nurse's ability to clearly communicate with the patient?

❖ Does the geriatric patient have impairment of vision or hearing that may hinder the assessment and advice to be given?

Assessment Using Decision Support Tools

Geriatric patients create special challenges for the telehealth nurse. Typical signs of illness in geriatric patients may be non-existent, wholly misleading, or present in a deceptively mild form.

Geriatric patients create special challenges for the telehealth nurse. First, when assessing older adults, the nurse must recognize that the decision support tools used for the younger population may not address the needs of older adults. Typical signs of illness in geriatric patients may be non-existent, wholly misleading, or present in a deceptively mild form (Beers, 2008).

Decision support tools should include symptoms related to the most common acute and chronic complaints of the geriatric patient. The four leading chronic health conditions in the geriatric population include (AoA, 2007):

✓ Hypertension	51%
✓ Arthritis	37%
✓ Heart disease	29%
✓ Eye disorders	25%

Careful assessment is particularly important in older adults, since the nurse needs to consider the possibility of more than one health problem. During the telehealth encounter, the nurse takes into account the normal aging process along with acute and chronic illness.

Identifying Warning Signs of Changing Status

The nurse must identify subtle changes in physical condition or behavior because they can act as early warning signs of changing health status in older adults. A urinary infection, sleep deprivation, dehydration, or constipation may present with any one or more of the following non-specific symptoms in older patients: malaise, decline in functional capacity, poor appetite, confusion, falls, urinary incontinence, fatigue, lethargy, weakness, anorexia, confusion, and dizziness (Beers, 2008). The onset of such symptoms, either abruptly or over a matter of days, should alert the nurse to the possibility of a developing acute illness.

Given subtle changes in older adults, the question for the nurse is how to assess for underlying problems. The nurse must develop a trusting relationship at the start of the interaction. Patient advocacy and early

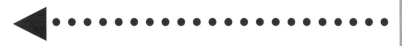

intervention by the nurse is a critical role. Identifying a problem early can minimize or even prevent serious complications in a patient who may lack the ability to snap back. Therefore, recognizing that there is a problem, asking questions, and seeking the answers to "why" may be the most important initial care for older adults who may exhibit subtle physical or behavior changes. Often, illness can be detected by verbal clues, such as the way the story is told, tempo of speech, tone of voice, lowered voice, and even tears (Beers, 2008). If an adult aged 65 years or older tells the nurse that he/she just doesn't feel good, the nurse must further assess to determine if there are any symptoms. This can be a long and tedious interaction, but is very important to the geriatric patient's well-being.

Atypical presentation of illness in the older adult may make accurate assessment difficult. Important markers of acute distress in older adults are outlined in the acronym *CLEAR*. The telehealth nurse should consider the CLEAR items below when assessing the geriatric patient (Linton & Lach, 2006).

- ❖ **C** ognitive changes and agitation could be caused by dementia, digoxin toxicity, infection, or pain.

- ❖ **L** oss of bladder control could be caused by infection, fecal impaction, or atrophic vaginitis.

- ❖ **E** ating and nutritional changes could be caused by anorexia due to medications, depression, or malignancies.

- ❖ **A** ctivity/energy changes could be caused by hyperthyroidism or hypothyroidism, congestive heart failure, medications, or electrolyte imbalances.

- ❖ **R** ecurrent falls could be caused by transient ischemic attacks, cardiac arrhythmias, or arthritic knees.

A comprehensive baseline assessment must be part of the telehealth nurse's role in order to meet the needs of geriatric patients. This assessment encompasses differentiation of age-related changes from pathological processes as well as atypical presentation of older adults. The comprehensive baseline assessment for the geriatric patient should also include assessment of medications and mental health issues, as well as being aware of impairments to assessment due to hearing and visual loss.

Assessment of Medications

Another area of special consideration with older adults is an accurate assessment of their medications and allergies. Multiple medications are a fact of life for older adults. Prescription and nonprescription drugs can exacerbate

> *Given subtle changes in older adults, the question for the nurse is how to assess for underlying problems. Recognizing that there is a problem, asking questions, and seeking the answers to "why" may be the most important initial care for older adults who may exhibit subtle physical or behavior changes.*

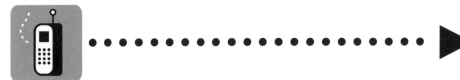

symptoms. Nurses must be careful to consider the role that medication plays as related to the symptoms of the patient.

Questions that the nurse may ask to determine the medication history include:

❖ Is the patient taking any prescription medication? If the patient is on prescription medication, have the patient name the medication, the dosage, and frequency of use.
❖ What over-the-counter medications is the patient taking (including the amount and how often)?
❖ Is the patient taking anything for pain?
❖ Does the patient take anything else to feel better (such as herbs, wine, etc.)?

Due to multiple chronic conditions, older adults may receive a variety of medications from different practitioners, none of whom are communicating with the others. Medication complications – both side effects and drug-drug interactions – are more common in older adults, mainly because of the high number of drugs used.

In the process of gathering this information from the patient, the nurse quickly gains an understanding about the patient's knowledge of his/her medications in a non-confrontational manner. *Polypharmacy medicine* is defined as the concurrent use of several different drugs. Due to multiple chronic conditions, older adults may receive a variety of medications from different practitioners, none of whom are communicating with the others. Medication complications – both side effects and drug-drug interactions – are more common in older adults, mainly because of the high number of drugs used. If the nurse has concerns regarding medications that the patient is taking, the nurse may ask the patient or a family member to bring in all the medications in the house (including the spouse's and other "borrowed" drugs) in a paper or plastic bag. This technique can be extraordinarily revealing and is recommended in making the initial evaluation for a new patient to a medical practice.

Persons ages 65 and older consume more prescriptions and over-the-counter (OTC) medications than any other age group (National Institute on Aging, 2005). The provider must know about OTC drugs taken because their overuse can have serious consequences (Beers, 2008). For a variety of reasons, the patient may be non-compliant with the administration of the OTC and prescribed medications. Non-compliance maybe due to the high cost of medications; older adults may have to make choices about taking the medication or taking it as prescribed. Another reason for non-compliance is that the patient may have problems following the treatment schedule, which may result in taking too may pills or forgetting to take the medication. Older adults may have a lack of knowledge about the dosage, purpose, side effects, or adverse reactions and instructions of the medication. For this reason, it is important to ask patients if there are any questions they would like to ask the doctor or nurse about their medications.

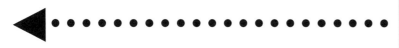

Assessment of the Medical History

The nurse may be unable to obtain an accurate assessment because the geriatric patient may be a poor historian. This can make collection of vital information a daunting process. Geriatric patients may feel awkward or embarrassed about sharing their problems or concerns. Additionally, the nurse needs to determine if the patient's inconsistent answers are due to the inability to remember or fear that telling the truth about a physical problem will result in being treated or hospitalized.

It is important to determine what is troubling the patient and to attempt to address the problem before continuing the assessment. Frequently, the older adult or a family member will dismiss new signs and symptoms as part of the normal aging process and not mention them to the nurse, thus disregarding a possible pathologic process. More time is needed to interview older patients because of their slower reaction time, poorer memory, diminished energy levels, more medications, greater number of psychosocial and physiologic problems, and longer life history (Beers, 2008).

There are several options for the nurse who is unable to obtain an accurate assessment. The first option would be to ask to speak to a family member or friend who is there with the patient. If the patient is alone, the nurse should ask permission to contact a family member who is supporting his/her care, and if granted, a telephone number. Let the patient know that he/she will be called back after the nurse talks with the family member. If the technology allows, the telehealth nurse should consider establishing a conference call including the patient and family member. When the nurse is not sure of the nursing assessment and which actions to take for the patient, the patient should come into the medical office or emergency department as appropriate for a medical assessment.

More time is needed to interview older patients because of their slower reaction time, poorer memory, diminished energy levels, more medications, greater number of psychosocial and physiologic problems, and longer life history.

Assessment of Mental Health Issues

Mental health problems may also interfere with the ability to clearly communicate a patient's problems and comply with advice given. A variety of conditions can impair cerebral circulation and cause disturbances in cognitive function. The following symptoms may be related to confusion and recognized by the nurse during the telehealth interaction: disorientation to time and place (but usually not of self), meaningless chatter, poor judgment, and altered memory span.

1 in 8 Americans over the age of 65 and nearly half of those over the age of 85 suffer from Alzheimer's disease. There are more than 5 million people in the United States living with Alzheimer's (Alzheimer's Association, 2007). The symptoms of this progressive, degenerative disease develop gradually and progress at different rates among affected individuals. Early in the disease, the patient may be aware of the changes in intellectual ability and become depressed or anxious. They may attempt to compensate by writing down information and attempt to structure routines. For example, the nurse

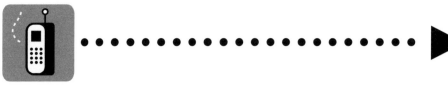

may ask the patient to write down the advice and then at the closure of the encounter, ask the patient to read the advice so that the nurse may evaluate the patient's understanding of the advice given.

Depression is one of the most common psychiatric disorders among the elderly (Beers, 2008). Depressive episodes may have been a life-long problem for some individuals, whereas other patients may experience depression as a new problem in old age. The nurse, by asking the older patient the simple question, "Do you often feel sad or depressed?" may be able to assess for depression. Asking the family member regarding subtle changes in personality, especially lack of enthusiasm and spontaneity, loss of sense of humor, and new forgetfulness may also indicate depression. Loss of interest in sex may be apparent only to a spouse or other sexual partner. Nurses also must be alert to loss of appetite, new sleep disturbances, and other signs and symptoms of depression (Beers, 2008). The patient's prescriptions should be reviewed to identify those that can cause symptoms of depression.

Depressed patients should be asked directly about suicidal thoughts and intentions (e.g., "Do you ever feel that life is not worth living? Have you thought of harming yourself?"). Asking about suicide does not increase the risk of suicide. Patients with suicidal thoughts should be asked about plans (e.g., "Have you planned how you would do it?"). Those with suicidal plans should be hospitalized immediately (Beers, 2008).

Impairment of the Assessment Due to Visual Deficits

A majority of older adults have sufficient vision to meet normal self-care demands with assistance of corrective lenses. Older adults with low or impaired vision can hinder the assessment of the telehealth nurse if they are unable to read the labels of medications or the thermometer. Geriatric patients may be hesitant or refuse to write down the advice or referral given because they know they will not be able to read their handwriting. Options for assisting patients with impaired vision are limited for the nurse. If the patient is unable to read the labels of medications, the patient should bring the medications in a brown or plastic bag to his/her health care provider to review at the next appointment. The nurse should ask permission to talk with someone else, either a family member or friend, to assist the patient in reading a medication label or thermometer. It may be necessary for a follow-up encounter if the patient is able to get someone to talk with the nurse regarding information that the patient is unable to read.

The telehealth nurse plays a preventive role by encouraging annual eye examinations. Prompt evaluation by a health care provider is required for any symptoms, which could indicate a visual problem. This may include burning, pain, blurred or double vision, redness of the conjunctiva, spots, headaches, flashes of light, and other changes in vision.

Depressed patients should be asked directly about suicidal thoughts and intentions. Asking about suicide does not increase the risk of suicide. Patients with suicidal thoughts should be asked about plans. Those with suicidal plans should be hospitalized immediately.

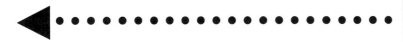

Impairment of the Assessment Due to Hearing Loss

Most geriatric patients have some degree of hearing loss that may cause hearing impairment. Therefore, good communication via telecommunications is another challenge for the telehealth nurse when talking with the hearing-impaired. Approximately one-third of Americans between the age of 65 and 74 have some hearing problems. One-half of people over age 85 and older have hearing loss. Whether hearing loss is small or great, it can worsen if left untreated. During the telephone interaction with the older adult, the nurse may determine that there is hearing loss when the patient responds inappropriately to questions, frequently asks the nurse to repeat the information, or the nurse realizes that the caller's voice tone is loud.

The following tips may assist the nurse when talking to the hearing-impaired (AoA, 2007):

❖ Speak in a normal tone without shouting or showing impatience.
❖ Speak clearly. Don't mumble or over-articulate.
❖ A woman's voice is often harder to hear than a man's because of its pitch. A woman might try to lower the pitch of her voice when talking to older adults to see if that helps.
❖ Speak slowly.
❖ Rephrase statements that may not have been heard or understood. Recognize that older people often can't hear and understand well when they are tired or ill.
❖ If the older person wears a hearing aid, ask if the hearing aid is on, if the volume can be increased, or if the batteries are working.
❖ If the older adult wears a hearing aid, try raising the pitch of your voice just slightly. If the older listener is not wearing an aid, try lowering the pitch of your voice.
❖ Avoid an abrupt change of subject or interjecting small talk into the conversation, as older adults often use context to understand what is being said.
❖ Pronounce words clearly. If the hearing-impaired individual has difficulty with letters and numbers say, "M as in Mary," "five six" instead of "fifty-six," etc.

The nurse must be patient; stay positive and relaxed. It is important to remember that hearing impairments do not indicate confusion and disorientation.

Assessment of Activities of Daily Living

When assessing older adults, activities of daily living (ADLs) often present the most accurate baseline picture of the patient. Physical functioning usually is measured by the ability to accomplish basic ADLs, including bathing, dressing, toileting, transferring, continence, and feeding.

When assessing older adults, activities of daily living (ADLs) often present the most accurate baseline picture of the patient. Physical functioning usually is measured by the ability to accomplish basic ADLs, including bathing, dressing, toileting, transferring, continence, and feeding.

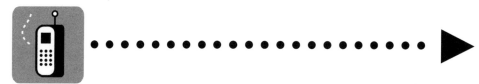

Other components of functional well-being are behavioral and social ADLs that require a higher level of cognition and judgment than physical activities. The instrumental activities of daily living (IADLs) include preparation of meals, shopping, light housework, financial management, medication, and use of the telephone. By asking the patient questions about ADLs and IADLs, the nurse will be able to determine his/her independence in getting out of bed, dressing, cooking, shopping, and other highly cognitive demands.

For example, a seemingly minor podiatry problem developing in the older adult who is already barely able to make it to the bathroom will render him or her dependent on others for essential daily functions. The nurse must recognize that function is of such importance because even a minor problem can affect all medical, nursing, and social decision-making for the geriatric patient.

Assessment of Developmental Characteristics and Aged-Related Physiological Changes

The telehealth nurse utilizes the knowledge of age-specific developmental characteristics for assessing and intervening for the geriatric patient. For example, the geriatric patient is adapting to physical changes that accompany aging, such as loose/wrinkled/dry skin, stiff/slow joints, and a bent/stooped posture. They may be facing changes in the level of independence and finances associated with retirement. It may be a time to be adjusting to the loss of loved ones and friends. Table 15-1 was adapted from *Gerontological Nursing* (Linton & Lach, 2006) and is an example of nursing actions in response to age-related changes. This is provided here only as an example of how a telehealth nurse might develop similar tolls in collaboration with his/her physician and is not endorsed by AAACN nor intended for clinical use.

The telehealth nurse utilizes the knowledge of age-specific developmental characteristics for assessing and intervening for the geriatric patient.

Table 15-1.
Summary of Selected Physiological Age-Related Changes and Nursing Actions

Age-Related Changes	Nursing Actions
Decrease in intracellular fluid	Assess for dehydration; instruct to maintain 1,500-ml fluid intake daily.
Reduction in subcutaneous fat	Assess and instruct to adjust room temperature to 70-75° F; provide warm clothing.
Lower oral temperature	Assess baseline norm for body temperature when patient is well to be able to identify manifestations of fever.

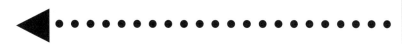

Reduction in cardiac volume	Instruct in allowing rest between activities; longer time frame required for heart rate to return to normal following stress.
Reduction in lung capacity	Recognize atypical signs and symptoms; can accompany less-effective gas exchange, respiratory infections, and cough response.
Brittleness of teeth	Encourage daily oral care and an annual visit to the dentist.
Decrease in taste sensations	Assess for over-consumption of sweets and salt.
Decreased esophageal and gastric motility	Assess for indigestion; advise patient not to lie down for at least one hour after meals.
Reduction in colonic peristasis	Assess for frequency, consistency, and amount of bowel movements; instruct in high fiber diet and prevention of constipation.
Decrease in size of renal mass, number of nephrons, glomerular filtration	Assess for adverse drug reactions; recognize renal lab result changes for BUN and creatinine.
Weaker bladder muscles	Assess for signs and symptoms of UTIs and incontinence.
Increased alkalinity of vaginal canal	Assess for signs and symptoms of vaginitis.
Atrophy of muscle; reduction in muscle strength and mass	Advise patient to avoid straining or overusing muscles; encourage regular exercise.
Decreased bone mass and mineral content	Instruct patient in safety measures to prevent falls and fractures; assess for and instruct in calcium intake.
Decreased visual accommodations; reduced peripheral vision; less effective vision in dark and dimly lit areas	Assess for and encourage annual eye exam; encourage use of night-lights.

Assessment for Identifying Elder Mistreatment

According to the National Center on Elder Abuse (NCEA), between 1 and 2 million elderly people ages 65 or older have been injured, exploited, or otherwise mistreated by someone on whom they depended on for care and protection.

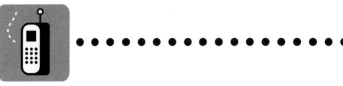

Data on elder abuse in domestic settings suggests that 1 in 14 (excluding incidents of self-neglect) come to the attention of authorities. It is estimated that for every 1 case that is reported, about 5 more go unreported (NCEA, 2005).

It is important for the nurse to be able to recognize signs and symptoms of neglect or abuse. Because direct observation is not available in telehealth nursing practice, a careful evaluation of physical and behavioral indicators of abuse or neglect is important. Abused geriatric patients and their caregivers frequently hide evidence of the problem, and if questioned, may deny it. Historical, psychological, and physical indicators may be used during the telehealth assessment to identify those patients who may be at risk for abuse.

Abused geriatric patients and their caregivers frequently hide evidence of the problem, and if questioned, may deny it.

Historical Indicators

❖ History of frequent changes in health care providers may be a way of trying to avoid detection of abuse. The nurse may detect this when asking the patient or family member, "Who is her primary care provider?" and the response is, "Mother goes to different offices or to no particular doctor."

❖ Delays between the onset of trauma or illness and the caregiver seeking assistance may indicate that the abuser thought the injury would resolve without medical treatment, thus avoiding possible detection of abuse. For example, the patient fell 5 days ago and the wrist is swollen and painful, and the skin is discolored. However, the caregiver states that he/she thought the wrist would improve in a few days without medical assistance.

❖ When the explanation of the patient or caregiver is implausible or vague, or when the severity of the injury does not fit the explanation given by the caregiver, it could be suggestive of elder abuse (Beers, 2008). For example, a family member seeks advice for cold symptoms. Near the end of the encounter, the nurse asks the family member, "Do you have any other questions?" and the reply is "Oh yes, dad fell and hurt his wrist several days ago. Can you give me advice to determine if it is broken or sprained?"

Psychological/Behavioral Indicators

The nurse must be aware of a variety of psychological and behavioral indicators that arouse suspicion of abuse while communicating with the patient or family member (Beers, 2008).

❖ If the patient is overly fearful or anxious during the telehealth interaction, it may indicate a fear of "saying the wrong thing."

❖ The patient expresses fears or anxiety about the relationship with the caregiver.

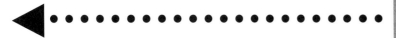

❖ The caregiver is excessively stressed by the care-giving responsibilities.
❖ The caregiver is unwilling to seek or accept outside assistance.
❖ The caregiver belittles the patient during the interaction with the nurse.

The nurse needs to use good communication skills to identify why the patient is fearful regarding the caregiver's behavior and then make the appropriate referral(s) to address the identified issues. If the caregiver expresses stress in caring for the patient, the nurse's role is to know what community resources are available for the caregiver and for the geriatric patient, such as self-help groups for the caregiver and adult day care centers for older adults. Additionally, when the caregiver expresses stress in caring for the patient, it is extremely important to explore with them what this statement means. The stress could be due to changes in the patient's mental or physical abilities, or the stress could be due to the caregiver's lack of coping mechanisms. It should be the nurse's responsibility to explore the issue with the patient.

Physical Indicators

In telehealth nursing, it is difficult for the nurse to assess if the physical problem is due to abuse unless the person informs the nurse. However, if the nurse has access to the patient's medical record, a pattern of injuries could be identified, such as frequent, repeated, or unusually placed injuries. Some signs of elder abuse include (Beers, 2008):

❖ Bruises, welts, or burns.
❖ Marks on wrists or ankles that suggest the use of restraints.
❖ Poor hygiene (such as general uncleanliness or inappropriate clothing).
❖ Skin turgor or signs of dehydration.
❖ Anxiety or depressed symptoms.
❖ Infestations.
❖ Abnormal gait.
❖ Unexplainable hair loss.
❖ Pressure sores or multiple skin lesions in various stages of evolution.
❖ Rectal or vaginal bleeding.

Nurses are federally mandated to report elderly abuse, and if abuse or neglect is suspected, the nurse is legally required to inform local or state authorities so that concerns can be investigated and the patient examined. If an elderly patient appears to be in imminent danger, the nurse should treat the situation as an emergency. The patient's safety must always be the first concern.

In telehealth nursing, it is difficult for the nurse to assess if the physical problem is due to abuse unless the caller informs the nurse. However, if the nurse has access to the patient's medical record, a pattern of injuries could be identified.

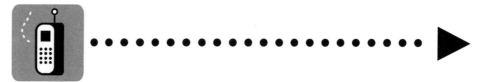

When suspicion of abuse or neglect is present, your documented telehealth interaction is very important. Note physical injuries and any patterns of injuries involved, as well as the patient's and caregiver's behavior. If the nurse hears the patient or caregiver mention abuse or neglect, this information must be documented. Indicate that it is a direct quote and give the source. Also document your plan of action.

TRANSPORTATION ISSUES

The final special consideration for the telehealth nurse is to assess for the availability of transportation should the patient need health services. Many elderly patients do not drive any longer and may not own a car. The group of drivers over age 70 is second only to the 16-20-year-old set in traffic deaths (WebMD, 2005). Lists should be available of alternative transportation resources available in the community. Managed care agencies may offer transportation to medical facilities as part of their benefit plan for geriatric participants. The nurse may need to assist the senior in identifying a family member, friend, or neighbor who could provide transportation for the patient to health services.

FOLLOW-UP ENCOUNTERS

In telehealth nursing, follow-up encounters are a vital part of evaluation in the nursing process. Follow-up encounters give the nurse the opportunity to obtain feedback, clarify or explain instructions, diminish risk management issues, and show caring and concern for the patient.

In telehealth nursing, follow-up encounters are a vital part of evaluation in the nursing process. Follow-up encounters give the nurse the opportunity to obtain feedback, clarify or explain instructions, diminish risk management issues, and show caring and concern for the patient. The nurse is able to verify compliance with the advice or information that was given to the geriatric patient. If the patient did not follow the advice, this gives the nurse the opportunity to investigate the reason for non-compliance and to address this issue.

For example, if the nurse is concerned about dehydration due to diarrhea or vomiting, the follow-up encounter is necessary to assess the amount of intake and output within a specific time frame and if the patient is following the advice given. From this follow-up interaction with the geriatric patient, the nurse will be able to determine if the patient needs to be seen to rule out fluid imbalance or is able to continue home care. Often, the older adult feels isolated and lonely, and the follow-up encounter demonstrates caring and concern.

TELEHEALTH SURVEILLANCE

Telehealth surveillance for older adults has continued to expand in communities. Two types of telehealth surveillance programs are home monitoring devices (with alarm systems) and reassurance lines. The purpose

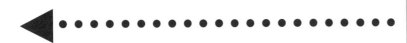

of these programs is to maintain independence, postpone admission to an assisted-living facility or nursing home, increase self-sufficiency, and reduce apprehension of the older adult and his/her family.

One type of alarm system is an electronic device placed in the home that automatically sets off an alarm at an emergency response center. The response center may be located in a hospital that will have a list of responders who will check on the older adult.

Another type of telehealth surveillance system provides personnel to call daily to check on the older adult. If there is no answer at the prearranged time, someone is sent for a home visit to assess the status of the patient.

Telehealth nurses play a vital role in the care plan for the elderly patient. For the patient to know that there is a nurse who can talk to them when they have concerns, is comforting and provides that extra support they may need.

SUMMARY

In 2006, there were 37.3 million people in the United States over the age of 65. There will be more than 71.5 million older adults in the United States by the year 2030 (AoA, 2007). Persons in this age group create special challenges for the telehealth nurse and require specific nursing knowledge to understand and meet their physical, mental, and social needs.

TIPS & PEARLS

☎ The nurse must understand the pathological changes brought on by aging. The patient may have atypical symptoms of illness, which makes it very difficult to perform an accurate assessment.

☎ The nurse should assess for polypharmacy, including over-the-counter medications and herbal remedies.

☎ Encounters with the elderly may take longer due to chronic conditions, more medications, poor history, and processing information more slowly.

There will be more than 71.5 million older adults in the United States by the year 2030. Persons in this age group create special challenges for the telehealth nurse and require specific nursing knowledge to understand and meet their physical, mental, and social needs.

References

Administration on Aging (AoA). (2007). *Statistics on the aging population.* Retrieved February 20, 2009, from http://www.aoa.gov

Alzheimer's Association. (2007). *Alzheimer's disease facts and figures.* Retrieved February 20, 2009, from http://www.alz.org/alzheimers_disease_facts_figures.asp

Beers, M.H. (2008). *The Merck manual of geriatrics* (3rd ed.) [updated online]. Retrieved February 20, 2009, from http://www.merck.com/mkgr/mmg/home.jsp

Linton, A.D., & Lach, H. (2006). *Matteson & McConnell's gerontological nursing: Concepts and practice* (3rd ed.). St. Louis, MO: Elsevier Science.

National Center on Elder Abuse (NCEA). (2005). *Fact sheet: Elder abuse prevalence and incidence.* Retrieved February 20, 2009, from http://www. ncea.aoa.gov/ncearoot/Main_Site/pdf/publication/FinalStatistics050331.pdf

National Institute on Aging. (2005). *Bound for your good health: A collection of age pages.* Gaithersburg, MD: Author.

WebMD. (2005). *Trading the car keys for a bus pass.* Retrieved February 20, 2009, from http://www.webmd.com

Answer/Evaluation Form
Continuing Nursing Education Activity
Telehealth Nursing Practice Essentials

AMBP9c11

Chapter 13: Clinical Knowledge – At-Risk Populations, and Chapter 14: Clinical Knowledge – Pediatric Population, and Chapter 15: Clinical Knowledge – Geriatric Population

This activity provides 1.4 contact hours of continuing nursing education (CNE) credit in nursing. (Contact hours calculated using a 60-minute contact hour.)

This test may be copied for use by others.

COMPLETE THE FOLLOWING:

Name: _____

Address: _____

City: _____ State: _____ Zip: _____

Telephone number: (Home)_____ (Work)_____

Email address:_____

AAACN Member Number and Expiration Date: _____

Processing fee: AAACN Member: $12.00
                 Nonmember: $20.00

Answer Form: (Please attach a separate sheet of paper.)
1. What did you value most about this activity?

_____

2. If you could imagine that you have fully integrated your learning into practice, what would be different about your present practice?

_____

Evaluation	Strongly disagree				Strongly agree
3. The offering met the stated objectives.					
a. Describe nursing actions related to interacting with patients who have at-risk conditions.	1	2	3	4	5
b. Explain challenges when interacting with at-risk patients within the telehealth environment.	1	2	3	4	5
c. Summarize strategies for implementing effective nursing actions when dealing with at-risk patients.	1	2	3	4	5
d. Describe the special considerations that need to be taken into account when caring for pediatric patients.	1	2	3	4	5
e. Explain challenges when interacting with pediatric patients and/or their families within the telehealth environment.	1	2	3	4	5
f. Summarize the essential components of an encounter with a pediatric patient.	1	2	3	4	5
g. Describe the importance of change in status of the geriatric patient and other indicators that the telehealth nurse should be aware of.	1	2	3	4	5
h. Explain challenges regarding transportation and the care of geriatric patients.	1	2	3	4	5
i. Summarize strategies for implementing effective nursing actions when dealing with geriatric patients.	1	2	3	4	5
4. The content was current and relevant.	1	2	3	4	5
5. The content was presented clearly.	1	2	3	4	5
6. The content was covered adequately.	1	2	3	4	5

7. How would you rate your ability to apply your learning to practice following this activity? (Check one)

☐ Diminished ability ☐ No change ☐ Enhanced ability

8. Time required to complete reading assignment and answer form: ___ minutes
Comments _____

_____

I verify that I have completed this activity:

_____
Signature

Objectives
This educational activity is designed for nurses and other health care professionals who provide telehealth care for patients. This evaluation is designed to test your achievement of the following educational activities.
1. Describe nursing actions related to interacting with patients who have at-risk conditions.
2. Explain challenges when interacting with at-risk patients within the telehealth environment.
3. Summarize strategies for implementing effective nursing actions when dealing with at-risk patients.
4. Describe the special considerations that need to be taken into account when caring for pediatric patients.
5. Explain challenges when interacting with pediatric patients and/or their families within the telehealth environment.
6. Summarize the essential components of an encounter with a pediatric patient.
7. Describe the importance of change in status of the geriatric patient and other indicators that the telehealth nurse should be aware of.
8. Explain challenges regarding transportation and the care of geriatric patients.
9. Summarize strategies for implementing effective nursing actions when dealing with geriatric patients.

Evaluation Form Instructions
1. To receive continuing nursing education (CNE) credit for individual study after reading the indicated chapter(s), please complete the evaluation form (photocopies of the answer form are acceptable). Attach separate paper.
2. Detach (or photocopy) and send the answer form along with a check, money order, or credit card payable to *AAACN* East Holly Avenue/Box 56, Pitman, NJ 08071-0056. You may also send this form as an email attachment to ambp401@ajj.com.
3. Answer forms must be postmarked by December 31, 2011. Upon completion of the answer/evaluation form, a certificate for 1.4 contact hours will be awarded and sent to you.

Payment Options
☐ Check or money order enclosed (payable in U.S. funds to AAACN)

☐ MasterCard ☐ VISA ☐ American Express

Credit Card #:_____

Expiration Date: _____ Security Code:_____

Card Holder (Please print):

_____

Signature:

_____

This educational activity has been co-provided by the American Academy of Ambulatory Care Nursing (AAACN) and Anthony J. Jannetti, Inc. (AJJ).
AAACN is a provider approved by the California Board of Registered Nursing, Provider Number CEP 5336.
AJJ is accredited as a provider of continuing nursing education by the American Nurses Credentialing Center's Commission on Accreditation.
This book was reviewed and formatted for contact hour credit by Sally S. Russell, MN, CMSRN, AAACN Education Director, and Maureen Espensen, MBA, BSN, RN, Editor.

American Academy of Ambulatory Care Nursing
East Holly Avenue/Box 56, Pitman, NJ 08071-0056
Phone: 800-AMB-NURS; Fax: 856-589-7463
Web: www.aaacn.org; Email: aaacn@ajj.com

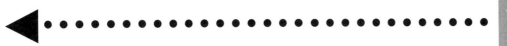

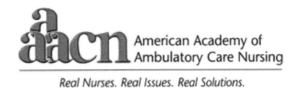
American Academy of
Ambulatory Care Nursing

Real Nurses. Real Issues. Real Solutions.

Glossary of Terms

Many terms in nursing and health care have multiple meanings and can be used in multiple contexts. Certain terms are defined to clarify the intent and application of these standards. Terms not defined are assumed either to have a generally acceptable meaning and interpretation, or to require contextual interpretation, depending on the setting and application.

A

Adverse event – Unnecessary patient injury, harm, pain, or suffering resulting from medical management (such as from medication or treatment).

Appropriateness – The degree to which the care and services provided are relevant to the patient's clinical needs, given the current state of knowledge.

Assessment – A systematic, dynamic process by which the registered nurse, through interaction with the patient, family, groups, communities, populations, and health care providers, collects and analyzes data. Assessment may include the following dimensions: physical, psychological, socio-cultural, spiritual, cognitive, functional abilities, developmental, economic, and lifestyle.

Availability – The degree to which the care and service are accessible and obtainable to meet the patient's needs.

C

Caregiver – Individual (for example, a family member, friend, or companion) over the age of 18 years who provides care and support.

Competency statements – Competencies define the behaviors and outcomes specific and necessary to provide efficient, effective, and evidenced-based care.

Continuity – Something that remains consistent or uninterrupted throughout the care process.

Continuity of care – An interdisciplinary process that includes patients, families, and significant others in the development of a coordinated plan of care. The process facilitates the patient's transition between settings and health care providers based on changing needs and available resources.

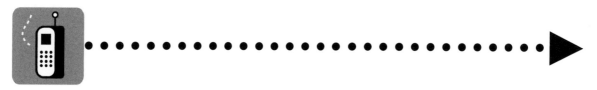

Criteria – Relevant, measurable indicators of the standards of practice and professional performance.

D

Decision support tools – A plan or guide for the assessment and management of a clinical problem to reduce the risk of omission and increase the predictability of desired clinical outcomes. The unique needs of patient preferences and his or her specific situation must be incorporated into their use in a practice setting. Protocols, guidelines, or algorithms may be referred to as decision support tools. Decision support tools are developed using scientifically valid and documented clinical principles and resources, clinical experience, and the needs of the setting in which they are used. They may be in hard copy or computerized format. They should be clinically reviewed annually and revised as needed.

E

Effective – Providing services based on scientific knowledge to all who could benefit and refraining from providing services to those not likely to benefit (avoiding underuse and overuse, respectively).

Efficacy – The potential, capacity, or capability to produce the desired effect or outcome, as already shown, such as through scientific research (evidence-based) findings.

Efficiency – The desired relationship between the outcomes (results of care) and the resources used to deliver patient care and services.

Efficient – Avoiding waste, including waste of equipment, supplies, ideas, and energy.

Encounter – Formally referred to as a "call" and now expanded to include any exchange of information through the use of an electronic technology (voice, fax, e-mail, IVR, Web, live text, video kiosk, or any other electronic connection).

Environment – A complex of external factors (objects, actions, or individuals) by which the person is surrounded or in which the action occurs.

Equitable – Providing care that does not vary in quality because of personal characteristics, such as gender, ethnicity, geographic location, and socioeconomic status.

Ergonomics – The scientific discipline concerned with the interactions between humans and other elements of a system, and the profession that applies theory, principles, data, and methods to system design in order to optimize human well-being and overall system performance.

Evidence-based nursing practice – The process by which nurses make clinical decisions using the best available research evidence, their clinical expertise, and patient preferences in the context of available resources.

Evidence-based practice literature reviews – The search and analysis of a body of research findings about a specific issue or topic.

Expected outcomes – End results that are measurable, desirable, and observable, and translate into observable behaviors.

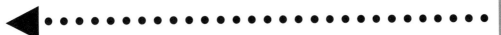

F

Family – Family members are defined by the patient in her or his own terms and may include individuals related by blood, marriage, or in self-defined relationships. (This definition is intended to include the family in nursing care as appropriate. It is not intended as a legal definition of *family*.)

H

Hazardous conditions – Any set of circumstances (exclusive of the disease, disorder, or condition for which the patient is undergoing care, treatment, and services) defined by the organization that significantly increases the likelihood of a serious adverse outcome.

Health care providers – Individuals with special expertise who provide health care services or assistance to patients. They may include nurses, physicians, psychologists, social workers, nutritionists/dieticians, and various therapists.

Health education – Teaching that is focused on the nurse's assessment of the patient's specific learning needs and is delivered at the patient's level of understanding.

Health information – Educational and informational resources designed to enhance the knowledge and understanding of health topics to promote wellness and self care.

I

Infection control – System designed for surveillance, prevention, and control of infection.

Interdisciplinary – Involving 2 or more academic subjects or fields of study and practice.

L

Leader – The person who has management, leadership, and/or oversight responsibilities for the telehealth nursing services. This person may or may not be a registered nurse.

Learning needs – The assessment of learning needs includes, but is not limited to, cultural and religious beliefs, emotional barriers, desire and motivation to learn, physical or cognitive limitations, and barriers to communication.

Literature reviews – The search and analysis of a body of research findings about a specific issue or topic.

M

Multidisciplinary – Studying or using several specialized subjects, expertise, or skills.

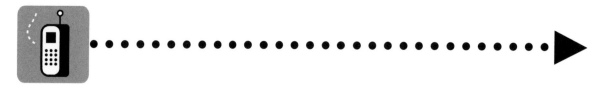

N

Nursing – The protection, promotion, and optimization of health and abilities, prevention of illness and injury, alleviation of suffering through the diagnosis and treatment of human response, and advocacy in the care of individuals, families, communities, and populations.

Nursing leader – The registered nurse who has management, leadership, and/or oversight responsibilities for telehealth nursing services.

O

Organization – Used interchangeably with *setting*; a broad term to describe the practice setting. This may be a physician's office, medical center, hospital, managed care facility, or pharmaceutical company.

Outcomes measurement – The collection and analysis of data using predetermined outcomes indicators for the purposes of making decisions about health care.

P

Patient – Recipient of nursing practice. The term *patient* is used to provide consistency and brevity, bearing in mind that other terms such as *client, individual, resident, family, groups, communities*, or *populations* might be better choices in some instances. When the patient is an individual, the focus is on the health state, problems, or needs of the individual. When the patient is a family or group, the focus is on the health state of the unit as a whole or the reciprocal effects of the individual's health state on the other members of the unit. When the patient is a community or population, the focus is on personal and environmental health and the health risks of the community or population.

Patient-centered – Providing care that is respectful of and responsive to individual patient preferences, needs, and values, and ensuring that patient values guide all clinical decisions.

Performance improvement – The continuous study and adaptation of a health care organization's functions and processes to increase the probability of achieving desired outcomes and to better meet the needs of individuals and other users of services.

Protected health information – Protected health information (PHI) under HIPAA includes any individually identifiable health information. "Identifiable" refers not only to data that is explicitly linked to a particular individual (that's identified information), but also includes health information with data items that reasonably could be expected to allow individual identification.

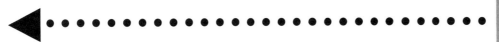

Q

Quality of care – The degree to which health services for individuals and populations increase the likelihood of desired health outcomes and are consistent with current professional knowledge.

Quality control – A process that consists of measuring performance, comparing performance against goals, and acting on the differences when performance falls short of defined goals.

R

Reliable – Instrument is consistent and dependable.
- Inter-rater reliability is used to assure an acceptable level of consistency when multiple individuals are collecting data.
- Test-retest reliability refers to the ability of the instrument to provide consistent results when administered multiple times.
- Internal consistency reliability refers to whether the individual items on an instrument all contribute positively to the concept being measured.

Research – Original investigation undertaken in order to gain knowledge and understanding. This includes:
- Work of direct relevance to the needs of commerce and industry, as well as to the public and voluntary sectors.
- Scholarship: The creation, development, and maintenance of the intellectual infrastructure of subjects and disciplines, in forms such as dictionaries, scholarly editions, catalogues, and contributions to major research databases.
- Invention and generation of ideas, images, performances, and artifacts (including design), where these lead to new or substantially improved insights.
- Use of existing knowledge in experimental development to produce new or substantially improved materials, devices, products, and processes, including design and construction.

Respect and caring – The degree to which those providing care and services do so with sensitivity and respect for the patient's needs, expectations, and individual differences, and the degree to which the individual or designee is involved in his or her own care and service decisions.

S

Safe – Avoiding injuries to patients from the care that is intended to help them.

Safety – The degree to which the risk of an intervention and risk in the care environment are reduced for a patient and other persons, including health care practitioners.

Self-efficacy – The belief and use of behaviors that one has mastery over the events of one's life and can meet challenges as they arise.

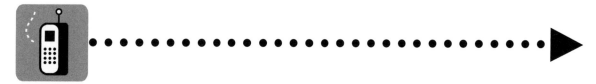

Setting – Used interchangeably with *organization*; a broad term to describe the practice setting of telehealth nursing. This may be a physician's office, medical center, hospital, managed care facility, or pharmaceutical company.

Spatial arrangements – A distribution of a particular landscape feature or features throughout a unit of space.

Staffing effectiveness – The number, competence, and skill mix of staff as related to the provision of needed services.

Standard – Authoritative statement enunciated and promulgated by the profession by which the quality of practice, service, or education can be judged.

Standards of care – Authoritative statements that describe a competent level of clinical nursing practice demonstrated through assessment, diagnosis, outcome identification, planning, implementation, and evaluation.

Standards of nursing practice – Authoritative statements that describe a level of care or performance common to the profession of nursing by which the quality of nursing practice can be judged. Standards of clinical nursing practice include both standards of care and standards of professional performance.

Standards of professional performance – Authoritative statements that describe a competent level of behavior in the professional role, including activities related to quality of care, performance appraisal, education, collegiality, ethics, collaboration, research, and resource utilization.

T

Tele (prefix) – At or over a distance.

Telecommunications – Use of the telephone, Internet, interactive video, remote sensory devices, or robotics to transmit information from one site to another.

Telehealth – The delivery, management, and coordination of health services that integrate electronic information and telecommunications technologies to increase access, improve outcomes, and contain or reduce costs of health care. *Telehealth* is an umbrella term used to describe the wide range of services delivered across distances by all health-related disciplines.

Telehealth nursing – The delivery, management, and coordination of care and services provided via telecommunications technology within the domain of nursing. *Telehealth nursing* encompasses all types of nursing care and services delivered across distances. It is a broad term encompassing practices that incorporate a vast array of telecommunications technologies (such as telephone, fax, electronic mail, Internet, video monitoring, interactive video) to remove time and distance barriers for the delivery of nursing care.

Telemedicine – The delivery, management, and coordination of care and services provided via telecommunications technology within the domain of medicine. *Telemedicine* is a broad term describing the subset of telehealth pertaining to the practice of medicine at a distance.

Telephone nursing – All care and services within the scope of nursing practice that are delivered over the telephone. *Telephone nursing* is a component of telehealth nursing practice restricted to the telephone.

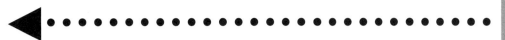

Telephone triage – An interactive process between the nurse and client that occurs over the telephone and involves identifying the nature and urgency of client health care needs and determining the appropriate disposition. *Telephone triage* is a component of telephone nursing practice that focuses on assessment, prioritization, and referral to the appropriate level of care.

Timeliness – The degree to which the needed care and services are provided to the patient at the most beneficial or necessary time.

Timely – Reducing waits and sometimes harmful delays for both those who receive and those who give care.

U

Unlicensed assistive personnel (UAP) – Applies to an unlicensed individual who is trained to function in an assistive role to the licensed nurse in the provision of patient/client activities as delegated by the nurse.

V

Valid – Instrument measures what it is supposed to measure. Generally determined by a panel of experts.

W

Web-based sources of evidence – Multiple sites on the World Wide Web that contain research-based evidence and commonly include:

- Guidelines and Best Practice Sites.
- National Guideline Clearinghouse: A program of the Agency for Healthcare Research and Quality (AHRQ); a database of evidence-based practice guidelines for nurses, physicians, and other health care providers (www.guideline.gov).
- The Joanna Briggs Institute: Affiliated with the Royal Adelaide Hospital in Australia; produces both best-practice information sheets and systematic reviews on topics of interest to nurses (www.joannabriggs.edu.au/).
- National Library of Medicine.
- MEDLINE: Electronic database of citations and abstracts. It indexes more than 4800 journals from more than 70 countries, from 1966 to the present (*Index Medicus* is the paper equivalent of MEDLINE). MEDLINE is available online at no cost through PubMed.
- PubMed: Web interface with a greater scope than MEDLINE, and is freely available on the Web (www.pubmed.gov).
- Systematic Literature Review Sites.

- *Online Journal of Clinical Innovations*: Electronic publication from CINAHL Information Systems (www.cinahl.com) that contains systematic reviews of the literature and other articles and abstracts (www.cinahl.com/cexpress/ojcionline3/index.html).
- The Sarah Cole Hirsh Institute for Best Nursing Practices Based on Evidence: Repository of systematic reviews of evidence-based practices at the Frances Payne Bolton School of Nursing, Case Western Reserve University. It publishes the reviews through the *Online Journal of Issues in Nursing* (http://fpb.case.edu/Centers/Hirsh/).

Adapted from:

American Academy of Ambulatory Care Nursing (AAACN). (2007). *Ambulatory care nursing administration and practice standards* (7th ed.). Pitman, NJ: Author.

American Academy of Ambulatory Care Nursing (AAACN). (2007). *Telehealth nursing practice administration and practice standards* (4th ed.). Pitman, NJ: Author.

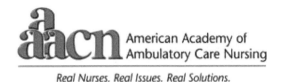

American Academy of
Ambulatory Care Nursing

Real Nurses. Real Issues. Real Solutions.

AAACN Telehealth Nursing Practice Core Course (TNPCC)
At *YOUR* Location

AAACN's Telehealth Nursing Practice Core Course (TNPCC) can be given at your location. AAACN will work closely with your practice facility to customize the logistics of the course as much as possible. The course is a one-day event offering **7.5 contact hours.**

The AAACN fee to present the course is $4,000 for the first 50 participants. The fee for additional participants is $50 per person. The fee includes **two** faculty honoraria, provision of contact hours, customized CNE certificates, a camera-ready course handout to be duplicated by your facility, and staff coordination.

As the hosting site, your facility would be responsible for:
♦ Speaker airfare and miscellaneous speaker expenses: transportation to/from airport, meals, etc.
♦ Securing faculty accommodations: two rooms for one night
   NOTE: two nights may be needed, depending on your accessibility to the airport
♦ Meeting room
♦ AV equipment: laptop computer with Power Point software, LCD projector, screen, microphone, and audio hook-up for the laptop (or CD player) for sound clips used of sample telephone conversations
♦ Food and beverage, if offered
♦ Promotion of the course
♦ Registration processing
♦ Handout duplication

We encourage participants to purchase the *Telehealth Nursing Practice Essentials* textbook to accompany the course and provide more in-depth reference material. We offer a quantity discount when 25 or more textbooks are ordered at one time.

For an additional $1,000, AAACN will provide a **site license** for the facility to post the review course audio and slides (the most recently recorded version) on their Local Area Network (LAN).

If you are interested in opening this course up to registered nurses in your community, you could recoup some of your costs through registration fees that you would determine. You might also consider obtaining local corporate sponsorship if that is applicable to your facility, or ask another nearby facility to co-sponsor the course and share the expenses. The AAACN fee would not change in these instances, unless the number of participants exceeded 50.

For further information or to schedule the course at your facility, contact AAACN using the information below.

American Academy of Ambulatory Care Nursing
East Holly Avenue/Box 56, Pitman, NJ 08071-0056
Phone: 800-262-6877, Fax: 856-589-7463, Email: reichartp@ajj.com
Web site: www.aaacn.org

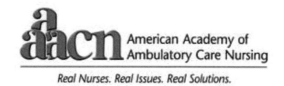

American Academy of
Ambulatory Care Nursing

Real Nurses. Real Issues. Real Solutions.

Fact Sheet

IDENTITY STATEMENT: The American Academy of Ambulatory Care Nursing (AAACN) is the association of professional nurses and associates who identify ambulatory care practice as essential to the continuum of accessible, high-quality, and cost-effective health care.

MISSION AND CORE PURPOSE: Advance the art and science of ambulatory care nursing.

CORE VALUES: The following values guide member and organization vision, actions, and relationships:
1) Responsible health care delivery for individuals and communities
2) Visionary and accountable leadership
3) Productive partnerships and alliances
4) Diversity
5) Continual advancement of professional ambulatory care nursing practice
6) Collaborative professional community

GOALS:
- ☎ **KNOWLEDGE** – AAACN will be the recognized source for knowledge in ambulatory care nursing.
- ☎ **EDUCATION** – Nurses will have the leadership skills and capabilities to articulate, promote, and practice nursing successfully in an ambulatory care setting.
- ☎ **ADVOCACY** – The health care community will recognize and value ambulatory care nursing.
- ☎ **COMMUNITY** – Ambulatory care nurses will have a supportive and collaborative community in which to share professional interests, experience, and practice.

ABOUT AAACN: AAACN (formerly the American Academy of Ambulatory Nursing Administration) was founded in 1978 as a not-for-profit, educational forum. In 1993, the organization's name was changed to the American Academy of Ambulatory Care Nursing (AAACN). Membership was broadened to include nurses in direct practice, education, and research roles, as well as those in management and administration. Today, membership is open to nurses and other professionals interested in ambulatory care nursing. Corporations and individual corporate representatives are also welcomed as members.

Ambulatory practice settings include universities, medical centers, HMOs, group practices, urgent care centers, physician office settings, hospital-based ambulatory care settings, military, community health and others. The Academy serves as a voice for ambulatory care nurses across the continuum of health care delivery and has membership in the Nursing Organizations Alliance (NOA). The Alliance provides a forum for nursing organizations to dialogue, collaborate, and facilitate policy formulation on professional practice and national health.

American Academy of Ambulatory Care Nursing
East Holly Avenue/Box 56, Pitman, NJ 08071-0056
Phone: 800-262-6877, Fax: 856-589-7463, Email: reichartp@ajj.com
Web site: www.aaacn.org

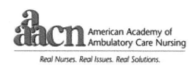

American Academy of
Ambulatory Care Nursing

Real Nurses. Real Issues. Real Solutions.

MEMBERSHIP BENEFITS: Academy membership benefits include discounted rates to the AAACN National Preconference and Conference, offering multiple practice innovations, distance learning programs, publications, and the ANCC ambulatory care nursing certification exam; industry exhibits and numerous networking opportunities; the bimonthly newsletter – *Viewpoint;* subscription to **one** of four journals – *Nursing Economic$, MEDSURG Nursing, Dermatology Nursing,* or *Pediatric Nursing*; opportunity to join a special interest group in the area of: Leadership, Patient Education, Pediatrics, Staff Education, Telehealth Nursing Practice, Veterans Affairs, and Tri-Service Military; awards and scholarship programs; access to national experts and colleagues through AAACN's online membership directory; monthly E-newsletter; email discussion lists; an Expert Panel; Web site (aaacn.org); and online Career Center.

AAACN PUBLICATIONS/EDUCATION RESOURCES:
- ➢ *Ambulatory Care Nurse Staffing: An Annotated Bibliography*
- ➢ *Ambulatory Care Nursing Administration and Practice Standards*
- ➢ *Ambulatory Care Nursing Certification Review Course Syllabus*
- ➢ *Ambulatory Care Nursing Certification Review Course CD-ROM*
- ➢ *Ambulatory Care Nursing Review Questions*
- ➢ *Core Curriculum for Ambulatory Care Nursing* (2nd Edition)
- ➢ *Guide to Ambulatory Care Nursing Orientation and Competency Assessment*
- ➢ *Telehealth Nursing Practice (TNP) Administration and Practice Standards*
- ➢ *Telehealth Nursing Practice Essentials Textbook*
- ➢ *Telehealth Nursing Practice Core Course (TNPCC)* CD-ROM
- ➢ *Telehealth Nursing Practice Resource Directory*

AAACN COURSES:
- • Ambulatory Care Nursing Certification Review Course*
- • Telehealth Nursing Practice Core Course (TNPCC)*
  *Both courses can be presented at your location.

ANNUAL CONFERENCE: AAACN provides cutting-edge information and education at its annual conference, usually held in the month of March or April. Nurses from across the country, as well as international colleagues, come together to network, learn from each other, and share knowledge and skills. Renowned speakers in the field of ambulatory care present topics of current interest offering over 30 contact hours. An Exhibit Hall featuring the products and services of vendors serving the ambulatory care and telehealth community provides information and resources to attendees.

LIVE AUDIO SEMINARS: Monthly continuing nursing education on timely topics is convenient for nurses and cost effective.

CERTIFICATION: AAACN values the importance of certification and promotes achieving this level of competency through its educational products to prepare nurses to take the ambulatory care nursing certification examination. AAACN strongly encourages all telehealth nurses to become certified in ambulatory care nursing. Because telehealth nurses provide care to patients who are in an ambulatory setting, they must possess the knowledge and competencies to appropriately provide ambulatory care. Ambulatory certification is and will continue to be the gold standard credential for any nursing position within ambulatory care.

CORPORATE COLLABORATIONS: Together, working with corporate colleagues, AAACN continues to advance the delivery of ambulatory care to patients. AAACN is open to alliances or collaborations with corporate industry to achieve mutual goals. Corporations are encouraged to contact the National Office to suggest ways in which AAACN can work with them to advance the practice of ambulatory care nursing.

For more information, call (800) AMB-NURS, fax (856) 589-7463,
email aaacn@ajj.com, or visit our Web site at www.aaacn.org.
East Holly Avenue/Box 56, Pitman, New Jersey 08071-0056

Corporate Sponsor Profile

AAACN would like to thank LVM Systems, Inc. for their sponsorship of this book.

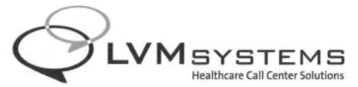

LVM Systems, Inc.
4262 E. Florian Avenue
Mesa, AZ 85206
Phone: 480-633-8200, ext. 223
Fax: 480-892-7016
E-mail: info@lvmsystems.com
Web site: www.lvmsystems.com

LVM Systems, Inc. develops call center software and related Internet products exclusively for the health care industry. LVM's primary niche: nurse triage, disease management, and referral/marketing services. They have proudly served this market for 20 years and have hundreds of health care organizations as clients. They offer both installed and hosted software solutions to meet their customers' individual circumstances of I.T. support, and capital versus operational budgets.

Proven Triage Content

The objective of a medical call center program is to provide sound clinical advice to callers. LVM utilizes protocols that are authored and supported by Barton Schmitt, MD, the renowned expert and pioneer in pediatric telephone triage, and David Thompson, MD, emergency and internal medicine physician. The protocol sets follow an identical structure and philosophy, resulting in a synergistic approach that reduces the length of calls.

Doctor's Office Calls

Doctor's Office Calls (DOC) extends the reach of telehealth nursing practice. DOC is an Internet-based triage product using the Schmitt-Thompson Office Protocols. It allows physician office staff to quickly assess the caller's symptoms and make the appropriate referral (see immediately, see later, or provide home care advice). DOC automatically documents the call interaction, saving staff time and enabling better tracking/reporting. Try it yourself at http://doc2.lvmsystems.com

Newsletter

To receive *Dialogue: Solutions for Your Healthcare Call Center* (free bimonthly newsletter), register at www.lvmsystems.com/form_dialogue.php

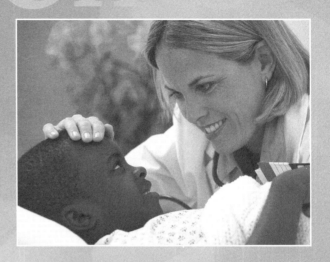
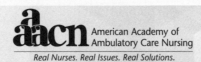

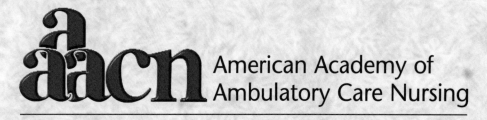

American Academy of Ambulatory Care Nursing

Real Nurses. Real Issues. Real Solutions.

1-800-AMB-NURS • Web site: www.aaacn.org • E-mail: aaacn@ajj.com

AAACN Membership Application

MTNP 09

Name: _____ Credentials: _____

Preferred Mailing Address (check one)

☐

Home Address: _____

City: _____ State: _____ Zip: _____

Home Phone: ( ) _____

☐

Employer: _____

Work Address: _____

_____

City: _____ State: _____ Zip: _____

Business Phone: ( ) _____ Fax #: ( ) _____

Preferred Daytime Phone: ❏ Home   ❏ Work

E-mail: _____

Please provide AAACN with your email address so that we can send you valuable information. AAACN will not sell or distribute email addresses to third parties.

Membership Fee

Dues and contributions are not deductible as a charitable organization, but may qualify as a business expense.

Categories of Membership* (Please check one)

☐ **Active (RN)** $130
Available to any registered nurse.

☐ **Active (RN)** $240
Pay 2 years – SAVE $20!

☐ **Affiliate** $105
Professional interested in ambulatory care nursing.

☐ **LPN/LVN** $105

☐ **Senior** $70
Active member for 3 years and reached age 62.

☐ **Student** $70
Course of study for initial licensure - enclose proof of enrollment.

☐ Check payable in US Funds to AAACN
   Charge my   ☐ Visa ☐ MasterCard ☐ AmEx

Card # __ __ __ __ - __ __ __ __ - __ __ __ __ - __ __ __ __

3 or 4 digit security code _____

Expiration Date _____ in the amount of $ _____

Name on card _____

Signature _____

Make checks payable to: AAACN • Fax this form to (856) 589-7463 or mail to: AAACN, Box 56, East Holly Ave., Pitman, NJ 08071-0056
phone: 856-256-2350; (800) AMB-NURSE; e-mail: aaacn@ajj.com; Web site: www.aaacn.org

---

Please circle one answer for each question.

1. Position
(1) Administrator/Director
(2) Manager/Supervisor
(3) Staff Nurse/Clinical Practitioner
(4) Educator
(5) Researcher
(6) Nurse Practitioner
(7) Consultant
(8) Other _____

2. Practice Setting
(1) University Hospital
(2) Group Practice/Health Center
(3) Community/Private Hospital
(4) Managed Care/HMO/PPO
(5) Military
(6) Free Standing Facility
(7) University/College/ Educational Institution
(8) Public Sector/Community Health Center/Public Health
(9) Other _____

3. Highest Level of Education Completed
(1) LPN/LVN
(2) Diploma—Nursing
(3) Associate Degree—Nursing
(4) Associate Degree—Other
(5) Bachelor's Degree—Nursing
(6) Bachelor's Degree—Other
(7) Master's Degree—Nursing
(8) Master's Degree—Other
(9) Doctorate Degree, Nursing
(A) Doctorate Degree, Other

4. If you are involved in clinical care, please circle the area that best describes your practice.
(1) Family Practice
(2) Internal Medicine
(3) Pediatrics
(4) Behavioral Health
(5) Obstetrics/Gynecology
(6) General Surgery
(7) Oncology
(8) Orthopaedics/Rehabilitation
(9) Ambulatory Surgery

(A) Telehealth
(B) Primary Care
(C) Medical Specialties
(D) Surgical Specialties
(E) Multispecialty Clinic
(F) Other _____

5. If you are in an administrative/ managerial position, please circle ONE area that best describes your area of responsibility.
(1) Physician Group Office Practice/Primary Care
(2) Hospital-based Emergency Services
(3) Urgent/Immediate Care Center
(4) Ambulatory Surgery
(5) Community/Public Health
(6) Employee/Occupational Health
(7) Specialty/Sub-specialty Physician Practice
(8) Oncology Clinic
(9) Triage
(A) Rehabilitation Outpatient
(B) Nurse-Managed Center

(C) Patient Education
(D) Staff Education
(E) Information Management

6. Are you Certified?
(1) Ambulatory Nursing ANCC
(2) Telehealth NCC
(3) Both

7. Choose membership in one special interest group (SIG).
(1) Pediatrics
(2) Telehealth Nursing Practice
(3) Staff Education
(4) Veterans Affairs
(5) Tri-Service Military
(6) Leadership
(7) Patient Education

8. Salary (Confidential)
(1) Less than $25,000
(2) $25,000 - $44,999
(3) $45,000 - $64,999
(4) $65,000 - $84,999
(5) $85,000 - $105,000
(6) more than $105,000

9. Select the journal you would like to receive as part of your membership benefits.
☐ NEC - Nursing Economic$
☐ DNJ - Dermatology Nursing
☐ PED - Pediatric Nursing
☐ MSJ - MEDSURG Nursing

10. How did you hear about AAACN?
(1) A member
(2) Web site
(3) Viewpoint
(4) Colleague
(5) AAACN Conference
(6) Another Conference
(7) AAACN Enews
(8) Certification organization

Date of birth _____

Who referred you to AAACN? _____

☐ AAACN occasionally makes available its members' information to organizations and vendors that provide products and services of value to the ambulatory care nursing community. If you prefer not to be included in these lists, please check the box provided.